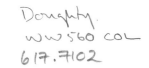

COLOR ATLAS OF THE EYE IN SYSTEMIC DISEASE

COLOR ATLAS OF THE EYE IN SYSTEMIC DISEASE

EDITORS

DANIEL H. GOLD, M.D.

Clinical Professor of Ophthalmology
University of Texas Medical Branch
Galveston, Texas

THOMAS A. WEINGEIST, M.D., Ph.D.

Professor and Head
Department of Ophthalmology
The University of Iowa
Iowa City, Iowa

With 198 Contributors

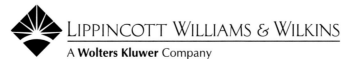

LIPPINCOTT WILLIAMS & WILKINS
A **Wolters Kluwer** Company
Philadelphia • Baltimore • New York • London
Buenos Aires • Hong Kong • Sydney • Tokyo

Acquisitions Editor: Jonathan Pine
Developmental Editor: Pamela Sutton
Production Editor: Maria Tortora
Manufacturing Manager: Colin Warnock
Cover Designer: Mark Lerner
Compositor: Maryland Composition

© 2001 by LIPPINCOTT WILLIAMS & WILKINS
530 Walnut Street
Philadelphia, PA 19106 USA
LWW.com

Printed in China

Library of Congress Cataloging-in-Publication Data

Color atlas of the eye in systemic disease / edited by Daniel H. Gold, Thomas
A. Weingeist ; with 198 contributors.
    p. ; cm.
  Includes bibliographical references and index.
  ISBN 0-397-51525-1 (alk. paper)
  1. Ocular manifestations of general diseases—Atlases. I. Gold, Daniel H., 1942- II.
  Weingeist, Thomas A.
    [DNLM: 1. Eye Manifestations—Atlases. 2. Eye Diseases—etiology—Atlases. WW 17
C7198 2000]
  RE65 .C65 2000
  617.7'1'0222–dc21

                                                                        00-044370

10 9 8 7 6 5 4 3 2 1

CONTENTS

CONTRIBUTING AUTHORS

Everett Ai, M.D. Department of Ophthalmology, California Pacific Medical Center, San Francisco, California

Daniel M. Albert, M.D., M.S. F.A. Davis Professor, Chair, and Lorenz E. Zimmerman Professor, Department of Opthalmology and Visual Sciences, University of Wisconsin Medical School, Madison, Wisconsin

Duncan P. Anderson, M.D. Associate Professor, Department of Ophthalmology, University of British Columbia, Vancouver, British Columbia, Canada; and, Department Chair, Department of Ophthalmology, St. Paul's Hospital, Vancouver, British Columbia, Canada

James J. Augsburger, M.D. Professor and Chairman, Department of Ophthalmology, University of Cincinnati, College of Medicine, Cincinnati, Ohio; and Ophthalmologist-in-Chief, The University Hospital, Cincinnati, Ohio

Susan Barkay, M.D. Former Chief, Department of Ophthalmology, Haemek Medical Center, Afula, Israel

Maria H. Berrocal, M.D. Assistant Professor, Department of Ophthalmology, University of Puerto Rico, Puerto Rico Medical Center—Medical Sciences, San Juan, Puerto Rico; and, Director, Vitreoretina Surgery, Mimiya Hospital, Santurce, Puerto Rico

Jose A. Berrocal, M.D. Department of Opthalmology, Mimiya Hospital, Santurce, Puerto Rico

Steven J. Blackwell, M.D., F.A.C.S. Professor, Department of Plastic Surgery, University of Texas Medical Branch, Galveston, Texas; and, Medical Director, Cleft and Craniofacial Project, Department of Plastic Surgery, John Sealy Hospital and Shriners Burns Hospital at Galveston, Galveston, Texas

Andrew N. Blatt, M.D. Department of Opthalmology, Washington University Medical School, St. Louis, Missouri

Charles J. Bock, M.D. Department of Ophthalmology, Duke University Medical Center, Durham, North Carolina

H. Culver Boldt, M.D. Associate Professor, Department of Ophthalmology, University of Iowa; and, Staff Physician, University of Iowa Hospitals, Iowa City, Iowa

Arnaldo F. Bordon, M.D. Assistant Doctor, Department of Ophthalmology, Universidade Federal de São Paulo, Brazil

David M. Brown, M.D. Clinical Instructor, Department of Ophthalmology, Baylor College of Medicine, Houston, Texas; and, Attending Surgeon, Department of Ophthalmology, Methodist Hospital, Houston, Texas

Jeremiah Brown, Jr., M.D. Director, Ophthalmology Research, U.S. Army Medical Research Department, Walter Reed Army Institute of Research, Brooks Air Force Base, Texas; and, Vitreoretinal Surgeon, Ophthalmology Service, Brooke Army Medical Center, Fort Sam Houston, Texas

Seymour Brownstein, M.D. Professor, Departments of Ophthalmology and Pathology, Faculty of Medicine, University of Ottawa, Ottawa, Ontario, Canada; and, Associate Ophthamologist and Pathologist, Departments of Ophthalmology and Pathology, University of Ottawa Eye Institute, The Ottawa Hospital—General Campus, Ottawa, Ontario, Canada

Helmut Buettner, M.D. Professor of Ophthalmology and Consultant, Department of Ophthalmology, Mayo Clinic and Medical School, Rochester, Minnesota

John D. Bullock, M.D., M.S., F.A.C.S. Professor of Physiology and Biophysics, Professor and Chair, Department of Ophthalmology, Wright State University School of Medicine, Dayton, Ohio

Ronald M. Burde, M.D. Professor of Opthalmology, Neurology, and Neurosurgery, Albert Einstein College of Medicine, Bronx, New York; and, Professor and Chairman, Department of Ophthalmology, Montefiore Medical Center, Bronx, New York

Capt. Frank K. Butler, Jr., M.D. Director of Biomedical Research, Naval Special Warfare Command, San Diego, California; and, Attending Physician, Department of Ophthalmology, Naval Hospital Pensacola, Pensacola, Florida

R. Jean Campbell, M.B, Ch.B. Professor Emeritus, Department of Pathology, Mayo Clinic, Rochester, Minnesota

Ronald E. Carr, M.D., M.Sci.Ophth. Professor, Department of Ophthalmology, New York University Medical Center, New York, New York

Gregory S. Carroll, M.D. Associate Professor, Department of Ophthalmology, University of Tennessee College of Medicine, Memphis, Tennessee

Robert J. Champer, M.D., Ph.D. Assistant Professor, Department of Surgery, East Tennessee State University, Johnson City, Tennessee

Wing-Kwong Chan, M.D. Senior Consultant and Head, Department of Refractive Surgery Service, Singapore National Eye Centre, Singapore

Devron H. Char, M.D. Director, The Tumori Foundation, California Pacific Medical Center—Davis Campus, San Francisco, California; and, Clinical Professor, Department of Ophthalmology, Stanford University Medical Center, Stanford, California

Kenneth C. Chern, M.D. Assistant Professor, Department of Ophthalmology, Boston University School of Medicine, Boston, Massachusetts

Hyong S. Choe, M.D. Department of Ophthalmology, University of Maryland, Baltimore, Maryland

Andrew E. Choy, M.D. University of California Los Angeles School of Medicine, Long Beach, California

Georgia A. Chrousos, M.D. Professor, Department of Ophthalmology, Georgetown University; and, Director, Pediatric and Neuro-ophthalmology, Department of Ophthalmology, Georgetown University Hospital, Washington, D.C.

Elaine L. Chuang, M.D. Associate Professor, Department of Ophthalmology, University of Washington School of Medicine, Seattle, Washington; and, Staff Ophthalmologist, Department of Veterans Affairs, Puget Sound Health Care System, Seattle, Washington

Gerhard Wolfgang Cibis, M.D. Clinical Professor of Ophthalmology, Department of Ophthalmology, University of Kansas and University of Missouri; and, Children's Mercy Hospital, Chief of Ophthalmology, Department of Surgery, Kansas City, Missouri

Alfred J. Cossari, M.D. Children's Eye Care, State University of New York, Port Jefferson, New York

Christopher R. Croasdale, M.D. Assistant Clinical Professor, Department of Ophthalmology and Visual Sciences, University of Wisconsin Medical School, Madison, Wisconsin; and, Attending Surgeon, Department of Surgery, St. Mary's Hospital Medical Center, Madison, Wisconsin

Juan Oscar Croxatto, M.D. Chairman, Department of Ophthalmic Pathology, Fundacion Oftalmologica Argentina, Bueno Aires, Argentina

Mary A. Curtis, M.D. Professor, Department of Pediatrics, University of Arkansas for Medical Sciences; and, Head, Departments of Clinical Genetics and Pediatrics, Arkansas Children's Hospital, Little Rock, Arkansas

Matthew D. Davis, M.D. Professor Emeritus, Department of Ophthalmology and Visual Sciences, University of Wisconsin Medical School, Madison, Wisconsin; and, University of Wisconsin Hospital and Clinics, Madison, Wisconsin

Jean-Jacques De Laey, M.D., Ph.D. Department of Ophthalmology, University Hospital, Ghent, Belgium

Kathleen B. Digre, M.D. Departments of Neurology and Ophthalmology, University of Utah, Salt Lake City, Utah

William J. Dinning, F.R.C.S., M.R.C.P., F.R.C.Ophth. Private Practice, London, England

Eric D. Donnenfeld, M.D. Assistant Clinical Professor, Department of Ophthalmology, North Shore University Hospital, Rockville Centre, New York; and, Co-Chairman, Department of Ophthalmology, Manhattan Eye and Ear, New York, New York

F. Jane Durcan, M.D. Associate Professor, Department Ophthalmology, University of Utah and University Hospital, Moran Eye Center, Salt Lake City, Utah

Frederick J. Elsas, M.D. Clinical Assistant Professor in Ophthalmology and Pediatrics, Department of Ophthalmology, University of Alabama at Birmingham, Birmingham, Alabama; and, Ophthalmologist-in-Chief, Department of Surgery, The Children's Hospital of Alabama, Birmingham, Alabama

Forrest D. Ellis, M.D. Department of Ophthalmology, Indiana University, Indianapolis, Indiana

R. Linsy Farris, M.D. Professor of Clinical Ophthalmology, Department Ophthalmology, College of Physicians and Surgeons of Columbia University; and, Attending, Department of Ophthalmology, Harlem Hospital, New York, New York

Andrew P. Ferry, M.D. Department of Ophthalmology, Virginia Commonwealth University, Richmond, Virginia

Timothy J. ffytche, LVO, F.R.C.S., F.R.C.Ophth. Consultant, Department of Ophthalmology, The Hospital of Tropical Diseases, London, England

Robert Folberg, M.D. Department of Ophthalmology, University of Iowa, Iowa City, Iowa

Joseph Z. Forstot, M.D., F.A.C.P., F.A.C.R. Departments of Internal Medicine and Rheumatology, Boca Raton Community Hospital, Boca Raton, Florida

S. Lance Forstot, M.D. Clinical Professor, Department of Ophthalmology, University of Colorado Medical School, Denver, Colorado

Thomas D. France, M.D. Professor, Department of Ophthalmology and Visual Science, University of Wisconsin and University of Wisconsin Hospital and Clinics, Madison, Wisconsin

Alan H. Friedman, M.D. Clinical Professor and Attending, Department of Ophthalmology and Pathology, Mount Sinai School of Medicine, New York, New York

Neil J. Friedman, M.D. Medical Staff, Department of Ophthalmology, Stanford Hospital, Stanford, California

William A. Gahl, M.D., Ph.D. Head, Section on Human Biochemical Genetics, Department of Heritable Disorders Branch, National Institute of Child Health and Human Development, National Institutes of Health, Bethesda, Maryland

Brenda L. Gallie, M.D. Professor, Departments of Ophthalmology and Molecular Medical Biophysics, University of Toronto; and, Head, Cancer Informatics, University Health Network, Princess Margaret Hospital, Toronto, Ontario, Canada

James A. Garrity, M.D. Professor, Department of Ophthalmology, Mayo Medical School, Rochester, Minnesota

Hanna J. Garzozi, M.D. Senior Lecturer, Department of Ophthalmology, Rappaport Faculty of Medicine, Bat-Galim, Haifa, Israel; and, Chairman, Department of Ophthalmology, Haemek Medical Center, Afula, Israel

Karen M. Gehrs, M.D. Clinical Assistant Professor of Ophthalmology, Department of Ophthalmology, University of Iowa; and, Staff Physician, Department of Ophthalmology, University of Iowa Hospitals, Iowa City, Iowa

David S. Gendelman, M.D. Clinical Instructor, Massachusetts Eye and Ear Infirmary, Boston, Massachusetts

Conrad L. Giles, M.D. Clinical Professor of Ophthalmology, Kresge Eye Institute, Wayne State University, Detroit, Michigan; and, Chief Emeritus, Department of Ophthalmology, Childrens Hospital of Michigan, Detroit, Michigan

Bernard F. Godley, M.D., Ph.D., F.A.C.S. Associate Professor, Department of Ophthalmology and Visual Sciences, University of Texas Medical Branch, Galveston, Texas

Daniel H. Gold, M.D. Clinical Professor, Department of Ophthalmology, University of Texas Medical Branch, Galveston, Texas

Rosalie B. Goldberg, M.D. Senior Associate, Associate Genetic Counselor, Department of Plastic Surgery and Molecular Genetics, Albert Einstein College of Medicine, Bronx, New York

Elizabeth M. Graham, F.R.C.P., F.R.C.Ophth. Consultant, Medical Eye Unit, St. Thomas' Hospital, London, England

Barrett G. Haik, M.D., F.A.C.S. Chair and Hamilton Professor, Department of Ophthalmology, University of Tennessee at Memphis, Memphis, Tennessee

Paul W. Hardwig, M.D. Assistant Professor, Department of Ophthalmology, Mayo Medical School, and Consultant, Mayo Medical Center, Department of Opthalmology, Rochester, Minnesota

Sohan Singh Hayreh, M.D., Ph.D., D.Sc., F.R.C.S., F.R.C.Ophth. Professor Emeritus, Department of Ophthalmology and Visual Sciences, College of Medicine, University of Iowa, The University of Iowa Hospitals and Clinics, Iowa City, Iowa

Thomas R. Hedges, Jr., M.D. University of Pennsylvania, Philadelphia, Pennsylvania

Thomas R. Hedges III, M.D. Professor, Departments of Ophthalmology and Neurology, Tufts University, Boston, Massachusetts; and, Director, Department of Neuro-Ophthalmology, New England Medical Center, Boston, Massachusetts

Craig J. Helm, M.D. Assistant Professor, Department of Ophthalmology, Eastern Virginia Medical School, Norfolk, Virginia

Elise Héon, M.D., F.R.C.S.C. Associate Professor, Department of Ophthalmology, University of Toronto, Toronto, Ontario, Canada; and, Staff Ophthalmologist/Ocular Geneticist, Department of Ophthalmology, The Hospital for Sick Children, Toronto, Ontario, Canada

David A. Hiles, M.D. Retired

William G. Hodge, M.D., M.P.H., F.R.C.S.C. Associate Professor, Department of Ophthalmology, University of Ottawa Eye Institute, Ottawa, Ontario, Canada

Edward J. Holland, M.D. Professor of Clinical Ophthalmology, Department of Ophthalmology, University of Cincinnati, Cincinnati, Ohio; and, Director of Cornea Services, Cincinnati Eye Institute, Cincinnati, Ohio

Gary N. Holland, M.D. David May II Professor of Ophthalmology, University of California Los Angeles School of Medicine, Chief, Cornea-External Ocular Disease and Uveitis Division, and Director, UCLA Ocular Inflammatory Disease Center, Jules Stein Eye Institute, Los Angeles, California

Rufus O. Howard, M.D., Ph.D. Yale University, New Britain, Connecticut

Scott W. Hyver, M.D. Medical Director, Department of Refractive Surgery, Aris Vision Institute, Atherton, California

Edsel B. Ing, M.D., F.R.C.S.(C.) Department of Neuro-Ophthalmology, Wayne State University, Detroit, Michigan

Alex E. Jalkh, M.D. Retina Associates, Harvard Medical School, Boston, Massachusetts

Darlene Skow Johnson, M.D. Massachusetts General Hospital, Boston, Massachusetts

Muriel I. Kaiser-Kupfer, M.D. Chief, Ophthalmic Genetics and Clinical Services Branch, National Eye Institute, National Institutes of Health, Bethesda, Maryland

Robert E. Kalina, M.D. Professor, Department of Ophthalmology, University of Washington, and Active Medical Staff, Department of Ophthalmology, University of Washington Medical Center, Seattle, Washington

Anastasios J. Kanellopoulos, M.D. Clinical Associate Professor, New York University Medical School, and Assistant Director of Residence Training, Manhattan Eye, Ear, and Throat Hospital, New York, New York

Aki Kawasaki, M.D. Clinical Assistant Professor, Department of Ophthalmology and Neurology, Indiana University Medical Center, Indianapolis, Indiana; and, Assistant Director, Department of Neuro-Ophthalmology, Midwest Eye Institute, Clarian Hospitals, Indianapolis, Indiana

Thomas P. Kearns, M.D. Consultant Emeritus, Department of Ophthalmology, Mayo Clinic, and Professor Emeritus, Department of Ophthalmology, Mayo Medical School, Rochester, Minnesota

Ronald V. Keech, M.D. Professor, Department of Ophthalmology, University of Iowa, Iowa City, Iowa

David Kendler, M.D. Clinical Assistant Professor, Department of Endocrinology, Vancouver Hospital and Health Sciences Centre, Eye Care Centre, Vancouver, British Columbia, Canada

Ali M. Khorrami Assistant Professor, Department of Ophthalmology, and Director, Residency Program in Ophthalmology, State University of New York, Syracuse, New York; and, Upstate Medical University of New York, Syracuse, New York

Marilyn C. Kincaid, M.D. (Retired) Clinical Professor, St. Louis University Eye Institute, St. Louis University, St. Louis, Missouri

Gordon K. Klintworth, M.D., Ph.D. Professor, Departments of Pathology and Ophthalmology, Duke University and Medical Center, Durham, North Carolina

David L. Knox, M.D. Associate Professor, Department of Ophthalmology, Wilmer Eye Institute, John Hopkins University, School of Medicine, Baltimore, Maryland

Douglas D. Koch, M.D. Professor and The Allen, Mosbacher, and Law Chair in Ophthalmology, Cullen Eye Institute, Baylor College of Medicine, Houston, Texas

Roger A. Kohn, M.D. University of California, Santa Barbara, California

Glenn Kolansky, M.D. Director, Advanced Dermatology Surgery and Laser Center, Tinton Falls, New Jersey

Jay H. Krachmer, M.D. Chairman, Department of Ophthalmology, University of Minnesota and Fairview University Medical Center, Minneapolis, Minnesota

Stephen P. Kraft, M.D., F.R.C.S.C. Associate Professor, Department of Ophthalmology, Faculty of Medicine, University of Toronto, Toronto, Ontario, Canada; and, Staff Ophthalmologist, The Hospital for Sick Children, Toronto, Ontario, Canada

Erik F. Kruger, M.D. New York Eye and Ear Infirmary, New York, New York

Baruch D. Kuppermann, M.D., Ph.D. Associate Professor, Department of Ophthalmology, University of California at Irvine, Irvine, California; and, Chief, Retina Service, Department of Ophthalmology, University of California Medical Center, Orange, California

H. Michael Lambert, M.D., F.A.C.S. Clinical Associate Professor, Department of Ophthalmology, Baylor College of Medicine, Houston, Texas; Clinical Associate Professor, Department of Surgery, Uniformed Services, University of Health Sciences, Bethesda, Maryland; and, Deputy Chief, Department of Ophthalmology, The Methodist Hospital, Houston, Texas

David A. Lee, M.D. Jules Stein Eye Institute, Los Angeles, California

Michael A. Lemp, M.D. Clinical Professor, Department of Ophthalmology, George Washington University, Washington, D.C.

Richard Alan Lewis, M.D. Professor, Departments of Ophthalmology, Pediatrics, Medicine, and Molecular Human Genetics, Baylor College of Medicine, Houston, Texas

Helen K. Li, M.D. Associate Professor and Director of Vitreoretinal Diseases and Surgery, Department of Ophthalmology and Visual Sciences, University of Texas Medical Branch, Galveston, Texas

Jacques Libert, M.D., Ph.D. Associate Professor and Chief, Department of Ophthalmology, Universite Libre De Bruxelles, Hopital Universitaire Saint-Pierre, Brussels, Belgium

Thomas J. Liesegang, M.D. Professor, Department of Ophthalmology, Mayo Clinic Jacksonville, Jacksonville, Florida; and, Division of Ophthalmology, St. Luke's Hospital, Jacksonville, Florida

Sornchai Looareesuwan, M.D., D.T.M.&H. Professor and Dean, Faculty of Tropical Medicine, Hospital for Tropical Diseases, Mahidol University, Bangkok, Thailand

Andrea L. Lusk, M.D. Department of Ophthalmology, University of Iowa, Iowa City, Iowa

David O. Magnante, M.D. Lafayette Eye Center, Lafayette, Indiana

Eric S. Mann M.D., Ph.D. Assistant Professor, Director of Vitreoretinal Diseases, Department of Ophthalmology, St. Louis University Eye Institute, St. Louis, Missouri

Ahmad M. Mansour, M.D. Clinical Professor, Department of Ophthalmology, American University of Beirut, Beirut, Lebanon

Curtis E. Margo, M.D., M.P.h. Watson Clinic, Department of Ophthalmology, Lakeland, Florida

Kathryn M. Brady-McCreery, M.D. Assistant Professor of Ophthalmology, Department of Ophthalmology, Baylor College of Medicine, Houston, Texas; and, Department of Pediatric Ophthalmology, Texas Children's Hospital, Houston, Texas

David M. Meisler, M.D. Consultant in Diseases of the Cornea and Anterior Segment, Cole Eye Institute, Cleveland Clinic Foundation, Cleveland, Ohio

Travis A. Meredith, M.D. Professor, Department of Ophthalmology, Washington University School of Medicine, St. Louis, Missouri

Joseph B. Michelson, M.D. Division of Ophthalmology, Scripps Clinic and Research Foundation, La Jolla, California

Marilyn T. Miller, M.D. Professor of Ophthalmology, Department of Ophthalmology and Visual Sciences, University of Illinois at Chicago, Chicago, Illinois

Manabu Mochziuki, M.D., Ph.D. Department of Ophthalmology, Kurume University School of Medicine, Kurume, Japan

Bartly J. Mondino, M.D. Professor and Chairman, Department Ophthalmology, and Director, Jules Stein Eye Institute, UCLA, School of Medicine, Los Angeles, California

Rafael Cordero Moreno, M.D. University of Central Venezuela, Caracas, Venezuela

Richard K. Neahring, M.D. Fellow Associate, Department of Ophthalmology and Visual Sciences, University of Iowa Hospitals and Clinics, Iowa City, Iowa; and, Associate Staff Physician, Department of Ophthalmology, Salem Hospital, Salem, Oregon

Ann G. Neff, M.D. Assistant Professor, Department of Ophthalmology, University of Miami, Coral Gables, Florida; and Assistant Professor, Department of Ophthalmology, Bascom Palmer Eye Institute, Miami, Florida

Guy W. Neff, M.D. Assistant Professor, Department of Hepatology, University of Miami, Coral Gables, Florida; and, Assistant Professor, Department of Hepatology, Jackson Memorial Hospital, Miami, Florida

Jeffrey A. Nerad, M.D. Professor of Ophthalmology and Director of Oculoplastic and Orbital Surgery, Department of Ophthalmology, University of Iowa, Iowa City, Iowa

Nancy J. Newman, M.D. Cyrus H. Stoner Professor of Ophthalmology, Neurology Instructor on Neurological Surgery and Lecturer on Ophthalmology, Harvard Medical School, Boston, Massachusetts; and, Director of Neuro-Ophthalmology, Emory University School of Medicine, Emory Eye Center, Atlanta, Georgia

Brian E. Nichols, M.D., Ph.D. Fellow, Pediatric Ophthalmology, Department of Ophthalmology, University of Iowa Hospitals and Clinics, Iowa City, Iowa

Kenneth G. Noble, M.D. Associate Professor of Clinical Ophthalmology and Attending, Department of Ophthalmology, New York University Medical Center, New York, New York

Reijo Norio, M.D. Professor, Department of Medical Genetics, The Family Federation of Finland Vaestoliitto, Helsinki, Finland

Robert A. Nozik, M.D. Clinical Professor, Department of Ophthalmology, University of California, Francis I. Proctor Foundation, San Francisco, California

James C. Orcutt, M.D., Ph.D. Professor, Department of Ophthalmology, Adjunct Professor, Department of Otolaryngology, University of Washington, Seattle, Washington; and, Specialist, Department of Ophthalmology, University of Washington Medical Center, Seattle, Washington

Juan Orellana, M.D. Mount Sinai Medical Center, New York, New York

Donald W. Park, M.D. Retinal Consultants of Arizona, Mesa, Arizona

James R. Patrinely, M.D. Cullen Eye Institute and Plastic Surgery, Baylor College of Medicine, Houston, Texas

Jacob Pe'er, M.D. Department of Ophthalmology, Hebrew University Hadassah Medical School, Jerusalem, Israel; and, Chairman, Department of Ophthalmology, Hebrew University Hospital, Hadassah University Hospital, Jerusalem, Israel

Jay S. Pepose, M.D., Ph.D. Professor of Clinical Ophthalmology, Department of Ophthalmology, Washington University School of Medicine, St. Louis, Missouri; and, Attending Ophthalmologist, Barnes-Jewish Hospital, St. Louis, Missouri

Henry D. Perry, M.D. Associate Professor, Department of Ophthalmology, Cornell University, Ithaca, New York; and, Chief, Corneal Service, Department of Ophthalmology, North Shore University Hospital, Manhasset, New York

Gholam A. Peyman, M.D. Professor, Department of Ophthalmology, Tulane University Medical School, New Orleans, Louisiana; and, Co-Director, Vitreo-Retinal Service, Department of Ophthalmology, Tulane University Hospital and Clinic, New Orleans, Louisiana

Daryl R. Pfister, M.D. Cornea and External Diseases of the Eye, Southwestern Eye Center, Mesa, Arizona

Timothy D. Polk, M.D. Parris-Castro Eye Care Center, Bel Air, Maryland

Jose S. Pulido, M.D., M.S. Professor and Head, Department of Ophthalmology and Visual Sciences, University of Illinois at Chicago, Chicago, Illinois

John J. Purcell, Jr., M.D. Associate Clinical Professor, Department of Ophthalmology, St. James University; and, Director, Department of Ophthalmology, St. Mary's Health Center, St. Louis, Missouri

Christina Raitta, M.D. Professor Emeritus, Department of Ophthalmology, University of Helsinki, Helsinki, Finland

Aref Rifai, M.D. Vitreoretinal Specialist, Center for Sight, Pensacola, Florida; and, Vitreoretinal Specialist, Department of Ophthalmology, Sacred Heart Hospital, Pensacola, Florida

Melvin I. Roat, M.D. Clinical Associate Professor, Department of Ophthalmology, University of Maryland, Baltimore, Maryland

Johane M. Robitaille, M.D. Assistant Professor, Department of Ophthalmology, Dalhousie University, Halifax, Nova Scotia, Canada; and, Department of Ophthalmology, IWK Grace Health Care Centre, Halifax, Nova Scotia, Canada

Merlyn M. Rodrigues, M.D. Department of Ophthalmology, University of Maryland, Baltimore, Maryland

Kenneth G. Romanchuk, M.D., F.R.C.S.C. Professor, Department of Ophthalmology, College of Medicine, University of Saskatchewan, Saskatoon, Saskatchewan, Canada; and, Active Staff, Eye Center, Saskatoon City Hospital, Saskatoon, Saskatchewan, Canada

Mark A. Ross Department of Neurology, University of Iowa, Iowa City, Iowa

Stuart T.D. Roxburgh Honorary Senior Lecturer, Department of Ophthalmology, University of Dundee, Dundee, United Kingdom; and, Consultant Ophthalmologist, Department of Ophthalmology, Ninewells Hospital and Medical School, Dundee, United Kingdom

Stephen R. Russell, M.D. Associate Professor, Director Vitreoretinal Service, Department of Ophthalmology and Visual Sciences, The University of Iowa, Iowa City, Iowa

Diva R. Salomao, M.D. Department of Pathology, University of Iowa, Iowa City, Iowa

Andrew P. Schachat, M.D. Karl Hagen Professor of Ophthalmology and Director, Retinal Vascular and Ocular Oncology Services, Johns Hopkins University, Baltimore, Maryland

Robert J. Schechter, M.D. Assistant Clinical Professor, Department of Ophthalmology, Jules Stein Eye Institute, University of California, Los Angeles School of Medicine, Los Angeles, California

Ernesto I. Segal, M.D. Department of Ophthalmology, University of Texas Medical Branch, Galveston, Texas

Val C. Sheffield, M.D. Department of Pediatrics, University of Iowa, Iowa City, Iowa

Carol L. Shields, M.D. Associate Professor, Jefferson Medical College, Thomas Jefferson University, Philadelphia, Pennsylvania; and, Attending Surgeon, Ocular Oncology Service, Wills Eye Hospital, Philadelphia, Pennsylvania

Jerry A. Shields, M.D. Professor of Ophthalmology, Jefferson Medical College, Thomas Jefferson University, Philadelphia, Pennsylvania; and, Director, Ocular Oncology Service, Wills Eye Hospital, Philadelphia, Pennsylvania

Stephen H. Sinclair, M.D. Clinical Professor, Department of Ophthalmology, Hahnemann University, Philadelphia, Pennsylvania; and, Active Staff, Department of Ophthalmology, Crozer Chester Medical Center, Upland, Pennsylvania

Harold Skalka, M.D. Nathan E. Miles Professor, Department of Ophthalmology, University of Alabama at Birmingham, Birmingham, Alabama; and, Department of Ophthalmology, Callahan Eye Foundation Hospital, Birmingham, Alabama

Richard J.H. Smith, M.D. Sterba Hearing Research Professor, Department of Otolaryngology, University of Iowa; and Vice Chairman, University of Iowa Hospitals and Clinics, Iowa City, Iowa

Richard S. Smith, M.D. Research Scientist, The Jackson Laboratory, Bar Harbor, Maine

Ronald E. Smith, M.D., D.Med.Sci. Professor, Department of Ophthalmology, University of Southern California, Los Angeles, California

Gilbert Smolin, M.D. Research Ophthalmologist, Department of Ophthalmology, Proctor Foundation, San Francisco, California; and, Clinical Professor, Department of Ophthalmology, University of California Medical School, San Francisco, California

Scott R. Sneed, M.D. Retinal Consultants of Arizona, Phoenix, Arizona

Peter L. Sonkin, M.D. Retina Vitreous Associates, Baptist Hospital North, Nashville, Tennessee

Edwin M. Stone, M.D. Professor, Department Ophthalmology, University of Iowa, Iowa City, Iowa

Mary Seabury Stone, M.D. Associate Professor, Departments of Dermatology and Pathology, University of Iowa, University of Iowa Health Care, Iowa City, Iowa

W.P. Daniel Su, M.D.

Alan Sugar, M.D. Professor, Associate Chair, Kellogg Eye Center, University of Michigan, Ann Arbor, Michigan

Joel Sugar, M.D. Department of Ophthalmology, University of Illinois, Chicago, Illinois

John E. Sutphin, M.D. Professor, Department of Ophthalmology and Visual Sciences, University of Iowa, Iowa City, Iowa

Paul M. Tesser, M.D., Ph.D. Eye Health Care Associates, Ltd., Florissant, Missouri

Zvi Tessler, M.D. Lecturer, Department of Medicine, Ben Gurion University, Beer-Sheva, Israel; and Senior Ophthalmologist, Department of Ophthalmology, Soroka Medical Center, Beer-Sheva, Israel

Andrea Cibis Tongue, M.D. Clinical Associate Professor of Ophthalmology, Casey Eye Institute, Portland, Oregon

Elise Torczynski, M.D. Professor, Departments of Ophthalmology and Pathology, Rush Medical College, Chicago, Illinois; and, Attending, Department of Ophthalmology, and Consultant, Department of Pathology, Rush Medical Center, Chicago, Illinois

Stefan D. Trocme, M.D. Associate Professor and Vice Chairman, Department of Ophthalmology, University of Texas Medical Branch, Galveston, Texas

David T. Tse, M.D., F.A.C.S. Professor, Department of Ophthalmology, Bascom Palmer Eye Institute, University of Miami School of Medicine, Miami, Florida

David L. Valle, M.D. Howard Hughes Medical Institute Research Laboratories, The John Hopkins School of Medicine, Baltimore, Maryland

Michael Varner, M.D. Department of Obstetrics and Gynecology, University of Utah, Salt Lake City, Utah

Carlos Vazquez-Fermin Department of Ophthalmology, University of Minnesota, Minneapolis, Minnesota

Joseph B. Walsh, M.D. Chair, Department of Ophthalmology, New York Medical College, Valhalla, New York; and, Chair, The New York Eye and Ear Infirmary, New York, New York

Frederick M. Wang, M.D. Clinical Professor, Department of Ophthalmology and Visual Science, Albert Einstein College of Medicine, Bronx, New York; and, Attending Surgeon, Department of Ophthalmology, New York Eye and Ear Infirmary, New York, New York

Raymond G. Watts, M.D. Associate Professor, Department of Pediatrics, University of Alabama, Birmingham, Alabama

Aaron Pererá Weingeist, M.D. Evergreen Eye Center, Washington, D.C.

Thomas A. Weingeist, M.D., Ph.D. Department Head and Professor, Department Ophthalmology, The University of Iowa, Iowa City, Iowa

Richard G. Weleber, M.D. Professor of Ophthalmology, Professor of Molecular and Medical Genetics, Casey Eye Institute, Oregon Health Sciences University, Portland, Oregon

Duane C. Whitaker, M.D. Professor, Department of Dermatology, University of Iowa, College of Medicine, Iowa City, Iowa

Michael Wiedman, M.D. Lecturer, Department of Medicine, Massachusetts Institute of Technology, Cambridge, Massachusetts; and, Board of Surgeons, Harvard Medical School, and Department of Ophthalmology, Massachusetts Eye and Ear Infirmary, Boston, Massachusetts

Kirk R. Wilhelmus, M.D., M.P.h. Professor, Department of Ophthalmology, Baylor College of Medicine, Houston, Texas

George A. Williams, M.D. Oakland University, Associated Retinal Consultants, Royal Oak, Michigan

W. Bruce Wilson, M.D. Clinical Professor of Ophthalmology, University of Colorado Medical Center, Denver, Colorado

William J. Wirostko, M.D.   Assistant Professor, Department of Ophthalmology, Vitreoretinal Section, Medical College of Wisconsin, Milwaukee, Wisconsin

Jonathan D. Wirtschafter, M.D., F.A.C.S.   Professor, Departments of Ophthalmology, Neurology, and Neurosurgery, University of Minnesota Medical School, Minneapolis, Minnesota; and Director, Neuro-Ophthalmology Service, Fairview—University Hospital, Minneapolis, Minnesota

Robert A. Wiznia, M.D.   Associate Clinical Professor, Department of Ophthalmology and Visual Science, Yale University School of Medicine, New Haven, Connecticut; and, Attending Surgeon, Department of Ophthalmology, Yale—New Haven Hospital, New Haven, Connecticut

Brian R. Wong, M.D.   Assistant Professor, Director of Ophthalmic Plastic and Reconstructive Surgery, Department Ophthalmology, University of Texas Medical Branch School of Medicine, University of Texas School of Medicine Hospitals, Galveston, Texas

Yuval Yassur, M.D.   Professor, Department of Ophthalmology, Sackler School of Medicine, Tel Aviv University, Tel Aviv, Israel; and, Chairman, Department of Ophthalmology, Rabin Medical Center, Petach-Tikva, Israel

Fiaz Zaman, M.D.   University of Texas Medical Branch, Galveston, Texas

Elaine Ziavras, M.D.   Clinical Assisstant Professor, Departments of Ophthalmology and Pediatrics, Georgetown University Medical Center; and, Pediatric Ophthalmology, Mid-Atlantic Permanente Medical Group, P.C., Largo Medical Center, Largo, Maryland

Marco A. Zarbin, M.D., Ph.D.   Professor and Chairman, Department of Ophthalmology, The University of Medicine and Dentistry of New Jersey—New Jersey Medical School, and Chief, Department of Ophthalmology, The University of Medicine and Dentistry of New Jersey—University Hospital, Newark, New Jersey

Ingrid E. Zimmer-Galler, M.D.   Assistant Professor, Department of Ophthalmology and Vitreoretinal Division, Wilmer Eye Institute, John Hopkins Medical Institutions, Baltimore, Maryland

PREFACE

"The eye is comparable to a small world," Rashi (Talmud Bechorot 16:a)

It has been ten years since the publication of our first text book, *The Eye in Systemic Disease.* We have been asked to create a new text that combines features of a color atlas with a quick reference, tabular format. This format inevitably involves a trade-off between depth of coverage and ease of accessibility of material. As we noted in the preface to the first book, no single text can encompass all of the entities that affect both the eye and the rest of the body. We have tried to include most of the major and more common systemic disorders with significant ocular manifestations, as well as other less common, but interesting ocular-systemic diseases.

Since any classification system is somewhat arbitrary, the issue of organizing the subject matter continues to be somewhat subjective. We have retained the basic structure of the original text because it follows the traditional clinical groupings of primary care medicine.

We wish to thank the many people who contributed to the creation of this book. Our thanks to the authors for their hard work in writing the individual chapters, and for their patience in waiting with us through the many and varied trials and tribulations in transforming this book from their manuscripts into the finished text. As always, our appreciation and gratitude go out to the staff members of the Department of Ophthalmology and Visual Sciences at the University of Iowa and the Eye Clinic of Texas for their support and enthusiasm in carrying out the innumerable tasks which went into the preparation of the book.

Even beyond the usefullness of the information contained in this book, we hope this *Color Atlas of the Eye in Systemic Disease* will be of value in stimulating the reader to think more broadly about the interconnectedness of the eye and the body. This miraculous organ, one inch long, packed with the most amazing structures and physiological wonders, has long been seen as a window to both the body and the soul. This book confirms the former, and defers to the poet and dreamer in all of us to explore the latter.

Daniel H. Gold, M.D.
Thomas A. Weingeist, Ph.D., M.D.

PART 1.   CARDIAC DISORDERS

Chapter 1
ENDOCARDITIS
Daniel H. Gold

I. GENERAL

1. Usually associated with underlying cardiac defect
2. Endothelial cell damage triggers local fibrin and platelet deposition—a nonbacterial thrombotic endocarditis.
3. Circulating microorganisms adhering to the fibrin–platelet vegetations produce infective endocarditis.
4. The organism's virulence and host's response combine to produce an acute, subacute, or chronic course.
5. Distant embolization of infected material causes most extracardiac complications.
6. Antigen–antibody complexes may cause immune complex vasculitis.
7. IV drug abusers and patients with prosthetic heart valves are at significant risk of developing endocarditis.

II. SYSTEMIC MANIFESTATIONS

1. Cardiac
   - Arrhythmias
   - Decreased myocardial perfusion
   - Pain
   - Palpitations
   - Heart murmur
   - Heart failure
2. Vascular
   - Arterial obstruction
   - Tissue infarction
   - Vasculitis
   - Aneurysms
3. Central nervous system
   - Strokes
   - Brain abscesses
   - Cerebral aneurysms
   - Suppurative meningitis
4. Musculoskeletal
   - Arthralgias/myalgias
   - Arthritis
   - Osteomyelitis
5. Renal
   - Focal or diffuse glomerulonephritis
   - Infarction
   - Abscess
6. Mucocutaneous
   - Petechial hemorrhages
   - Osler's nodes
   - Janeway's lesions
7. Nonspecific
   - Fever
   - Chills
   - Malaise
   - Abscesses
   - Arterial obstruction

III. OCULAR MANIFESTATIONS

1. Conjunctiva
   - Hemorrhages
2. Retina
   - Hemorrhages (usually superficial)
   - Roth's spot (white-centered hemorrhage)
   - Branch retinal artery occlusion
   - Central retinal artery occlusion
   - Cotton-wool spots
3. Neuroophthalmologic
   - Secondary to central nervous system involvement
   - Visual field defect
   - Cranial nerve palsies
   - Diplopia
   - Nystagmus
   - Papilledema
4. Nonspecific
   - Intraocular infection with
     - Acute endophthalmitis
     - Focal retinitis
     - Choroiditis
     - Vitritis
     - Uveitis

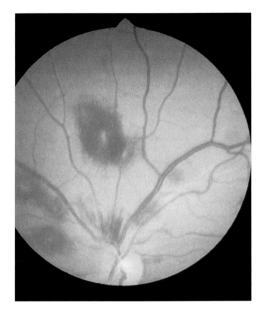

FIGURE 1.1. White-centered retinal hemorrhages in infective carditis. Courtesy of Joseph B. Walsh, MD.

SUGGESTED READINGS

Gold DH. Endocarditis. In: Gold DH, Weingeist TA, eds. *The Eye in Systemic Disease.* Philadelphia: JB Lippincott; 1990:3–5. *A general review of the ocular manifestations of endocarditis.*

Munier F, Othenin-Girard P. Subretinal neovascularization secondary to choroidal septic metastasis from acute bacterial endocarditis. *Retina* 1992;12:108–112.

Terpenning MS. Infective endocarditis. *Geriatr Med Clin* 1992;8:903–912.

Tunkel AR, Kaye D. Neurologic complications of infective endocarditis. *Neurol Clin* 1993;11:419–440.

Wilson WR, Steckelberg JM, eds. Infective endocarditis. *Infect Dis Clin North Am* 1993;7:1–170. *A good review of the pathogenesis and treatment of infectious endocarditis.*

PART 2. CHROMOSOMAL DISORDERS

Section A. Deletion Syndromes

Chapter 2

DELETION OF THE LONG ARM OF CHROMOSOME 13

Elise Héon
Brenda L. Gallie
Edwin M. Stone

I. GENERAL

1. The spectrum of disorders resulting from deletions of the long arm of chromosome 13 varies according to the site and extent of the deletion.
2. Deletions of chromosome 13q may lead to multisystem syndromes or anomalies such as retinoblastoma.
3. The retinoblastoma gene is located at 13q14, near the esterase D gene.
4. 5% of retinoblastoma are caused by chromosomal deletions of the 13q14 region.
5. 100% of these are transmissible in an autosomal dominant fashion.
6. These germline mutations in the retinoblastoma gene increase the risk of second malignancy.
7. The retinoblastoma gene (*RB1*) has been cloned and molecular diagnosis is now available.
8. The gene for Wilson's disease also lies at 13q14. Homozygous deletions can occasionally occur and cause this hepatolenticular degeneration with autosomal recessive inheritance.
9. Genetic counseling is indicated in the presence of a 13q deletion.

II. SYSTEMIC MANIFESTATIONS

1. General
   - Low birth weight
   - Decreased levels of esterase D activity (band 13q14)
2. Facial characteristics
   - "Greek" profile (band 13q33)
   - Broad nasal bridge
   - Large malrotated ears
   - Asymmetry of face
   - Short philtrum
   - Small chin
   - Rabbit incisors (forward and slanted)
3. Skeletal
   - Absent thumbs (band 13q21)
   - Agenesis of first metacarpal, fifth toe
   - Fusion of fourth and fifth metacarpal
   - Supernumery rib
   - Lumbosacral agenesis
4. Genital
   - Hypospadias
   - Epispadias
   - Undescended testis
   - Bifid uterus
5. Renal
   - Aplasia or hypoplasia of kidney
   - Tubular dysfunction (Wilson's disease)
6. Cardiac
   - Atrial or ventricular septal defects
7. Hepatic
   - Cirrhosis (Wilson's disease)
8. Neurologic
   - Mental retardation
   - Microcephaly (arhinecephaly, holoprosencephaly, aplasia of the falx cerebri, agenesis of the corpus collosum) (band 13q21-qter)
   - Progressive neuronal degeneration; failure of motor but not sensory functions (Wilson's disease)

III. OCULAR MANIFESTATIONS

1. General
   - Hypertelorism
   - Microphthalmia (band 13q22 or q31-qter)
   - Ptosis
   - Leucocoria
2. Retina
   - Retinoblastoma (usually bilateral) (band 13q14)
   - Choroidal coloboma (band 13q22 or q31-qter)
3. Anterior segment
   - Iris coloboma (band 13q22 or q31-qter)
   - Corneal opacities
   - Kayser-Fleisher ring (Wilson's disease; at the level of Descemet)
   - Cataracts

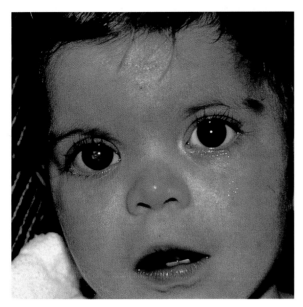

FIGURE 2.1. Unilateral leukokoria in a child with bilateral retinoblastoma and a 13:14 translocation (the breakpoint involving the region of the *RB1* gene).

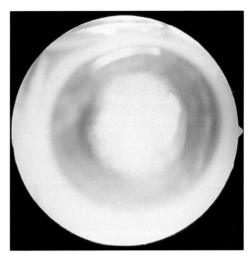

FIGURE 2.2. Photograph of the right eye with retinoblastoma causing a retinal detachment and glaucoma.

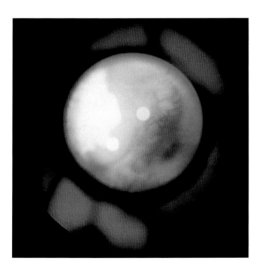

FIGURE 2.3. Photograph of the left eye with retinoblastoma extending to the ora serrata and secondary glaucoma. Both eyes were enucleated as primary procedure.

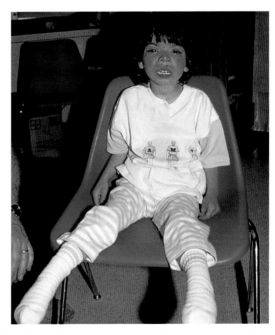

FIGURE 2.4. Photograph of the child shown in Figs 2.1–2.3 at age 6. This patient is mentally retarded, bilaterally enucleated, and has hypertelorism, a hypoplastic philtrum, and motility problems.

SUGGESTED READINGS

Bull P, Thomas GR, Rommens J, et al. The Wilson gene is a putative copper transporting P-type ATPase similar to the Menkes gene. *Nat Genet* 1993;5:327–337.

Buyse ML. *Birth Defect Encyclopedia.* Cambridge, MA: Blackwell Scientific Publications; 1990:366–368.

Friend S, Bernards R, Rogeli S, et al. A human DNA segment with properties of the gene that predisposes to retinoblastoma and osteosarcoma. *Nature* 1986;323:643.

Liberfarb R, Bustos T, Miller W, et al. Incidence and significance of a deletion of chromosome band 13q14 in patients with retinoblastoma and in their families. *Ophthalmology* 1984;91:1695–1699.

Niebuhr E. Partial trisomies and deletions of chromosome 13. In: Yunis JJ, ed. *New Chromosomal Syndromes.* New York: Academic Press; 1977:273–295.

Section B. Sex Chromosome Disorders

Chapter 3

TURNER'S SYNDROME

Elaine Ziavras
Georgia A. Chrousos

I. GENERAL

1. A chromosomal disorder in which phenotypic females have complete or partial monosomy of chromosome X
2. 1/3,500 female newborns has the 45,X karyotype. There is high lethality prenatally (present in 9% of spontaneous abortions).
3. 40% with the Turner's phenotype are mosaics, resulting in a broad spectrum of phenotypic features.
4. Karyotypes vary from those with a structural alteration of the X chromosome to mosaicism involving one or more cell lines with abnormal number or structure (*eg*, X/XX, X/XXX, isochromosome for the long arm of X, deletions of parts of Xp or Xq, and ring X chromosomes).
5. The cardinal features are short stature and gonadal dysgenesis with primary amenorrhea.
6. In most cases the ovaries consist of only a streak of connective tissue and therefore secondary sex characteristics do not develop.

II. SYSTEMIC MANIFESTATIONS

1. Nonspecific
   - Short stature
   - Tendency to become obese
   - Generally normal intelligence
2. Genitourinary
   - Ovarian dysgenesis with hypoplasia—"streak ovaries"
   - Female external genitalia
3. Endocrine
   - Primary amenorrhea
   - Sexual infantilism
   - Sterility
   - Thyroid disorders
   - Diabetes mellitus
4. Cardiac
   - Coarctation of the aorta
   - Aortic stenosis
5. Vascular
   - Peripheral lymphedema—usually congenital with residual puffiness
   - Hypertension (primary)
6. Musculoskeletal
   - Cubitus valgus (reduced carrying angle at elbow)
   - Short neck
   - Shield chest (with widely spaced nipples)
   - Pectus excavatum
   - Short metacarpals or metatarsals
7. Mucocutaneous
   - Loose skin—webbed neck
   - Unusual dermatoglyphics (high ridge count)
   - Low nuchal hairline
   - Hypoplastic, hyperconvex nails
   - Pigmented nevi
8. Ear/nose/throat
   - Anomalous auricles
   - Micrognathia
   - Narrow maxilla
   - High palate
9. Renal
   - Horseshoe kidney
   - Double or cleft renal pelvis
10. Neurologic
    - Perceptive hearing impairment

III. OCULAR MANIFESTATIONS

1. Ocular motility
   - Strabismus (33%)
   - Esotropia four times more common than exotropia
2. Lids
   - Ptosis (16%)
   - Epicanthus (blepharalis or inversus)
   - Antimongoloid slanting
3. Orbit
   - Hypertelorism
4. Nonspecific
   - Red-green color deficiency (10%, similar to normal male population)
5. Conjunctiva/sclera
   - Telangiectasia of conjunctival vessels
   - Conjunctival cysts
   - Blue sclerae
6. Neuroophthalmologic
   - Periodic alternating nystagmus
7. Cornea
   - Microcornea
   - Corneal nebulae
   - Keratoconus
8. Lens
   - Cataract
9. Uvea
   - Brushfield spots
   - Iris nevi

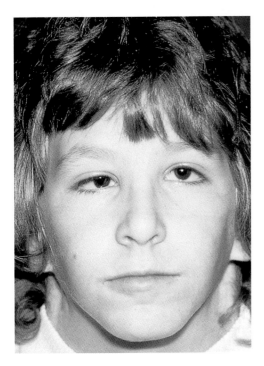

FIGURE 3.1. Characteristic facial features of a patient with Turner's syndrome. Note right ptosis and esotropia, as well as epicanthus, webbed neck, and low-set ears. From Chrousos GA, Ross JL, Chrousos G, et al. Ocular findings in Turner syndrome. A prospective study. *Ophthalmology* 1984;91:926–928.

SUGGESTED READINGS

Chrousos GA, Ross JL, Chrousos G, et al. Ocular findings in Turner syndrome. A prospective study. *Ophthalmology* 1984;91:926–928.

Jones KL. *Smith's Recognizable Patterns of Human Malformation,* 4th ed. Philadelphia: WB Saunders; 1988:74–79.

Lessell S, Forbes AP. Eye signs in Turner's syndrome. *Arch Ophthalmol* 1966;76:211–213.

Thompson MW. The sex chromosomes and their disorders. In: Thompson JS, Thomson MW, eds. *Genetics in Medicine.* Philadelphia: WB Saunders; 1986:144–145.

Traboulsi EI, Chrousos GA. Turner's syndrome gonadal dysgenesis. In: Gold DH, Weingeist TA, eds. *The Eye in Systemic Disease.* Philadelphia: JB Lippincott; 1990:26–27.

Section C. Trisomy Syndromes

Chapter 4

TRISOMY 18

Rufus O. Howard

I. GENERAL

1. This congenital chromosomal disease involves all body tissues.
2. Multiple anomalies arise from abnormal gene dosage—an extra complement of normal genes on chromosome 18.
3. The majority of affected individuals die in utero and are aborted spontaneously. There are three liveborn females for every male. Approximately 90% die by 1 year of age. The rare survival to the teens or early twenties is at least partially attributed to mosaicism.
4. An effect of maternal age is observed; this anomaly occurs more frequently in older mothers.
5. Although a clinical diagnosis may be inferred at birth on the basis of neonatal features, an exact diagnosis can be made with a chromosome determination. If this anomaly arises because of translocation, the chromosomes of the parents should be examined to see if one is a balanced translocation carrier with a high risk for recurrence in future pregnancies. This condition can be identified by amniocentesis.

II. SYSTEMIC MANIFESTATIONS

1. Cardiac
   - Ventricular septal defect, auricular septal defect, patent ductus arteriosus, patent foramen ovale, bicuspid aortic and/or pulmonic valves, nodularity of valve leaflets, pulmonic stenosis, atrial septal defect, abnormal mitral valve coarctation of the aorta, aorta from right ventricle, left superior vena cava, transposition of great vessels, hypoplasia of left atrium, overriding aorta, tetralogy of Fallot, dextrocardia
2. Pulmonary
   - Malsegmentation, absence of lung, short trachea, tracheoesophageal fistula, muscular defects of diaphragm with eventration of the diaphragm
3. Renal
   - Horseshoe kidney, double ureter, hydronephrosis, polycystic kidney, unilateral absence or hypoplastic kidney, ectopic kidney
4. Gastrointestinal
   - Meckel's diverticulum, heterotopic pancreatic or splenic tissue, omphalocele, incomplete rotation of colon, malposed or funnel-shaped anus, imperforate anus, hypoplastic gallbladder, biliary atresia, bile duct stenosis, pyloric stenosis
5. Genitourinary
   - Males: cryptorchidism, hypospadias, bifid scrotum
   - Females: hypoplasia of labia majora with prominent clitoris, uterus bicornis, uterus bicollis, ovarian hypoplasia
6. Neurologic
   - Hypotonic at birth, followed by hypertonia after neonatal period, facial palsy, hydrocephaly, meningomyelocele, deficiency in myelination, defect in corpus callosum, abnormal gyri, arhinecephaly, cyst of cisterna magna, small brain, heterotopic ganglion cells/abnormal stratification of cerebellum
7. Musculoskeletal
   - Hypoplasia of skeletal muscle, prominent occiput, short sternum, reduced ossification centers, small pelvis, limited hip abduction, clenched hand with tendency for overlapping of index finger over third, fifth finger over fourth, hypoplasia of nails, especially fifth fingers and toes, short hallux, inguinal/umbilical hernia, diastasis recti, talipes equinovarus, rocker-bottom feet

1. Lids
   - Discontinuous eyebrows, trichiasis, ankyloblepharon filiforme adnatum, slanted or narrow palpebral fissures, epicanthal folds, ptosis, abnormally thick lids, abnormally long or sparse lashes, inability to close lids, blepharophimosis
2. Cornea
   - Opacity, absent Bowman's layer and Descemet's membrane, hypercellularity of stroma, short radius of corneal curvature
3. Uvea
   - Iris stromal hypoplasia, vacuolization of iris pigment epithelium, coloboma of posterior pole, hypoplastic ciliary processes
4. Lens
   - Cataract, posterior migration of lens epithelium
5. Retina
   - Decreased ganglion cells, retinal folds/dysplasia, optic pit, hypoplasia of optic nerve, Bergmeister's papilla, decreased mature melanosomes in retinal pigment epithelium, persistent hyaloid artery
6. Orbit
   - Shallow orbits, hypoplastic orbital ridges, hypertelorism, hypotelorism
7. Neuroophthalmology
   - Strabismus, abnormal extraocular movement, decreased response to visual stimuli, nystagmus, anisocoria, decreased myelination of optic nerve
8. Nonspecific
   - Cebocephaly, microphthalmos, cyclopia, glaucoma, blue sclera, nictitating membrane, conjunctiva overriding the cornea

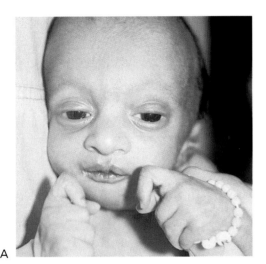 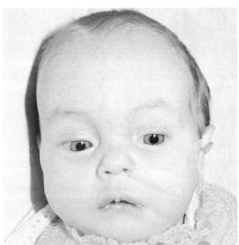

A   B

FIGURE 4.1. (**A** and **B**) The facial features of two children with trisomy 18 are strikingly similar.

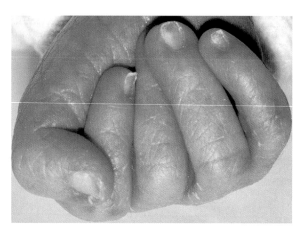

FIGURE 4.2. The index finger may overlap the third and the fifth finger may overlap the fourth.

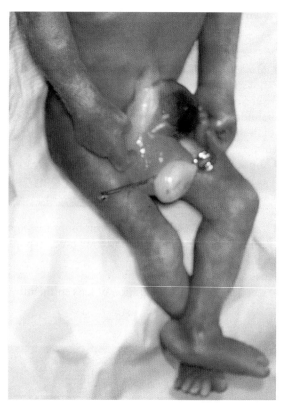

FIGURE 4.3. An omphalocoele and rocker-bottom feet are characteristic findings.

SUGGESTED READINGS

Calderone JP, Chess J, Borodic G, Albert DM. Intraocular pathology of trisomy 18 (Edwards's syndrome): Report of a case and review of the literature. *Br J Ophthalmol* 1983;67:162–169. *Comprehensive summary of ocular clinical and histopathologic abnormalities.*

Edwards JH, Harnden DG, Cameron AH, et al. A new trisomic syndrome. *Lancet* 1960;1:787. *Initial case report.*

Jones KL. *Smith's Recognizable Patterns of Human Malformation.* Philadelphia: WB Saunders; 1988:16–17. *Concise clinical summary of more than 130 defects from multiple case reports.*

Warkany J. *Congenital Malformations.* Chicago: Yearbook Medical Publishers; 1971:303–310. *Excellent review of clinical and pathologic findings.*

Chapter 5
TRISOMY 21
Thomas D. France

I. GENERAL

1. Associated with trisomy of chromosome 21 but may include a translocation or a mosaic form

2. Most common type of mental retardation with an estimated 11,000 affected infants born each year

II. SYSTEMIC MANIFESTATIONS

1. Cardiac
- Congenital heart defects in 40%

2. Pulmonary
- Increased respiratory infections

3. Genitourinary
- Poor genital development

4. Gastrointestinal
- 12% with TEF, pyloric stenosis, etc. (requiring immediate surgical intervention)

5. Neurologic
- Early onset of Alzheimer's disease

6. Hematologic
- Increased incidence of leukemia

7. Endocrine
- Hypothyroidism
- Diabetes mellitus

8. Musculoskeletal
- Muscle flaccidity
- Short stature

9. Mucocutaneous
- Palmar creases

III. OCULAR MANIFESTATIONS

1. Lids
- Epicanthal folds
- Fissure slanted upward about 10°
- Fissure shorter than normal
- Blepharitis

2. Lacrimal system
- Nasolacrimal duct obstruction

3. Cornea
- Keratoconus in 15%

4. Iris
- Brushfield spots/speckles
- 90% have blue or gray color
- Increased sensitivity to cycloplegic agents (atropine, etc.)

5. Lens
- Cortical, flakelike opacities in 10% to 50%

6. Optic nerve
- Increased vascularity

7. Neuroophthalmologic
- Nystagmus, may be vertical, horizontal, or torsional

8. Ocular motility
- Strabismus in 21% to 44%
- Esotropia most common

9. Nonspecific
- High refractive errors
- Myopia greater than 5 D
- Astigmatism greater than 3 D in 25%
- Abnormal head position (secondary to nystagmus, strabismus, etc.)

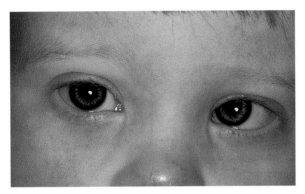

FIGURE 5.1. Two-year-old child with Down syndrome. Note epicanthal folds, short palpebral fissures of normal height, and esotropia.

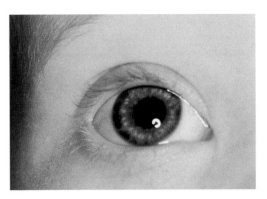

FIGURE 5.2. Brushfield spots in typical blue/gray iris.

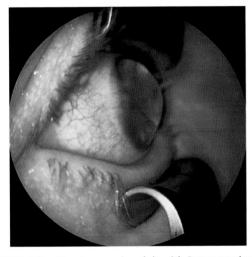

FIGURE 5.3. Keratoconus in adult with Down syndrome.

SUGGESTED READINGS

Patterson D. The causes of Down syndrome. *Sci Am* 1987;257:52–60.
Shapiro MB, France TD. The ocular features of Down's syndrome. *Am J Ophthalmol* 1985;99:659–633.

PART 3. COLLAGEN DISORDERS

Chapter 6

ANKYLOSING SPONDYLITIS

S. Lance Forstot
Joseph Z. Forstot

I. GENERAL

1. Prevalence of ankylosing spondylitis (AS) is 1% to 2%.
2. Etiology is unknown.
3. Sex distribution
   - Male more than female
   - Males more progressive spine disease (3:1)
4. Age at onset
   - $\geq$ 20 years
   - 20–30 years age group peak
5. Serology
   - HLA-B27 positivity, 90%
   - normal white population, 7% positive
   - normal African-American population, 4% positive
   - AS white, 90% positive
   - AS African-American, 60% positive
   - HLA-B27 positive population, 20% develop AS
   - Rheumatoid factor, negative
6. Pathology (enthesopathy)
   - Inflammation develops at the site of the enthesis or ligamentous insertion into bone.

II. SYSTEMIC MANIFESTATIONS

1. Musculoskeletal
   - Sacroiliitis—symmetrical
   - Joint—oligoarthropathy; asymmetrical; large joints; lower extremity greater than upper extremity
   - Spine—total involvement (ascending); fusion (end-stage)
   - Plantar spurs
2. Pulmonary
   - Upper lobe fibrosis
   - Chest wall restriction due to thoracic spine fusion
3. Cardiac
   - Aortic regurgitation
   - Cardiomegaly
   - Conduction defects
4. Neurologic
   - Cauda equina syndrome (rare)
   - Cord compression if fracture of fused cervical spine

III. OCULAR MANIFESTATIONS

1. Uveitis
   - Acute onset
   - Anterior—iritis
   - Active inflammation—unilateral, rarely active bilateral
   - Discrete episodes may alternate between eyes
   - Occurs in 20% to 40% of patients with AS
2. Cataract
   - Secondary to recurrent iritis or recurrent treatment with steroids

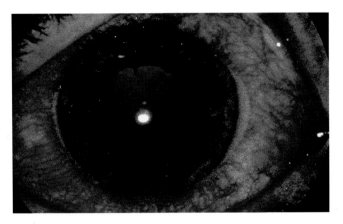

FIGURE 6.1. Acute anterior iritis with posterior synechiae. Courtesy of Syntex.

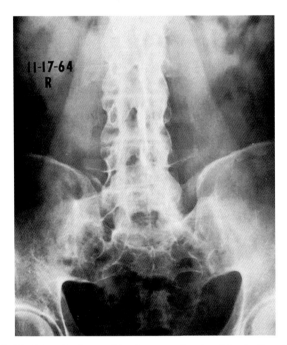

FIGURE 6.2. Radiographic changes of spine (classic "bamboo spine").

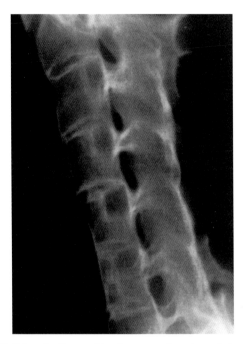

FIGURE 6.3. Radiographic changes of neck vertebra—total neck fusion. Courtesy of Syntex.

SUGGESTED READINGS

Khan MA. Ankylosing Spondylitis. In: Klipped JH, Weyand CM, Wortmann RL, eds. *Primer on the Rheumatic Diseases*. Atlanta: Arthritis Foundation; 1997: 180–183.

McGuigan AF, Edmonds JP. The immunopathology of ankylosing spondylitis—a review. *Semin Arthritis Rheum* 1985;15:81–105.

Wollheim FA. Ankylosing spondylitis. In: Kelly WN, Harris ED Jr, Ruddy S, Sledge CB, eds. *Textbook of Rheumatology*, 4th ed. Philadelphia: WB Saunders; 1993: 943–960.

Chapter 7

GIANT CELL ARTERITIS (TEMPORAL ARTERITIS)

Jeremiah Brown, Jr
Sohan Singh Hayreh

I. GENERAL

1. Demographic and epidemiologic data
   - A disease of persons aged 55 years and over, with mean age 75 years
   - More common in women (73%) than men (27%)
   - Higher incidence in individuals of northern European origin; rare in African-Americans and Asians
   - Genetic component confirmed by linkage to HLA-DR4
2. Pathophysiology
   - Giant cell arteritis is an autoimmune syndrome affecting medium-sized and large arteries.
   - Clonal expansion of infiltrating T cells can be demonstrated, consistent with an autoimmune etiology.
   - Interferon-γ is produced by a subset of infiltrating T cells.
   - Tissue and circulating macrophages secrete interleukin-6, a stimulant of acute phase reactants.
   - Tissue-infiltrating macrophages also produce nitric oxide synthetase.
   - The media of the arterial wall is the primary focus of the inflammatory response. Giant cells may be found.
   - Patchy infiltrates of inflammatory cells extend into the intima and adventitia.
   - Necrosis of the media and fragmentation of the internal elastic lamina may lead to aneurysm formation.
   - Intimal hyperplasia results in vascular occlusion and tissue ischemia.

II. SYSTEMIC MANIFESTATIONS

1. Symptoms
   - Headache (56%)
   - Anorexia, weight loss (52%)
   - Jaw claudication (48%)
   - Malaise (38%)
   - Myalgia (29%)
   - Fever (26%)
   - Temporal artery abnormality (tender, prominent, nonpulsatile cord) (20%)
   - Scalp tenderness (18%)
   - Neck pain (16%)
   - Fatigue and night sweats may also be present.
   - Occult giant cell arteritis (in 21% of patients with ocular manifestations) has no systemic symptoms at all.
2. Systemic vascular disorders
   - Arteries involved
     - Any of the medium-sized and large arteries may be affected, including:
       - Aorta and all its major branches
       - Pulmonary artery
       - Coronary artery
       - Internal and external carotid arteries
       - Vertebral artery
       - Subclavian artery
       - Axillary artery
       - Brachial artery
       - Celiac artery
       - Mesenteric artery
       - Renal artery
       - Femoral artery
       - Popliteal artery
   - Systemic manifestations due to
     - Vasoocclusive events (most common)
     - Aneurysm formation and dissection
     - Central nervous system
       - Euphoria
       - Hallucinations
       - Stroke
     - Gastrointestinal
       - Bowel perforation, necrosis
       - Diverticular abscess
       - Elevated hepatic enzymes
     - Musculoskeletal
       - Claudication
     - Hematologic
       - Elevated erythrocyte sedimentation rate
       - Elevated C-reactive protein
       - Normochromic or slightly hypochromic anemia
     - Cardiac
       - Myocardial infarction
     - Otologic
       - Otalgia with vertigo
       - Deafness
     - Dermatologic
       - Necrosis and ulceration

1. Present in 50% of patients with giant cell arteritis
2. Symptoms (in one or both eyes)
   - Amaurosis fugax (31%)
   - Visual loss of variable amount (98%)
   - Diplopia (6%)
   - Eye pain (8%)
3. Ocular vascular disorders
   - Arteries involved
     - Posterior ciliary arteries *invariably*
     - Cilioretinal artery (22%)
     - Central retinal artery (14%)
     - Ophthalmic artery rarely
   - Ophthalmic manifestations (due to vasoocclusive disorders)
     - Optic nerve ischemic disorders
       - Amaurosis
       - Anterior ischemic optic neuropathy (AION; 81%)
       - Posterior ischemic optic neuropathy (7%)
     - Retinal ischemic disorders
       - Amaurosis fugax
       - Central retinal artery occlusion (14%)
       - Cilioretinal artery occlusion (22%)
       - Cotton-wool spots (33%)
     - Choroidal ischemic disorders
       - Choroidal infarcts resulting in chorioretinal scars
     - Extraocular motility disorders
       - Palsies of oculomotor cranial nerves
       - Ischemia of extraocular muscles
       - Internuclear ophthalmoplegia
     - Anterior segment disorders
       - Anterior segment ischemia
       - Scleritis and episcleritis
       - Marginal corneal ulceration
       - Neovascular glaucoma
     - Pupillary abnormalities
       - Relative afferent pupillary defect from visual loss in one eye
       - Horner's syndrome
     - Ocular ischemia from ophthalmic artery occlusion
     - Orbital disorders
       - Orbital pseudotumor

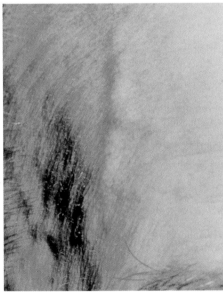

FIGURE 7.1. A prominent, tender temporal artery found in a patient with giant cell arteritis.

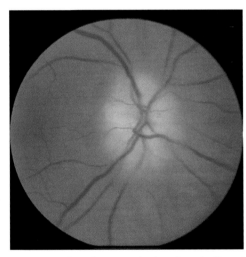

FIGURE 7.2. Fundus photograph showing chalky white disc edema, typically seen in arteritic AION.

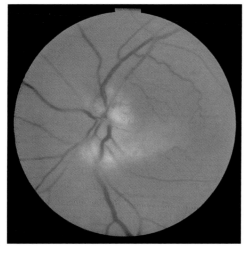
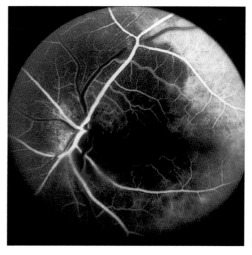

A

B

FIGURE 7.3. Left eye of a 63-year-old woman with arteritic AION and associated cilioretinal artery occlusion. (**A**) Fundus photograph shows segmental chalky white disc edema and a patch of retinal infarction in the distribution of a cilioretinal artery. (**B**) Fluorescein fundus angiogram shows normal filling of the central retinal artery and of the choroid supplied by the lateral posterior ciliary artery. There is no filling of the choroid and optic disc supplied by the medial posterior ciliary artery and the cilioretinal artery. **A** reproduced from Hayreh (1990). **B** reproduced from Hayreh SS. Ischemic optic neuropathy. *Int Ophthalmol* 1978;1:9–18.

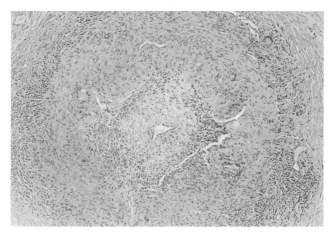

FIGURE 7.4. Temporal artery biopsy specimen demonstrates lymphocyte infiltration, giant cells within the intima and media, and intimal hyperplasia with constriction of the lumen. Photomicrograph courtesy of Robert Folberg, MD.

SUGGESTED READINGS

Hayreh SS. Ophthalmic features of giant cell arteritis. *Clin Rheumatol* 1991;5:431–459. *A review of ocular manifestations of giant cell arteritis.*

Hayreh SS, Podhajsky PA, Raman R, Zimmerman B. Giant cell arteritis: Validity and reliability of various diagnostic criteria. *Am J Ophthalmol* 1997;123:285–296. *A study of diagnostic criteria for giant cell arteritis in 363 patients with temporal artery biopsy over 21 years and followed prospectively.*

Hayreh SS, Podhajsky PA, Zimmerman B. Ocular manifestations of giant cell arteritis. Validity and reliability of various diagnostic criteria. *Am J Ophthalmol* (in press). *A study of ocular manifestations in 170 patients with giant cell arteritis over 22 years and followed prospectively.*

Hayreh SS, Podhajsky PA, Zimmerman B. Occult giant cell arteritis: Ocular manifestations. *Am J Ophthalmol* (in press). *A study of incidence and ocular manifestations in patients with occult giant cell arteritis over 22 years and followed prospectively.*

Hayreh SS. Anterior ischaemic optic neuropathy: Differentiation of arteritic from non-arteritic type and management. *Eye* 1990;4:25–41. *Good discussion of the clinical features suggestive of arteritic AION and management of giant cell arteritis.*

Weyland CM, Bartley GB. Giant cell arteritis: New concepts in pathogenesis and implications for management. *Am J Ophthalmol* 1997;123:392–395. *Very complete editorial discussing the current research into the pathogenesis of giant cell arteritis.*

Weyland CM, Hickok KC, Hunder GG, Goronzy JJ. The HLA-DRB1 locus as a genetic component in giant cell arteritis: Mapping of a disease-linked sequence motif to the antigen-binding site of the HLA-DR molecule. *J Clin Invest* 1992;90:2355–2361. *This study demonstrates linkage of giant cell arteritis with the B1*0401 and B*0404/8 variants of the HLA-DR4 haplotype.*

Chapter 8
POLYARTERITIS NODOSA

John J. Purcell, Jr.

I. GENERAL

1. Immune complexes damage small- and medium-sized arteries.
2. Etiology is unknown.
3. May be acute, subacute, or chronic
4. More frequent in men
5. Clinical manifestations are protean with single or multiple organs involved.

II. SYSTEMIC MANIFESTATIONS

1. Cutaneous
   - Cutaneous or subcutaneous nodules
   - Osler's nodes
   - Urticaria
   - Petechiae
   - Purpura
   - Hemorrhagic bullae
2. Renal
   - Glomerulonephritis
   - Renal infarcts
   - Hypertension
   - Hemorrhagic cystitis
3. Pulmonary
   - Arteries of smaller branches of the pulmonary artery may be involved.
4. Musculoskeletal
   - Arthralgias/myalgias
5. Gastrointestinal
   - Abdominal pain
   - Nausea
   - Vomiting
   - Diarrhea
   - Intestinal bleeding
   - Hepatomegaly
6. Neurologic
   - Peripheral neuritis
   - Central nervous system involvement
7. Nonspecific
   - Fever
   - Weight loss
   - Leukocytosis
   - Malaise

III. OCULAR MANIFESTATIONS

1. Retina
   - Edema
   - Cotton-wool spots
   - Retinal hemorrhages
   - Irregular caliber vessels
   - Branch and central retinal artery occlusion
2. Optic nerve
   - Papillitis
   - Papilledema
3. Neuroophthalmologic
   - Extraocular muscle palsies
   - Amaurosis
   - Homonymous hemianopsia
   - Horner's syndrome
   - Nystagmus
   - Cogan's syndrome
4. Uvea
   - Iridocyclitis
5. Conjunctiva/sclera
   - Necrotizing scleritis
   - Conjunctival edema and necrosis
6. Cornea
   - Keratitis
   - Corneal ring ulcer
7. Orbit
   - Exophthalmos

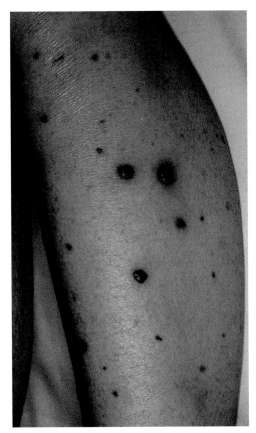

FIGURE 8.1. Nodular, painful, hemorrhagic skin lesion in a patient with polyarteritis nodosa.

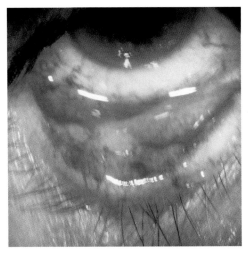

FIGURE 8.2. Areas of conjunctival edema and necrosis in polyarteritis nodosa.

SUGGESTED READINGS

Parker CW. *Clinical Immunology.* Philadelphia: WB Saunders; 1980:478.

Purcell JJ Jr, Birkenkamp R, Tsai CC. Conjunctival lesions in periarteritis nodosa, a clinical and immunopathologic study. *Arch Ophthalmol* 1984;102:736–738.

Sams WJ, Clayrian HN, Kohler PF. Human necrotizing vasculitis: Immunoglobulins and complement in vessel walls of cutaneous lesions and normal skin. *J Invest Dermatol* 1975;64:441.

Chapter 9

REITER'S SYNDROME

Christopher R. Croasdale
Edward J. Holland

I. GENERAL

1. The "classic triad" consists of arthritis, conjunctivitis, and urethritis; the most common manifestations include arthritis, eye inflammation (conjunctivitis or iridocyclitis), urethritis, and mucocutaneous lesions.
2. A presumptive diagnosis can be made based on findings of a seronegative, oligoarticular arthritis with urethritis or cervicitis.
3. The pathogenesis is not fully understood; immune-related mechanisms are involved, and 75% to 90% of patients are HLA-B27 positive.
4. Genitourinary (postvenereal: *Chlamydia trachomatis* and *Ureaplasma urealyticum*) and gastrointestinal (post-dysenteric: *Yersinia enterocolitica, Salmonella* spp, *Shigella* spp, and *Campylobacter jejuni*) infections may lead to Reiter's syndrome; in individual positive for HLA-B27 the risk is 20% to 35%.

II. SYSTEM MANIFESTATIONS

1. Rheumatologic
   - Typically acute, oligoarticular, asymptomatic arthritis
   - Tenosynovitis
   - Dactylitis
   - Sacroiliitis
   - Plantar fasciitis
   - Periostitis of the calcaneus
2. Genitourinary
   - Either sex: intermittent urethritis
   - Women: cervicitis, nonspecific vaginitis
   - Men: prostatitis, cystitis, urethral strictures, circinate balanitis
3. Mucocutaneous
   - Keratoderma blennorrhagicum
   - Superficial lesions of the oral mucosa (aphthous stomatitis) and glans penis (circinate balanitis)
   - Nail abnormalities including subungual pustules and hyperkeratosis
4. Cardiac (less common)
   - Pericarditis, myocarditis
   - Aortic insufficiency
   - Cardiac conduction defects
5. Systemic
   - Amyloidosis
6. Nonspecific
   - Fevers
   - Weight loss

III. OCULAR MANIFESTATIONS

1. Conjunctiva/sclera
   - Conjunctivitis (30–60%), often mild with mucopurulent discharge (culture negative); most patients often do not seek attention and the inflammation usually resolves without treatment in 7 to 10 days.
2. Uvea
   - A nongranulomatous iridocyclitis is the second most common ocular manifestation (15–25%); episodes typically present with mild to moderate inflammation and often show rapid progression to severe inflammation with posterior synechia, and in some cases, hypopyon formation.
   - Posterior uveitis has been reported, but is less common.
3. Cornea
   - Keratitis described as diffuse punctate epithelial erosions with anterior stromal infiltrates and micropannus

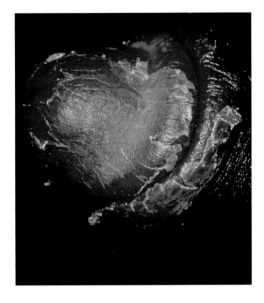

FIGURE 9.1. Reiter's syndrome with balanitis. Courtesy of C. Crutchfield, MD.

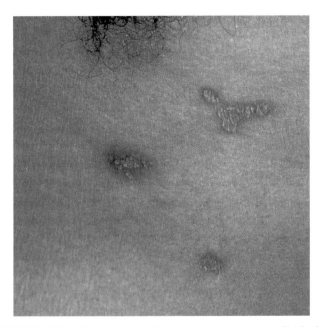

FIGURE 9.2. Keratoderma blennorrhagicum in an individual with Reiter's syndrome. Courtesy of C. Crutchfield, MD.

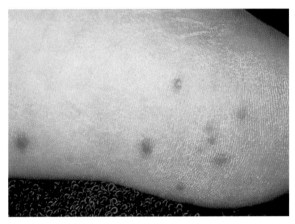

FIGURE 9.3. Keratoderma blennorrhagicum. Courtesy of C. Crutchfield, MD.

SUGGESTED READINGS

Gerber RC. Diagnosis and management of Reiter's syndrome. *Compr Ther* 1984;10:51–57.

Keat A. Reiter's syndrome and reactive arthritis in perspective. *N Engl J Med* 1983;309:1606–1615.

Lee DA, Barker SM, Su WPD, et al. The clinical diagnosis of Reiter's syndrome: Ophthalmic and nonophthalmic aspects. *Ophthalmology* 1986;93:350–356.

Mielants H, Veys EM. Reiter's syndrome and reactive arthritis. *N Engl J Med* 1984;320:1539.

Chapter 10

RELAPSING POLYCHONDRITIS

Eric S. Mann

I. GENERAL

1. Age of onset at diagnosis is approximately 40 to 60 years but may occur at any age with equal sex distribution but no familial predisposition. The disease has been found in all races but predominantly in whites.
2. Ocular manifestations occur in approximately 60% of cases and may be the first manifestation of the disease in 19%.
3. Pathogenesis reveals a genetically determined, aberrant autoimmune response to type II collagen present in sclera and cartilage.
4. Immune-mediated activation and release of degradative enzymes results in recurrent episodes of painful inflammation involving various cartilaginous (eg, ear and nose) and other connective tissue structures throughout the body.
5. Diagnostic criteria include three or more of the six following signs: (1) recurrent chondritis of both auricles, (2) nasal chondritis, (3) nonerosive, inflammatory polyarthritis, (4) ocular inflammation, (5) laryngeal and/or tracheal chondritis, and (6) cochlear or vestibular damage. One sign with a positive biopsy or chondritis in two or more separate anatomic locations that is responsive to corticosteroids or dapsone have also been used as diagnostic criteria.
6. The 5- and 10-year survival rates following diagnosis are 74% and 55%, respectively, with infection and systemic vasculitis the most frequent causes of death.

II. SYSTEMIC MANIFESTATIONS

1. Cardiac
   - Aortic and mitral valve insufficiency
   - Myocarditis
   - Cardiac conduction defects and arrhythmia
2. Vascular
   - Vasculitis
   - Aortitis
   - Aortic aneurysms
   - Thrombosis
3. Pulmonary
   - Laryngeal or tracheobronchial chondritis
4. Renal
   - Proteinuria
   - Microscopic hematuria
   - Glomerulonephritis
5. Neurologic
   - Cerebellar dysfunction
   - Seizure
   - Paresthesia
   - Cerebral vasculitis (arteritis)
   - Stroke
   - Cranial neuropathies
   - Organic brain syndrome
   - Aseptic meningitis
6. Hematologic
   - Antiphospholipid antibodies
   - Elevated erythrocyte sedimentation rate
   - Normochromic/normocytic anemia
   - Leukocytosis, thrombocytosis, and polyclonal hypergammaglobulinemia
7. Musculoskeletal
   - Facial deformities
   - Peripheral inflammatory nonerosive polyarthritis
   - Associated autoimmune disease (eg, rheumatoid arthritis, lupus)
8. Mucocutaneous
   - Superficial thrombophlebitis
   - Palpable purpura
   - Livedo reticularis
   - Erythema nodosum and multiforme
   - MAGIC (mouth and genital ulcers with inflamed cartilage) syndrome
9. Ear/nose/throat
   - Auricular chondritis (drooping, "cauliflower" ear)
   - Auditory dysfunction (conductive or neurosensory hearing loss)
   - Vestibular dysfunction (tinnitus, vertigo)
   - Nasal chondritis ("saddle nose" deformity)
   - Acute airway collapse (10% of all deaths)
10. Nonspecific
    - Fever, myalgia, and weight loss
    - Headache
    - Confusion
    - Hallucinations

1. Lids
   - lid edema
   - tarsitis
2. Lacrimal system
   - Dacryocystitis
3. Conjunctiva/sclera
   - Conjunctivitis
   - Episcleritis
   - Anterior (diffuse, necrotizing, and nodular) and posterior scleritis
   - Scleromalacia and corneoscleral perforation
4. Cornea
   - Peripheral ulcerative keratitis
   - Peripheral corneal infiltrates/thinning/pannus formation
   - Descemetocele
   - Keratitis sicca
5. Uvea
   - Iridocyclitis
6. Lens
   - Cataract

7. Vitreous
   - Vitritis
8. Retina
   - Vasculitis
   - Exudative retinal detachment
   - Vein occlusion
   - Choroiditis
9. Optic nerve
   - Ischemic optic neuropathy
   - Optic neuritis
   - Papilledema
10. Orbit
    - Ptosis
    - Proptosis
    - Inflammation
11. Neuroophthalmology
    - Diplopia
    - Nystagmus
12. Ocular motility
    - Extraocular muscle paresis

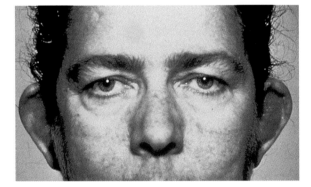

FIGURE 10.1. Floppy ears with bilateral external ear chondritis. This 55-year-old woman also experienced unilateral hearing loss, hoarseness, and costochondritis. Courtesy of Thomas Liesegang, MD.

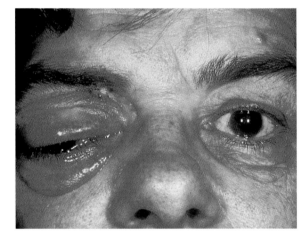

FIGURE 10.2. Proptosis in relapsing polychondritis simulating orbital pseudotumor with unilateral lid, conjunctival, and orbital edema. These clinical features resolved with systemic corticosteroid therapy. Courtesy of Thomas Liesegang, MD.

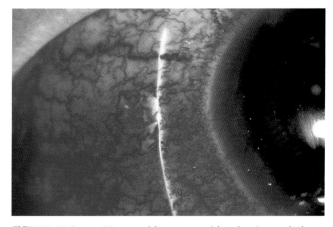

FIGURE 10.3. A 37-year-old woman with relapsing polychondritis and anterior scleritis, which responded promptly to systemic steroids and nonsteroidal therapy. Courtesy of Alan Sugar, MD.

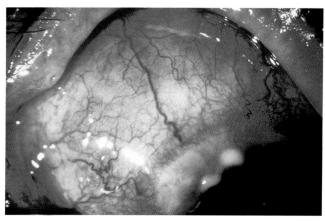

FIGURE 10.4. Anterior nodular scleritis with scleral keratitis and areas of corneal infiltration with later corneal thinning. Courtesy of Thomas Liesegang, MD.

SUGGESTED READINGS

Hoang-xuan T, Foster CS, Rice BA. Scleritis in relapsing polychondritis: Response to therapy. *Ophthalmology* 1990;97:892–898.

Hochberg MC. Relapsing polychondritis. In: Kelley WN, Ruddy S, Harris, Jr. ED et al., eds. *Textbook of Rheumatology*. Philadelphia: WB Saunders Co., 1997:1404–1408.

Isaak BL, Liesegang TL, Michet CJ Jr. Ocular and systemic findings in relapsing polychondritis. *Ophthalmology* 1986;93:681–689.

Margagal LE, Donoso LA, Goldberg RE, et al. Ocular manifestations of relapsing polychondritis. *Retina* 1981;1:96–99. *Excellent reviews of ocular and systemic manifestations.*

Massry GG, Chung SM, Selhorst JB. Optic neuropathy, headache, and diplopia with MRI suggestive of cerebral arteritis in relapsing polychondritis. *J Neurophthalmol* 1995;15:171–175.

Priori R, Paroli MP, Luan FL, et al. Cyclosporin A in the treatment of relapsing polychondritis with severe eye involvement (letter). *Br J Rheumatol* 1992;32:352. *Excellent reviews of treatment and management.*

Chapter 11
ADULT RHEUMATOID ARTHRITIS

Daryl R. Pfister
Jay H. Krachmer

I. GENERAL

1. A chronic multisystem inflammatory disease characterized by progressive polyarthropathy
2. Onset usually in the third to fourth decade affecting women three times more than men
3. Variable course with onset often heralded by constitutional symptoms including fever, malaise, and weight loss followed by arthropathy
4. Diagnosis based on clinical criterion
5. Rheumatoid factor (RF; an IgM immunoglobulin reactive to autologous IgG) positive in 70% of patients with rheumatoid arthritis
6. Systemic symptoms more common in RF positive patients or those with severe joint disease
7. Initial insult appears to be a synovial membrane microvascular event causing edema, vessel occlusion, and neutrophilic infiltration.
8. Hyperplasia and hypertrophy of synovial tissue invades the joint space and a mononuclear cell infiltrate invades the normally acellular synovial stroma (T and B lymphocytes and plasma cells).
9. Progressive joint destruction occurs from degradative neutrophil enzymes and disruption of local joint structures by granulation tissue.
10. Histology shows fibrinoid necrosis in tissues surrounded by palisades of connective tissue, granulation tissue, and lymphocytes/plasma cells.

II. SYSTEMIC MANIFESTATIONS

1. Musculoskeletal
   - Insidious destructive polyarthropathy affecting any joint, but most common in proximal interphalangeal (swan neck deformity) and metacarpophalangeal joints (ulnar deviation)
   - Carpel tunnel syndrome
   - Joint effusions
   - Arthralgias
   - Popliteal cyst (Baker's cyst)
2. Vascular
   - Vasculitis—usually insidious and may manifest in other systems, rarely fulminant causing death
   - Compression of vertebral artery causing syncope
3. Central nervous system
   - Strokes (vasculitis)
   - Syncope (vascular compression)
   - Subluxation of odontoid process with severe nerve damage
4. Mucocutaneous
   - Subcutaneous nodules/granulomas of extensor surfaces
   - Cutaneous ulcerations
   - Raynaud's phenomenon
5. Cardiovascular
   - Myocardial infarctions (vasculitis)
   - Pericarditis—frequent autopsy finding (40%)
   - Granulomas
6. Gastrointestinal
   - Visceral ischemia (vasculitis)
   - Bowel infarction (vasculitis)
7. Pulmonary
   - Pleurisy with or without pleural effusions
   - Rheumatoid nodules
   - Interstitial fibrosis
   - Pulmonary hypertension
8. Hematologic
   - Anemia
   - Leukopenia
   - Lymphadenopathy
9. Renal
   - Renal tubular disease
   - Glomerulonephritis
10. Nonspecific
    - Fever
    - Malaise
    - Weight loss

III. OCULAR MANIFESTATIONS

1. Lacrimal gland
   - Keratoconjunctivitis sicca
2. Cornea
   - Filamentary keratitis
   - Punctate epithelial erosions
   - Corneal ulcers
   - Sclerokeratitis
   - Vascularization/pannus
   - Sclerosing keratitis
   - Peripheral corneal furrowing
   - Keratolysis
3. Sclera/episclera
   - Episcleritis

- Scleritis
  - Anterior—diffuse and nodular
  - Necrotizing with inflammation
  - Necrotizing without inflammation (scleromalacia perforans)
    - Staphylomas
4. Nonspecific
   - Papillary conjunctival reaction
   - Conjunctivitis
   - Staphylococcal blepharitis
   - Uveitis
   - Uveal effusions
   - Exudative retinal detachments

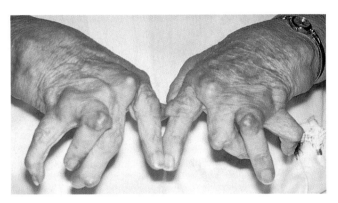

FIGURE 11.1. Characteristic joint deformities of the hands in long-standing rheumatoid arthritis showing ulnar deviation of the metacarpophalangeal joints and rheumatoid nodules on the extensor surfaces of several fingers.

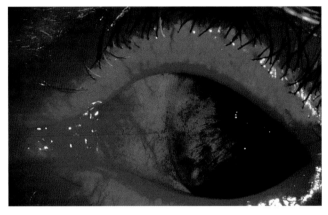

FIGURE 11.2. Sjögren's syndrome showing corneal filaments with punctate corneal and conjunctival rose bengal staining.

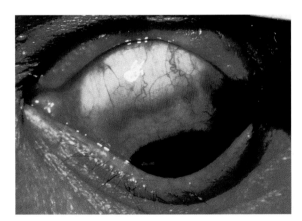

FIGURE 11.3. Scleromalacia perforans with uveal pigment visible through the thin and uninflamed sclera.

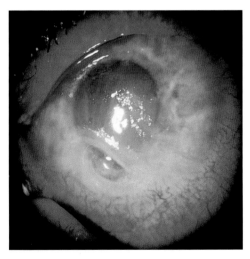

FIGURE 11.4. Peripheral keratolysis with corneal perforation secondary to rheumatoid arthritis.

SUGGESTED READINGS

Nelson JD. Diagnosis of keratoconjunctivitis sicca. *Int Ophthalmol Clin* 1994;34:37–56.

Rodnan GP, Schumacher HR, Zavifler NJ, eds. *Primer on the Rheumatic Diseases,* 8th ed. Atlanta, GA: Arthritis Foundation; 1983:38–46.

Rovin JB, Schanzlin DJ, Verity SM, et al. Peripheral corneal disorders. *Surv Ophthalmol* 1986;31:1–36.

Whitson WE, Krachmer JH. Adult rheumatoid arthritis. In: Gold DH, Weingeist TA, eds. *The Eye in Systemic Disease.* Philadelphia: JB Lippincott; 1990:61–64. *A general review of ocular and systemic manifestations of rheumatoid arthritis.*

Chapter 12
JUVENILE RHEUMATOID ARTHRITIS

Conrad L. Giles

1. Juvenile rheumatoid arthritis (JRA) expresses itself in five distinct subgroups: systemic, rheumatoid factor (RF)-negative polyarticular, RF positive–polyarticular, early onset pauciarticular, and later onset pauciarticular.

2. The pauciarticular subgroups are most frequently associated with ocular disease.

3. The correlation between JRA activity and the severity of eye disease is inconsistent.

4. The prognosis of both the systemic disease (JRA) and its ocular manifestations is significantly improved with early diagnosis and careful monitoring.

II. SYSTEMIC MANIFESTATIONS

SUBGROUPS OF JRA

Subgroup	Ratio Girls/Boys	Age at Onset	Joints Affected	Serology Genetic	Extraarticular Manifestations
1. Systemic onset	8:10	Any	Any	ANA negative RF negative	High fever, rash, organomegaly, polyserositis, leukocytosis, growth retardation
2. Rheumatoid factor–negative, polyarticular	8:1	Any	Any	ANA 25% RF negative	Low-grade fever, mild anemia, malaise, growth retardation
3. Rheumatoid factor–positive, polyarticular	6:1	Late childhood	Any	ANA 75% RF 100%	Low-grade fever, anemia, malaise, rheumatoid nodules
4. Pauciarticular early onset	8:1	Early childhood	Few large joints (hips and sacroiliac joints spared)	ANA 50% RF negative	Few constitutional complaints, chronic iridocyclitis in 50%
5. Pauciarticular	1:10	Late childhood	Few large joints (hip and sacroiliac involvement common)	ANA negative RF negative HLA-B27 75%	Few constitutional complaints, acute, iridocyclitis in 5–10% during childhood

ANA, antinuclear antibodies; RF, rheumatoid factor

III. OCULAR MANIFESTATIONS

1. Early onset pauciarticular JRA
- Normal external appearance
- Biomicroscope necessary to make diagnosis of iritis in most patients
- Low or normal intraocular pressure
- Early to moderate cataract formation at time of initial diagnosis
- Extensive posterior synechiae (adhesions between lens and iris) commonly seen
- Band keratopathy common
- Management of cataract is surgical and usually successful.
- Glaucoma may initially respond to medical therapy but 50% of the patients will require surgery with resultant guarded prognosis.

2. Later onset JRA
- Conjunctiva
  - Markedly injected
- Anterior chamber
  - Marked acute inflammatory response
- Lens
  - Seldom cataractous unless iritis is recurrent
- Intraocular pressure
  - Usually low at onset, seldom elevated even with recurrent disease
- Complications less common than with inflammation in early onset JRA

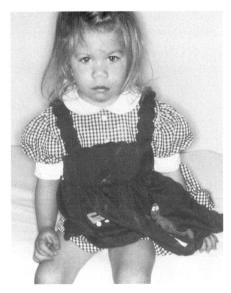

FIGURE 12.1. Girl, aged 2½ years, with pauciarticular JRA exhibiting signs of an acute inflammatory process involving both knees.

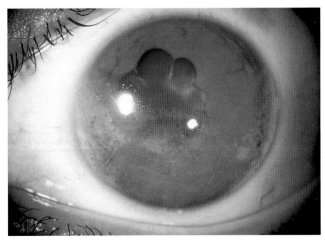

FIGURE 12.2. External photograph of the right eye in a 6-year-old African-American girl with posterior synechiae formation resulting in a scalloped pupil and early band keratopathy in the interpalpebral area of the cornea.

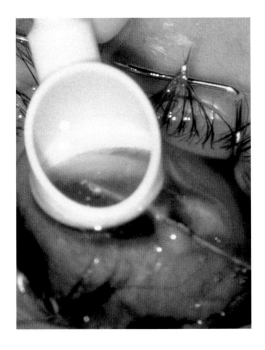

FIGURE 12.3. Trabeculodialysis procedure seen intraoperatively in patient with uncontrolled secondary glaucoma.

SUGGESTED READINGS

Giles CL. Juvenile rheumatoid arthritis and the eye. In: Gold DH, Weingeist TA, eds. *The Eye in Systemic Disease.* Philadelphia: JB Lippincott; 1990;64–67.

Kanski JJ. Anterior uveitis in juvenile rheumatoid arthritis. *Arch Ophthalmol* 1977;95:1794–1797.

Schaller JG. The seronegative spondyloarthropathies of childhood. *Clin Orthop* 1979;143:76–79.

Wolf MD, Litcher PR, Ragsdale CG. Discussion by Smith RE. Prognostic factors in the uveitis of juvenile rheumatoid arthritis. *Ophthalmology* 1987;94:1242–1247.

Chapter 13
SJÖGREN'S SYNDROME
R. Linsy Farris

I. GENERAL

1. An autoimmune disorder in which dry eyes and dry mouth are associated with a connective tissue disease. The presence of any two of the three—dry eye, dry mouth, or connective tissue disease—establishes the diagnosis.
2. Lymphocytic infiltration of lacrimal and salivary glands and organ-directed autoimmune actvity occur with autoimmune features such as hyperglobulinemia and autoantibodies.
3. A predilection for postmenopausal women
4. Primary Sjögren's or sicca complex is a dry mouth (xe-rostomia) and dry eyes (xerophthalmia) in the absence of a connective tissue disorder.
5. Secondary Sjögren's includes the full triad of dry eyes, dry mouth, and a connective tissue or collagen disease such as rheumatoid arthritis, scleroderma, or systemic lupus erythematosus.
6. Organ-directed autoimmune activity produces a wide spectrum of extraglandular features in the lung, kidney, skin, stomach, liver, muscle, thyroid, nerves, and bone marrow.

II. SYSTEMIC MANIFESTATIONS

1. Oral and dental
   - Xerostomia
   - Tongue ulcers and fissures
   - Lip and buccal membrane ulcers
   - Halitosis
   - Caries
   - Periodontal disease
   - Parotid gland enlargement
   - Salivary gland pain
2. Ear/nose/throat
   - Dysphagia
   - Hoarseness
   - Thrush
   - Nasal dryness and crusts
   - Ear canal dryness
3. Vascular
   - Vasculitis
   - Skin changes
     - Purple discolorations
     - Pink hivelike welts
   - Leg ulcers
4. Musculoskeletal
   - Polymyositis
   - Myopathy
   - Muscle weakness
   - Myalgia
   - Arthralgia
5. Central nervous system
   - Paralysis
   - Disordered thinking
   - Loss of speech
   - Muscle weakness
   - Headaches
6. Hematologic
   - Lymphadenopathy
   - Pseudolymphoma
   - Lymphoma
   - Hypergammaglobulinemia
   - Cryoglobulinemia
   - Splenomegaly
   - Leukemia
   - Angioblastic lymphadenopathy
   - Myeloma
   - Aplastic anemia
   - Lymphopenia and neutropenia
7. Mucocutaneous
   - Raynaud's phenomenon
   - Hyperglobulinemic purpura
   - Leg ulcers
   - Mouth dryness
   - Vaginal dryness
   - Nasopharyngeal dryness
   - Anorectal dryness
8. Gastrointestinal
   - Dysphagia
   - Gastric achlorhydria
   - Atrophic gastritis
   - Achalasia
   - Celiac disease
9. Hepatobiliary
   - Hepatitis
   - Pancreatitis
   - Biliary cirrhosis
   - Sclerosing cholangitis
10. Renal
    - Renal tubular acidosis
    - Interstitial nephritis
    - Glomerulonephritis
11. Endocrine
    - Thyroiditis
    - Diabetes
12. Pulmonary
    - Pulmonary fibrosis
    - Pseudolymphoma with nodular infiltrates
    - Pleural effusion
    - Pulmonary hypertension
    - Bronchitis
    - Lymphocytic interstitial pneumonia

13. Nonspecific
  - Fatigue
  - Fever
  - Rheumatoid factor

- Antinuclear antibodies
- Ro/SS-A, La/SS-B autoantibodies
- HLA-DR3 positive

III. OCULAR MANIFESTATIONS

1. Tear film
  - Deficient inferior marginal tear strip
  - Excess debris
  - Excess mucus
  - Increased viscosity

2. Lids
  - Excess debris and foam
  - Excess oiliness
  - Occluded meibomian glands

3. Conjunctiva
  - Dryness
  - Redness
  - Prolapse
  - Hemorrhages
  - Ulceration
  - Folliculosis
  - Symblepharon

4. Cornea
  - Dryness
  - Keratinization

- Ulceration
- Vascularization
- Keratitis

5. Symptoms
  - Foreign body sensation
  - Blurred vision
  - Photophobia
  - Eye awareness
  - Pain
  - Blepharospasm

6. Positive tests
  - Schirmer equals or is less than 5 mm/5 min
  - Rose Bengal staining 4 or more
  - Decreased tear lysozyme and lactoferrin
  - Shortened tear film break-up time
  - Elevated tear osmolarity
  - Impression cytology
    - Decreased goblet cells
    - Squamous metaplasia

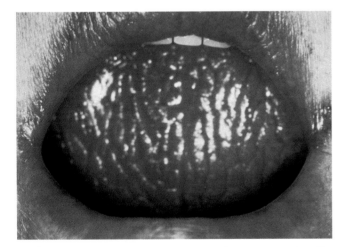

FIGURE 13.1. Dry mouth and dry eye without a connective disorder is considered primary Sjögren's or sicca complex. Patients require frequent ingestion of liquids and have difficulty speaking, chewing, swallowing, and wearing dentures. Note dry fissured tongue.

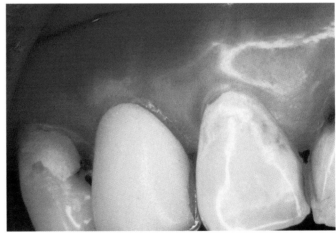

FIGURE 13.2. Gum disease and caries accompany a dry mouth and are worsened by the use of lozenges containing sugar. A positive labial gland biopsy of minor salivary glands demonstrates lymphoid infiltrates.

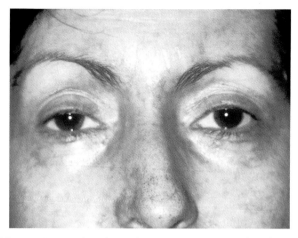

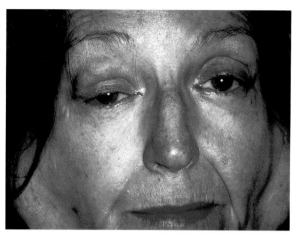

FIGURE 13.3. Scleroderma is a connective tissue disorder that qualifies a patient with dry mouth or dry eye for the diagnosis of secondary Sjögren's syndrome. Scleroderma is often associated with tightness of the eyelids and narrowing of the palpebral tissues. Rheumatoid arthritis, lupus, and positive blood tests for rheumatoid factor, antinuclear antibody, SS-A, and SS-B indicate a systemic autoimmune disorder.

FIGURE 13.4. Parotid gland enlargement occurs in approximately 50% of patients with Sjögren's syndrome and may fluctuate in size and be accompanied by fever, tenderness, and erythema.

SUGGESTED READINGS

Farris RL. Sjögren's syndrome. In: Gold DH, Weingast TA, eds. *The Eye in Systemic Disease.* Philadelphia: JB Lippincott; 1990:70–71. *A general review of the ocular and systemic manifestations of Sjögren's syndrome.*

Farris RL, Stuchell RN, Nisengard R. Sjögren's syndrome and keratoconjunctivitis sicca. *Cornea* 1991;10:207–209. *A study of the incidence of autoantibodies SS-A and SS-B in dry eye patients presenting to ophthalmologists contrasted to studies of dry eye populations presenting to rheumatologists.*

Fox RI, Howell FV, Bone RC, Michelson P. Primary Sjögren's syndrome: Clinical and immunopathologic features. *Semin Arthritis Rheum* 1984;14:77–105. *A good review with 177 references.*

Harris E, ed. *The Sjögren's Syndrome Handbook.* Jericho, NY: Sjögren's Syndrome Foundation; 1989. *An excellent book for both nonprofessionals and professionals compiled by having specialists describe in layman's language the various medical conditions and therapies.*

Chapter 14
SYSTEMIC LUPUS ERYTHEMATOSUS

Bernard F. Godley

I. GENERAL

1. A multisystem inflammatory disease characterized by diverse, asynchronous clinical manifestations and a relapsing course
2. Occurs primarily in women of childbearing age
3. Etiology is multifactorial with an undefined genetic predisposition.
4. Circulating antibodies to components of the cell nucleus are almost invariably present as well as other autoantibodies.
5. Autoantibodies, immune complexes, and complement pathway activation are associated with the diverse multiorgan clinical manifestations.
6. Defective immune regulation results in polyclonal B-cell hyperactivity and T-cell functional impairment.
7. A mild form of lupus may be induced by drugs such as chlorpromazine, hydralazine, methyldopa, isoniazid, and procainamide.

II. SYSTEMIC MANIFESTATIONS

1. Cardiac
   - Pericarditis
   - Myocarditis
2. Vascular
   - Vasculitis
   - Hypertension
   - Thromboses
3. Pulmonary
   - Pleural effusion
   - Pneumonitis
   - Diffuse interstitial fibrosis
4. Renal
   - Nephrotic syndrome
   - Proteinuria
   - Nephritis
   - Hematuria
   - Renal failure
5. Genitourinary
   - Recurrent abortions
6. Neurologic
   - Depression
   - Psychosis
   - Organic brain syndrome
   - Seizures
   - Cranial and peripheral neuropathies
   - Transverse myelitis
   - Idiopathic intracranial hypertension
7. Hematologic
   - Normochromic, normocytic anemia
   - Hemolytic anemia
   - Neutropenia
   - Lymphocytopenia
   - Thrombocytopenia
8. Musculoskeletal
   - Myalgias
   - Arthritis
   - Tenosynovitis
   - Myositis
9. Mucocutaneous
   - Malar facial rash
   - Discoid skin lesions
   - Alopecia
   - Photosensitivity
   - Mucosal ulcers
10. Nonspecific
   - Peritonitis
   - Fever
   - Malaise

III. OCULAR MANIFESTATIONS

1. Lids
   - Subcutaneous nodules
2. Conjunctiva/sclera
   - Scleritis
3. Cornea
   - Keratoconjunctivitis sicca
4. Retina
   - Cotton-wool spots
   - Intraretinal hemorrhages
   - Macular ischemia
   - Roth spots (white-centered hemorrhages)
   - Vasculitis
   - Central serous chorioretinopathy
   - Hard exudates
   - Arteriolar occlusion
   - Retinal neovascularization
5. Optic nerve
   - Anterior/posterior optic neuropathy
6. Orbit
   - Myositis
7. Neuroophthalmologic
   - Gaze palsies
   - Internuclear ophthalmoplegia
   - Papillitis
   - One-and-a-half syndrome

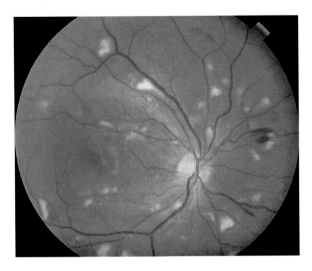

FIGURE 14.1. Right fundus of a 25-year-old woman with an acute exacerbation of systemic lupus erythematosus shows cotton-wool spots and retinal hemorrhages.

SUGGESTED READINGS

Cunningham ET Jr, Alfred PR, Irvine AR. Central serous chorioretinopathy in patients with systemic lupus erythematosus. *Ophthalmology* 1996;103:2081–2090.

Gold DH, Morris DA, Henkind P. Ocular findings in systemic lupus erythematosus. *Br J Ophthalmol* 1972;56:800–804.

Jampol LM, Jabs DA, Gold DH, et al. Ocular complications of acquired diseases of connective tissue. In: Singerman LJ, Jampol LM, eds. *Retinal and Choroidal Manifestations of Systemic Disease.* Baltimore: Williams & Wilkins, 1991:1–16.

Keane JR. Eye movement abnormalities in systemic lupus erythematosus. *Arch Neurol* 1995;52:1145–1149.

Pisetsky DS, Gilkeson G, St. Clair EW. Systemic lupus erythematosus. Diagnosis and treatment. *Med Clin North Am* 1997;18:113–128.

Serop S, Vianna RN, Claeys M, De Laey JJ. Orbital myositis secondary to systemic lupus erythematosus. *Acta Ophthalmol* 1994;72:520–523.

Spalton DJ. Systemic lupus erythematosus. In: Gold DH, Weingeist TA, eds. *The Eye in Systemic Disease.* Philadelphia: JB Lippincott, 1990:72–74.

Steinberg AD, Klinman DM. Pathogenesis of systemic lupus erythematosus. *Rheum Dis Clin North Am* 1988;14:25–41.

Tan E, Cohen A, Fries J, et al. The 1982 revised criteria for the classification of systemic lupus erythematosus. *Arch Rheum* 1982;25:1271–1277.

Chapter 15
WEGENER'S DISEASE

Ernesto I. Segal

1. Classic triad is necrotizing granulomatous lesions of the upper and lower respiratory tracts, focal necrotizing vasculitis, and glomerulonephritis.
2. A limited form of Wegener's granulomatosis has minimal renal involvement.
3. The cause is unknown. A hypersensitivity to an unidentified antigen is suspected, but no antigen–antibody complexes have been found. Experimental evidence suggests an abnormality in the cell-mediated immunity.
4. Antineutrophil cytoplasmic antibodies (ANCA) are present in 60% to 96% of the patients with Wegener's disease. It is more sensitive for the active generalized disease (88% of the patients) than in the active localized disease or in the remission phase of the disease (44% of the patients).
5. Histopathology involves mainly the collagen and blood vessels. Vasculitis lesions are characterized by fibrinoid degeneration of the arteries, arterioles, and occasionally of the venules. The granulomas have a central necrotizing focus, surrounded by fibrohistiocytes and multinucleated giant cells.
6. The fourth to fifth decade of life is the most frequent age of onset, there is no sex predominance, and the course of the disease is variable from 5 months to years, with treatment.
7. The mechanism of ocular involvement is scleritis, vasculitis-related damage to the retina and optic nerve, and granulomatous inflammation in the orbit and adnexae.
8. Current treatment consists of the combined used of systemic cytotoxic drugs (especially cyclophosphamide) and corticosteroids, with improvement in approximately 91% of the patients and complete remission in 75%. The overall mortality rate is 13%.

II. SYSTEMIC MANIFESTATIONS

1. Pulmonary
   - Multiple bilateral infiltrates, nodules, or cavities
   - Pleuritis
   - Hemoptysis
   - Cough
2. Ear/nose/throat
   - Mucosal inflammation and ulceration
   - Epistaxis
   - Sinusitis
   - Secondary bacterial infections
   - Secondary structural destruction and deformities
   - Midface granulomas
   - Pharyngitis
   - Tracheitis
3. Renal
   - Proteinuria
   - Hematuria
   - Focal or diffuse glomerulonephritis
   - Renal failure
4. Cardiac
   - Pericarditis
   - Coronary vasculitis
5. Neurologic
   - Mononeuritis multiplex
   - Cranial neuritis
   - Meningocerebral inflammation
   - Secondary central nervous system infections
6. Skin
   - Palpable purpura
   - Ulcers
   - Papules and vesicles
   - Subcutaneous nodules
7. Musculoskeletal
   - Arthritis
   - Arthralgias, myalgias
8. Hematologic
   - Chronic anemia
   - Eosinophilia
   - Granulomatous vasculitis in the liver, spleen, and lymph nodes
9. Vascular
   - Necrotizing vasculitis of the arteries and arterioles
10. Nonspecific
    - Fever
    - Weight loss

1. Lids
- Painful ptosis
- Edema
- Nodules

2. Conjunctiva/sclera
- Anterior scleritis (mainly diffuse anterior or necrotizing)
- Posterior scleritis
- Episcleritis
- Conjunctival inflammation

3. Cornea
- Marginal ulcerative keratitis (necrotizing sclerokeratitis)
- Exposure keratopathy (secondary to severe exophthalmos)

4. Intraocular pressure
- Secondary neovascular glaucoma (in patients with severe retinal vasculitis)

5. Retina and vitreous
- Vasculitis: perivascular sheathing
- Cotton-wool spots
- Superficial and intraretinal hemorrhages
- Vasoocclusive disease: central retinal and branch retinal artery occlusion, branch retinal vein occlusion
- Secondary retinal neovascularization and vitreous hemorrhage

6. Optic nerve
- Anterior ischemic optic neuropathy
- Optic disc vasculitis

7. Orbit and lacrimal system (most common)
- Exophthalmos
- Granulomatous inflammation (usually an extension from the sinuses)
- Orbital celullitis
- Orbital pseudotumor
- Dacryocystitis
- Nasolacrimal duct obstruction

8. Neuroophthalmologic
- Compressive optic neuropathy (secondary to orbital pathology)
- Ocular motility restriction
- Cranial nerves palsies
- Diplopia

9. Nonspecific
- Posterior uveitis
- Loss of vision from vasculitis or compressive optic neuropathy

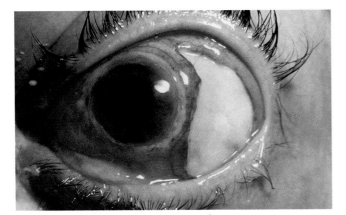

FIGURE 15.1. Scleral ulcer in patient with Wegener's granulomatosis. Note necrotic white area temporally.

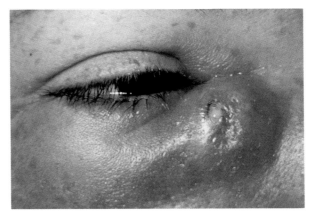

FIGURE 15.2. Dacryocystitis in patient with Wegener's granulomatosis. Note fistula draining to skin.

SUGGESTED READINGS

Grove AS Jr. Wegener's disease. In: Gold DH, Weingeist TA, eds. *The Eye in Systemic Disease.* Philadelphia: JB Lippincott; 1990:74–76.

Hoffman GS, Kerr GS, Leavitt RV, et al. Wegener granulomatosis: An analysis of 158 patients. *Ann Intern Med* 1992;116:488–498.

Jabs DA. Rheumatic diseases. In: Ryan SJ, ed. *Retina,* vol 2. St. Louis: Mosby; 1994:1434–1435.

Jakobiec FA, Jones IS. Orbital inflammation. In: Tasman W, Jaeger EA, eds. *Duane's Clinical Ophthalmology,* vol 2. Philadelphia: JB Lippincott; 1993:30–34.

Leavitt RV, Fauci AS, Bloch DA, et al. The American College of Rheumatology 1990 criteria for the classification of Wegener's granulomatosis. *Arthritis Rheum* 1990;33:1101.

Newman NJ, Slamovits TL, Friedland S, et al. Neuro-ophthalmic manifestations of meningocerebral inflammation from the limited form of Wegener's granulomatosis. *Am J Ophthalmol* 1995;120:613–621.

Power WJ, Rodriguez A, Neves RA, et al. Disease relapse in patients with ocular manifestations of Wegener granulomatosis. *Ophthalmology* 1995;102:154–160.

Wolff S, Fauci A, Horn R, et al. Wegener's granulomatosis. *Ann Intern Med* 1974;81:513.

PART 4.   ENDOCRINE DISORDERS

Chapter 16

DIABETES MELLITUS

Matthew D. Davis

I. GENERAL

1. Definition: Deficiency in production, secretion, or action of insulin, causing intolerance to ingested carbohydrate and consequent hyperglycemia
2. Insulin-dependent diabetes mellitus (IDDM; juvenile onset, type 1)
   - Caused by severe loss of insulin-producing cells of pancreas (beta cells), thought to be secondary to inflammation caused by autoimmune reaction or viral infection
   - Clinical characteristics
     - Abrupt onset (polyuria, thirst, weight loss) usually before age 20 to 30 years
     - Permanent dependence on insulin injections to prevent acidosis, dehydration, and death in hyperglycemic coma
3. Non–insulin-dependent diabetes mellitus (NIDDM; adult onset, type 2)
   - Causal mechanisms unclear
     - Abnormalities of insulin secretion or resistance to its action in peripheral tissues
     - Strong genetic component (concordance in identical twins approaches 100% versus probably 50% or less in IDDM)
   - Clinical characteristics
     - Typically discovered during intercurrent illness or on routine examination after age 40 years. Occasionally symptoms of a chronic complication of presumably long-standing undetected diabetes lead to the diagnosis.
     - Most patients are obese.
     - Ketoacidosis and coma do not occur.

II. SYSTEMIC MANIFESTATIONS

1. Although pathogenetic mechanisms are not well understood, data from the Diabetes Control and Complications Trial (DCCT) demonstrate that in patients with IDDM development of most complications can be inhibited substantially by very careful control using self-monitoring of blood glucose levels and multiple daily insulin injections. Similar studies in the United Kingdom and Japan have found that good control is also a benefit in NIDDM.
2. Nephropathy
   - Diffuse and nodular deposits of basement membrane-like material in the mesangial region of the glomerulus cause occlusion of glomerular capillaries and renal failure.
   - More common in IDDM, with 30% to 40% of these patients eventually developing end-stage renal disease
   - Renal transplantation is usually successful.
3. Neuropathy
   - Pathogenesis is not well understood.
   - Types
     - Distal symmetrical polyneuropathy most common (pain, impaired touch or pain sensation beginning in lower extremities)
     - Autonomic neuropathy (impotence, gastrointestinal disturbances, neurogenic bladder, orthostatic hypotension)
     - Cranial nerve palsies are due to vascular occlusions, not neuropathy, and typically recover spontaneously (sixth nerve, third nerve with pupil spared).
     - Treatment unsatisfactory
4. Accelerated atherosclerosis
   - Pathogenesis not well understood
   - Myocardial infarction, cerebrovascular accidents, and vascular occlusions in the smaller arteries of the lower legs and feet leading to gangrene and amputation are particularly common in NIDDM but also occur in IDDM
   - Relationship to diabetic control less clear than for other complications

III. OCULAR MANIFESTATION

1. Retinopathy
   - Causal mechanisms
     - Earliest anatomic abnormalities are loss of intramural pericytes of retinal capillaries, closure of capillaries, and microaneurysm formation.
     - Pathogenesis is unclear (theoretical causes suggested for capillary closure include excess wear and tear related to deficient autoregulation and thrombosis related to increased red blood cell aggregation or platelet adhesiveness; causes suggested for microaneurysms include vasoproliferation, weakening of capillary wall, and increased intraluminal pressure).
   - Natural course
     - Microaneurysm formation
     - Excess permeability of microaneurysms and capillaries, leading to hard exudates and retinal thickening (edema)
     - Capillary closure, indicated by cotton-wool patches, capillary dropout on fluorescein angiography and, when advanced, by dark red blot hemor-

rhages and finally by "featureless retina" and small white arteriolar branches

- Proliferation
  - Within the retina, intraretinal microvascular abnormalities (IRMA) and venous beading
  - On the surface of the disc and retina, new vessels (source of vitreous hemorrhage) and fibrous proliferations
- Contraction of fibrous proliferations and vitreous, leading to displacement, distortion, or detachment of the retina
- Role of blood glucose control
  - In the DCCT, long-term risk of retinopathy progression in patients with IDDM reduced about 5-fold in group assigned to careful control (which had, on average, lower hemoglobin A_{lc} by 2 percentage points).
  - When severe nonproliferative diabetic retinopathy (NPDR) (Fig. 16.1) or proliferative diabetic retinopathy (PDR) (Fig. 16.2) is already present in patients with long-standing poor control, rapid change to good control may be accompanied by sight-threatening progression of retinopathy.
- Treatment of macular edema
  - Indicated when retinal thickening (edema) or hard exudate involve or threaten the center of the macula (Fig. 16.3)
  - Focal or grid photocoagulation
    - Efficacy in slowing further visual loss is well documented, but improvement is infrequent.
    - Repeated treatments often needed
  - Systemic treatment. Clinical impression suggests that lowering elevated lipids, controlling hypertension, and combating fluid retention with diuretics or salt restriction may be helpful in some patients.
- Treatment of very severe NPDR (Fig. 16.2) or high-risk PDR (Fig. 16.3)
  - Scatter (panretinal) photocoagulation should be considered when retinopathy approaches the high-risk stage (ie, in the very severe nonproliferative or early proliferative stages) and should generally be carried out promptly when the high-risk stage is present.
  - Goals are regression of existing new vessels and prevention of additional new vessels.
  - Efficacy in reducing risk of severe visual loss is well documented.

2. Anterior segment neovascularization and neovascular glaucoma
   - Unusual before stage of very severe NPDR or PDR
   - Prompt retinal scatter photocoagulation may stop progression to otherwise intractable angle closure glaucoma.
3. Corneal epithelium is vulnerable to damage and healing after trauma is often slow.
4. Sixth and pupil-sparing third nerve palsies from ischemic events; spontaneous recovery is usual.
5. Cataract. Snowflake occasionally in young with very poor control, otherwise indistinguishable from age-related cataract (but occur earlier). Extraction is sometimes followed by retinopathy progression or anterior segment neovascularization.
6. Orbital cellulitis from *Mucor* species in patients in ketoacidosis

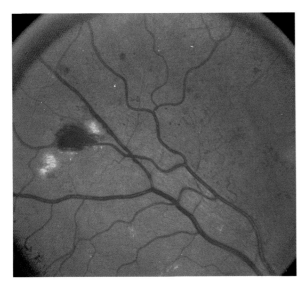

FIGURE 16.1. Very severe NPDR. On the left side of the figure are two prominent cotton-wool spots (soft exudates) with a large blot hemorrhage between them. Venous beading is present where the superior branch of the superior temporal vein passes by the upper exudate. On the right side of the figure is a faint soft exudate with many prominent IRMA near it. This eye is classified as very severe NPDR on the basis of the extensive IRMA and obvious venous beading. Courtesy of the ETDRS Research Group.

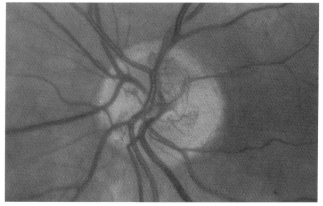

FIGURE 16.2. Standard photograph 10A of the Modified Airlie House Classification, defining the lower margin of the moderate category for new vessels on or within 1 disc diameter (dd) of the disc (NVD). New vessels cover about one-quarter the area of this disc, which is a little larger than average. New vessels equaling or exceeding those in this photograph are sufficient to place an eye in the high-risk category (without regard to the size of the disc). Eyes with NVD less than shown, or with new vessels elsewhere, that is, > 1 dd from the disc (NVE), when accompanied by vitreous or preretinal hemorrhage also belong to the high-risk category. Courtesy of the DRS Research Group.

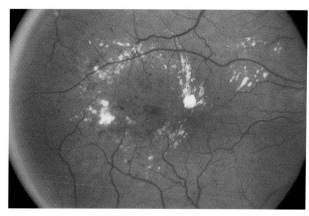

FIGURE 16.3. A hard exudate ring about 1.5 dd in diameter is centered about 1.0 dd supertemporal to the center of the macula in this right eye. Part of the ring is a plaque of hard exudate just above the center of the macula. Within the ring many large microaneurysms can be seen, some with visible walls. They are slightly out of focus because the retina here is thickened (edematous) and the camera is focused on the surrounding retina. With stereoscopic viewing retinal thickening was obvious and could be seen to extend into the center of the macula. Courtesy of the ETDRS Research Group.

SUGGESTED READINGS

Davis MD. Diabetic retinopathy: A clinical overview. *Diabetes Care* 1992;15:1844–1874. *General summary.*

Diabetes Control and Complications Trial Research Group. The effect of intensive diabetes treatment on the progression of diabetic retinopathy in insulin-dependent diabetes mellitus. *Arch Ophthalmol* 1995;113:36–51. *One of two DCCT reports on retinopathy.*

Diabetic Retinopathy Study Research Group. Photocoagulation treatment of proliferative diabetic retinopathy. Clinical application of Diabetic Retinopathy Study (DRS) findings. Diabetic Retinopathy Study Report 8. *Ophthalmology* 1981;88:583–600. *Summary of DRS results.*

Early Treatment Diabetic Retinopathy Study Research Group. Photocoagulation for diabetic macular edema. Early Treatment Diabetic Retinopathy Study Report Number 4. *Int Ophthalmol Clin* 1987;27:265–272. *ETDRS technique for treatment of macular edema and results.*

Early Treatment Diabetic Retinopathy Study Research Group. Early photocoagulation for diabetic retinopathy. ETDRS Report Number 9. *Ophthalmology* 1991;98:766–785. *Principal ETDRS report.*

Early Treatment Diabetic Retinopathy Study Research Group. Fundus photographic risk factors for progression of diabetic retinopathy. ETDRS Report Number 12. *Ophthalmology* 1991;98:823–833. *Classification of diabetic retinopathy.*

Chapter 17

HYPERTHYROIDISM AND HYPOTHYROIDISM

Devron H. Char

I. GENERAL

1. Thyroid-related orbitopathy is the most common etiology for either unilateral or bilateral proptosis in adult patients.
2. Approximately 66% of thyroid orbitopathy cases present within an 18-month interval around the time of discovery of systemic hyperthyroidism.
3. Women more commonly develop thyroid orbitopathy as compared to men.
4. Shared orbital-thyroid antigens are important in pathophysiology.
5. More than 90% of hyperthyroid patients have subtle, transient eye changes.
6. Only 5.2% of hyperthyroid patients develop severe enough eye changes to require corticosteroids, radiation, or surgery.
7. Smokers have an increased risk of severe thyroid orbitopathy.
8. Family history is often positive for thyroid disease.

II. SYSTEMIC MANIFESTATIONS

1. Cardiac
   - Rhythm abnormalities depending on thyroid status and age
2. Vascular
   - Thyroid storm
3. Central nervous system
   - Change in autonomic function and reflexes
   - Emotional alterations
   - Tremor
   - Periodic paralysis (almost entirely in Asian patients)
   - Change in libido
   - Occasional association with myasthenia gravis
   - Myxedema coma in elderly
4. Musculoskeletal
   - Weakness
   - Osteoporesis
   - Bone pain
5. Renal
6. Mucocutaneous
   - Hair changes
   - Dermopathy
7. Nonspecific
   - Heat intolerance
   - Altered bowel habits: diarrhea or constipation
   - Weight change
   - Jaundice in thyroid storm

III. OCULAR MANIFESTATIONS

1. Lids
   - Puffiness
   - Eyelid retraction
   - Eyelid lag on downgaze (von Graefe's sign)
2. Lacrimal system—excessive lacrimation
3. Conjunctiva/sclera
   - Staining due to exposure
   - Increased vascularity over insertion of extraocular muscles
4. Cornea
   - Exposure due to either excessive proptosis, eyelid retraction, or restriction of inferior recti with subsequent loss of Bell's phenomena
   - Rarely, a variant that simulates superior limbic punctate keratopathy
5. Intraocular pressure (Braley's sign) increased when measured in upgaze as compared to normal position
6. Uvea
7. Lens
8. Vitreous
9. Retina
   - Rarely choroidal striae with severe compression and proptosis
10. Optic nerve
    - Compression of apical portion of optic nerve by enlarged extraocular muscles
    - Evidence of optic nerve swelling on fundus examination of approximately 50% of compressive optic neuropathy patients
11. Orbit
    - Typical pattern, muscles: inferior recti, medial recti, less commonly superior recti, obliques. Relative sparing of the muscle tendons of extraocular muscle involvement noted on imaging
    - Increased orbital fat (may occur alone in 9% of cases)
    - Compressive optic neuropathy in 2% of cases
12. Neuroophthalmologic
    - Compressive optic neuropathy
    - Combined syndromes, *ie,* myasthenia gravis and Graves' disease
    - Restrictive myopathy
13. Ocular motility
    - Restrictive myopathy most commonly involves the inferior or medial recti muscles.
    - Superior and lateral recti and the oblique muscles are less frequently affected.

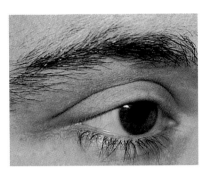

FIGURE 17.1. The patient complained of a loss of lashes from the right upper eyelid for over 2 years. There was no history of intraocular inflammation. There was a loss of approximately 50% of lashes from the lid, with poliosis of the remaining lashes.

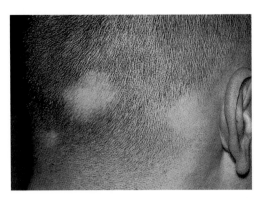

FIGURE 17.2. The patient's scalp shows areas of patchy alopecia and whitening of the remaining hair. The patient had previously undergone treatments for alopecia areata with intralesional corticosteriod injections without success. Metabolic evaluation revealed undiagnosed primary hyperthyroidism.

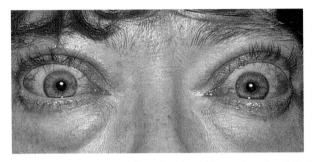

FIGURE 17.3. Patient with active thyroid-associated ophthalmopathy. Features exhibited include conjunctival hyperemia, periorbital edema, upper lid retraction, and exophthalmos. Courtesy of Mr. Peter Fells, Moorfields Eye Hospital, London.

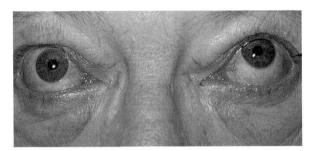

FIGURE 17.4. Patient in the quiescent cicatricial phase of thyroid-associated ophthalmopathy. There is limited upgaze in the right eye due to fibrosis of the inferior rectus muscle. Courtesy of Mr. Peter Fells, Moorfields Eye Hospital, London.

SUGGESTED READINGS

Bahn RS, Heufelder AE. Pathogenesis of Graves' ophthalmopathy. *N Engl J Med* 1993;329:1468–1475.

Char DH. *Thyroid Eye Disease.* Boston: Butterworth Heinemann; 1997.

Greenspan F, ed. Thyroid diseases. *Med Clin North America* 1991; 75.

Jaume JC, Portolano S, Prummel MF, et al. Molecular cloning and characterization of genes for antibodies generated by orbital tissue-infiltrating B-cells in Graves' ophthalmopathy. *J Clin Endocrinol Metab* 1994;78:348–352.

Chapter 18
PARATHYROID DISORDERS

Yuval Yassur
Zvi Tessler

I. GENERAL: HYPERPARATHYROIDISM

Parathyroid hormone (PTH) regulates calcium metabolism in the body (together with vitamin D and calcitonin) and participates in systemic phosphorus homeostasis.

1. Occurs between third and seventh decade
2. The primary form is the result of adenoma (80%), hyperplasia (15%), or carcinoma (4%).
3. Secondary and tertiary forms are the consequence of chronic renal failure, phosphate retention, compensatory hypocalcemia, and a resultant overproduction of PTH.
4. Elevated PTH increases calcium recruitment from renal tubules, intestine, and bone.
5. The systemic and ocular signs are caused mainly by the hypercalcemia with contributions by hypophosphatemia and elevated PTH.

II. SYSTEMIC MANIFESTATIONS: HYPERPARATHYROIDISM

1. Renal
   - Stones
   - Tubular acidosis
2. Musculoskeletal
   - Bone demineralization
   - Muscle weakness
   - Muscle atrophy
   - Chondrocalcinosis
   - Arthritis
3. Central nervous system
   - Lethargy
   - Depression
   - Psychosis
4. Gastrointestinal
   - Abdominal pain
   - Peptic ulcers
   - Pancreatitis
5. Cardiac—electrocardiographic
   - Shortened QT
   - Prolonged PR
   - First-degree block
6. Skin
   - Necrosis
7. Vascular
   - Hypertension

III. OCULAR MANIFESTATIONS: HYPERPARATHYROIDISM

1. Conjunctiva/sclera
   - Calcifications
   - Redness
   - Grittiness
2. Cornea
   - Calcifications
   - Band keratopathy
3. Orbit
   - Brown tumor

I. GENERAL: HYPOPARATHYROIDISM

1. Due to PTH deficiency (true hypoparathyroidism) or PTH resistance (pseudohypoparathyroidism)
2. May be idiopathic, the consequence of thyroidectomy, or the result of inherited target organ resistance
3. Results in hypocalcemia and hyperphosphatemia
4. The systemic and ocular signs are attributed to hypocalcemia.

II. SYSTEMIC MANIFESTATIONS: HYPOPARATHYROIDISM

1. Neurologic
   - Paresthesias
   - Chvostek's sign
   - Trousseau's sign
   - Laryngospasm
   - Dysphagia
   - Dyspnea
   - Tetany
2. Central nervous system
   - Anxiety
   - Confusion
   - Psychosis
   - Mental retardation
   - Seizures
   - Increased intracranial pressure
   - Brain calcifications

3. Mucocutaneous
   - Enamel hypoplasia
   - Coarse hair/alopecia
   - Brittle nails
   - Monilial infections (nails/oral mucosa)
4. Musculoskeletal
   - In pseudohypoparathyroidism
     - Short stocky build
     - Short metacarpus/metatarsus
5. Cardiac
   - Prolonged QT
   - Congestive heart failure
6. Nonspecific
   - Weakness
   - Fatigue

III. OCULAR MANIFESTATIONS: HYPOPARATHYROIDISM

1. Conjunctiva/cornea
   - Keratoconjunctivitis
   - Stromal vascularization
   - Photophobia
   - Blepharospasm

2. Lens
   - Cataract
3. Neuroophthalmologic
   - Papilledema

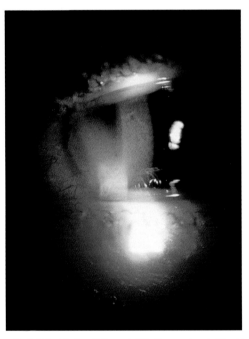
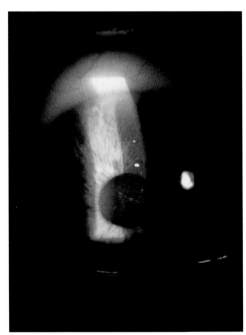

A
B

FIGURE 18.1. **(A)** and **(B)** Corneal calcifications in the shape of band keratopathy in hyperparathyroidism.

SUGGESTED READINGS

Hyperparathyroidism

Heath H III. Clinical spectrum of primary hyperparathyroidism: Evaluation with changes in medical practice and technology. *J Bone Miner Res* 1991;6(suppl 2):S63–S70.

Potts JT Jr, Fradkin JE, Aurbach GD, et al. Proceedings of the NIH Consensus Development Conference on Diagnosis and Mananagement of Asymptomatic Primary Hyperparathyroidism. *J Bone Miner Res* 1991;6(suppl 2):S1–S165.

Rao DS. Primary hyperparathyroidism: Changing patterns in presentation and treatment decisions in the eighties. *Henry Ford Hosp Med J* 1985;33:194–197.

Hypoparathyroidism

Basser LS, Neale FC, Ireland AW, et al. Epilepsy and electroencephalographic abnormalities in chronic surgical hypoparatyroidism. *Ann Intern Med* 1969;71:507–515.

Brickman AS. *Diagnosis, Classification and Treatment of Hypoparathyroid Disorders.* Nutley, NJ: Hoffman-La Roache; 1982.

Phillipson B, Angelin B, Chrisstenson T, et al. Hypocalcemia with zonular cataract due to idiopathic hypoparathyroidism. *Acta Med Scand* 1978;203:223.

Chapter 19

MULTIPLE ENDOCRINE NEOPLASIA SYNDROME

R. Jean Campbell

1. The term multiple endocrine neoplasia (MEN) denotes a genetically determined syndrome that is characterized by the independent appearance of benign or malignant tumors of the endocrine glands. Occasionally, changes of neural, muscular, and connective tissue also occur. Tumor growth is universally bilateral and multicentric.

2. Subgroups of the syndrome are identified according to the organs that are involved:
   - Type 1 (MEN 1) Wermer's disease
   - Type 2 (MEN 2)
       MEN 2A Sipple's syndrome
       MEN 2B

3. Tumor types include
   - Medullary carcinoma of the thyroid
   - Pheochromocytoma of the adrenal medulla
   - Focal nodular hyperplasia, parathyroids, adrenals
   - Carcinoid bronchus, intestine
   - Polyps, stomach
   - Schwannoma, peripheral nerves
   - Lipomas, hibernomas, numerous sites

4. Autosomal dominant pattern of inheritance. Genetic linkage studies have mapped the MEN type 2 loci to a small interval on chromosome 10q 11.2.
   - MEN 2B is also associated with mutation of the RET protooncogene.

II. SYSTEMIC MANIFESTATIONS

Organs Affected	Disease
Pituitary, pancreas, parathyroid	Type 1 Wermer's syndrome Pituitary tumors Pancreatic islet cell tumor Parathyroid hyperplasia
Thyroid, adrenal, parathyroid	Type 2A Sipple's syndrome Medullary carcinoma Pheochromocytoma Parathyroid hyperplasia
Thyroid, adrenal, parathyroid	Type 2B
Gastrointestinal tract	Medullary thyroid carcinoma
Ocular manifestations	Pheochromoctyoma Ganglioneuromas

III. OCULAR MANIFESTATIONS

1. Conjunctiva
   - Neuromas of palpebral conjunctiva result in thickened eyelids.
2. Cornea
   - Bundles of enlarged nerves are most obvious at the corneoscleral junction.
   - Nerves are evident throughout the cornea on slit-lamp examination.
3. Intraocular
   - Large nerve bundles present in the iris, ciliary body.
   - Increased numbers of ganglion cells present in trabecular meshwork, iris root, and ciliary body.

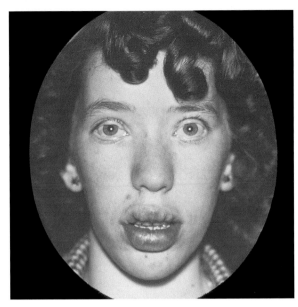

FIGURE 19.1. Note thickened, partially everted upper eyelids due to palpebral conjunctival neuromas. Upper and lower lips are thickened by mucosal neuromas.

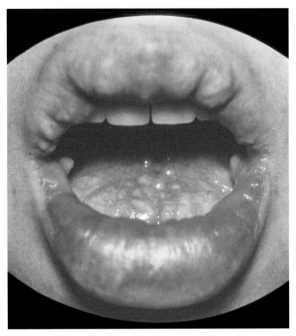

FIGURE 19.2. Multiple neuromas thicken the lips and produce characteristic tumefactions at the angles of the mouth.

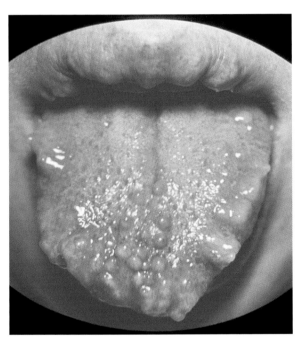

FIGURE 19.3. Tongue is irregularly thickened by submucosal neuromas.

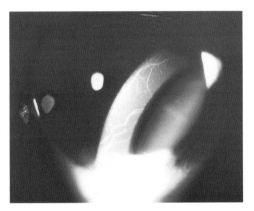

FIGURE 19.4. Slit-lamp appearance of prominent corneal nerves.

SUGGESTED READINGS

Campbell RJ. Multiple endocrine neoplasia syndrome. In: Gold DH, Weingeist TA, eds. *The Eye in Systemic Disease.* Philadelphia: JB Lippincott; 1990:91–93. *A review of the ocular manifestation of multiple endocrine neoplasia syndrome type 2B.*

Carlson KM, Dou S, Chi D, et al. Single missense mutation in the tyrosine kinase catalytic domain of the RET protooncogenesis associated with multiple endocrine neoplasia type 2B. *Proc Natl Acad Sci USA* 1994;91:1579–1583. *A report of the sequence differences in germ line mutation ATG-ACG in MEN 2B in 34 unrelated individuals with its effect on the oncogenic activity on the RET protein.*

Hofstra RM, Landsvater RM, Ceccherini L, et al. A mutation in the RET protooncogene associated with multiple endocrine neoplasia type 2B and sporadic medullary carcinoma. *Nature* 1994;367:375–376. *A review of the three clinically distinct MEN 2 syndromes with information of the germ line mutations.*

Raue F, Zink A. Clinical features of multiple endocrine neoplasia type 1 and type 2. (Review) *Horm Res* 1992;38 (suppl 2):31 35. *A general review of the clinical manifestations of the MEN syndrome.*

Chapter 20

PITUITARY DISORDERS

Duncan P. Anderson
David Kendler

1. Pituitary adenoma comprises 10% to 15% of surgical intracranial tumors and 6% to 23% in unselected autopsy series.
2. Histologically benign: microadenoma less than 10 mm, macroadenoma greater than 10 mm.
3. Symptoms of headache are variable; more common with macroadenoma.
4. Minority of presentations: ocular manifestations from mechanical compression of visual sensory pathways and ocular motor nerves.
5. Majority of presentations are hormonal excess. Hormonal deficiencies from tumor mass effect luteinizing hormone (LH), follicle-stimulating hormone (FSH) deficiency most common followed by growth hormone (GH), thyroid-stimulating hormone (TSH), adrenocorticotropic hormone (ACTH), and prolactin (PRL); children often present with growth arrest or delayed puberty.
6. Evaluation includes endocrine assay, neuroophthalmic examination, and neuroimaging of pituitary (computed tomography/magnetic resonance imaging of sella turcica).
7. Management goal is to normalize hormonal function, eliminate mass effect. May be accomplished by medical, surgical, or radiotherapy modalities.

II. SYSTEMIC MANIFESTATIONS

Adenoma Type	PRL	GH	ACTH	LH/FSH	TSH	Pleuri	Null
Hormone secreted	Prolactin	Growth hormone	Adrenocorticotrophic hormone	Luteinizing/follicle-stimulating hormone (gonadotropins)	Thyroid-stimulating hormone	Multiple hormones, often GH/PRL	Not yet identified
Old term	Chromophobe	Eosinophilic	Basophilic				
Frequency	27%	13%	10%	9%	1%	9%	31%
Hormone excess: clinical manifestations	Amenorrhea Decreased libido Infertility Galactorrhea Gynecomastia	Gigantism or acromegaly: Bony/other tissue hypertrophy (eg, hand, foot, jaw) Sweating Diabetes mellitus Hypertension	Cushing's disease: Obesity Hypertension Diabetes mellitus Striae Weakness Infection Psychosis	None	Hyperthyroid: Weight loss Tremor Sweating Tachycardia Weakness Diarrhea	Variable	None
Hormone deficiency: clinical manifestations	Deficient lactation	Growth arrest Deficient lactation	Addison's disease: Hypotension Fatigue Weakness Hypoglycemia	Amenorrhea Decreased libido Infertility	Hypothyroid: Weight gain Coarse hair Cold intolerance Constipation	Variable	None
Immunoassays	PRL	Insulinlike growth factor (IGF-I) GH	Cortisol ACTH	Estradiol Progesterone Testosterone FSH LH	T$_3$ T$_4$ TSH	Variable Alpha-subunit (of TSH, LH, FSH)	None
Therapy	Bromocriptine Somatostatin-analogue Pituitary surgery Radiotherapy	Pituitary surgery Somatostatin-analogue Radiotherapy	Pituitary surgery Adrenalectomy Mitotane Somatostatin-analogue Radiotherapy	Pituitary surgery Somatostatin-analogue Radiotherapy	Pituitary surgery Thyroidectomy Radiotherapy	Pituitary surgery Somatostatin-analogue Radiotherapy	Pituitary surgery Somatostatin-analogue Radiotherapy

III. OCULAR MANIFESTATIONS: SUPERIOR TUMOR EXTENSION

Structure Compressed	Visual Acuity	Visual Field	Pupils	Discs
Optic nerve	Reduced ipsilateral Normal contralateral	Ipsilateral central scotoma +/− contralateral superotemporal defect ("junction scotoma")	Ipsilateral relative afferent defect ("Marcus-Gunn pupil")	Ipsilateral temporal pallor
Optic chiasm	Normal or mildly reduced unilateral or bilateral	Bitemporal hemianopia or hemianopic scotomas	Bilateral hemi-afferent defects ("Wenicke's hemianopic pupil")	Bilateral horizontal bow-tie pallor
Optic tract	Normal or reduced ipsilateral	Contralateral incongruous homonymous hemianopia	Bilateral hemi-afferent defects +/− unilateral relative afferent defect	Ipsilateral general pallor and contralateral bow-tie pallor

III. OCULAR MANIFESTATIONS: LATERAL TUMOR EXTENSION

Structure Compressed	Signs and Symptoms
3rd nerve	Exotropia, ptosis, mydriasis
4th nerve	Hypertropia (worse in down gaze)
6th nerve	Esotropia (worse at distance)
5th nerve	Face pain, hypesthesia, neurotrophic keratitis
Sympathetic nerves	Horner syndrome—ptosis and miosis
Cavernous sinus	Proptosis, orbit congestion, venous congestion

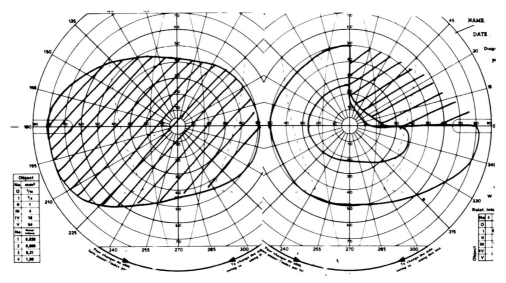

FIGURE 20.1. Junction scotoma. Compression of left posterior optic nerve causes ipsilateral visual loss and contralateral superotemporal visual field defect.

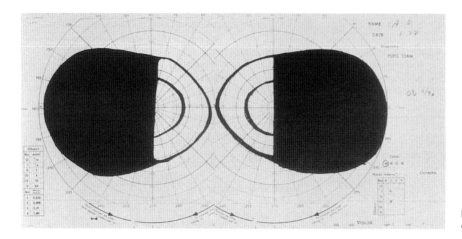

FIGURE 20.2. Bitemporal hemianopia—compression of chiasm.

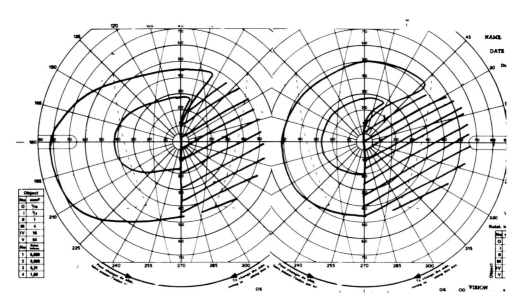

FIGURE 20.3. Incongruous right homonymous hemianopia—compression of left optic tract.

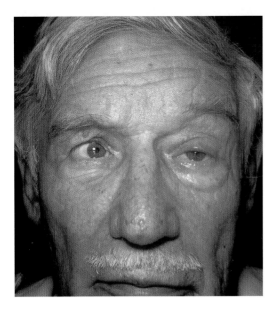

FIGURE 20.4. Left cavernous sinus syndrome. Lateral extension into cavernous sinus causes combined oculosympathetic and cranial nerve III, IV, V, VI involvement with proptosis, and orbital congestion.

SUGGESTED READINGS

Anderson DP, Faber P, Markovitz S. Pituitary tumors and the ophthalmologist. *Ophthalmology* 1983;90:1265–1270.

Burde RB, Savino PJ, Trobe JD. *Clinical Decisions in Neuro-Ophthalmology.* St. Louis: CV Mosby; 1992:74–87.

Kovaks K, Horvath E. In: Hartmann WH, ed. *Atlas of Tumor Pathology.* Fascicle 21. 2nd Series. Washington, DC: Armed Forces Institute of Pathology; 1986:1–264.

Kovaks K, Horvath E. Pathology of pituitary tumors. *Endocrinol Metab Clin North Am* 1987;16:529–551.

Wilson CB. A decade of pituitary microsurgery. *J Neurosurg* 1984;61:814–833.

PART 5. GASTROINTESTINAL DISORDERS

Chapter 21

GARDNER'S SYNDROME

Robert J. Champer
James C. Orcutt

I. GENERAL

1. Autosomal dominant inheritance (chromosome 5) with variable penetrance
2. Syndrome originally described as consisting of intestinal polyposis, soft tissue tumors, and benign osseous growths
3. Prevalence of adenocarcinoma nearly 100% by age 50
4. Identification of individuals with cutaneous, osseous, and ophthalmic findings of Gardner's syndrome enables early detection of intestinal polyposis and treatment prior to malignant transformation.

II. SYSTEMIC MANIFESTATIONS

1. Gastrointestinal
   - Intestinal polyposis
   - Adenocarcinoma of the colon
2. Musculoskeletal
   - Osteomas of skull and facial bones
   - Mandibular osteomas in 70%
   - Multiple carious teeth in 50%
   - Multiple impacted, supernumerary teeth
   - Fibrosarcomas
3. Dermatologic
   - Epidermoid cysts
   - Desmoid tumors, lipomas, leiomyomas, neurofibromas, incisional fibromas
   - Pigmented spots on torso and limbs
4. Endocrine
   - Thyroid carcinoma
5. Nonspecific
   - Retroperitoneal mixed tumors
   - Mesenteric fibrous tumors

III. OCULAR MANIFESTATIONS

1. Retina
   - Multiple foci of retinal pigment epithelium hypertrophy in both eyes
   - Lesions may range from darkly pigmented to completely depigmented, and vary from 0.1 mm to several millimeters
2. Lids
   - Epidermoid cysts
3. Orbit
   - Orbital osteomas arising from ethmoid or frontal bone

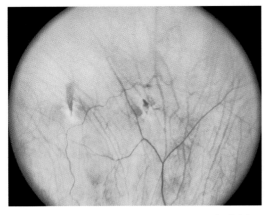

FIGURE 21.1. Congenital retinal pigment epithelial hypertrophy in the left eye of a patient with Gardner's syndrome.

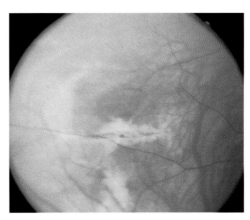

FIGURE 21.2. Congenital retinal pigment epithelial hypertrophy in the right eye of the patient described in Fig. 20.1.

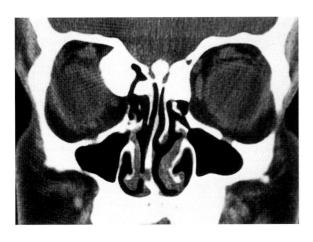

FIGURE 21.3. Orbital osteoma. Computed tomography scan of a 30-year-old woman with Gardner's syndrome demonstrating an osteoma of the left orbit arising from the ethmoid bone. The patient had a mandibular osteoma removed 6 years earlier and has undergone prophylactic colectomy. Two additional osteomas project into the ethmoid sinuses.

SUGGESTED READINGS

Awan KJ. Familial polyposis and angioid streaks in the ocular fundus. *Am J Ophthalmol* 1977;83:12–125.

Blair NP, Trempe CL. Hypertrophy of the retinal pigment epithelium associated with Gardner's syndrome. *Am J Ophthalmol* 1980;90:661–667.

Gardner EJ. Follow-up study of a family group exhibiting dominant inheritance for a syndrome including polyps, osteomas, fibromas, and epidermal cysts. *Am J Hum Genet* 1953;14:376.

Romania Z, Zakov ZN, McGannon E, et al. Congenital hypertrophy of the retinal pigment epithelium in familial adenomatous polyposis. *Ophthalmology* 1989;96:879–884.

Traboulsi EI, Krush AJ, Gardner EJ, et al. Prevalence and importance of pigmented ocular fundus lesions in Gardner's syndrome. *N Engl J Med* 1987;316:661–667.

Traboulsi EI, Murphy SF, de la Cruz Z, et al. A clinicopathologic study of the eyes in familial adenomatous polyposis with extracolonic manifestations (Gardner's syndrome). *Am J Ophthalmol* 1990;110:550–561.

Whitson WE, Orcutt JC, Walkinshaw MD. Orbital osteoma in Gardner's syndrome. *Am J Ophthalmol* 1986;101:236–241.

Chapter 22
HEPATIC DISEASE
Kenneth G. Romanchuk

I. GENERAL

1. Alagille's syndrome is prolonged neonatal jaundice thought to be autosomal dominant.

II. SYSTEMIC MANIFESTATIONS

1. Gastrointestinal
- Chronic familial intrahepatic cholestasis with a paucity of intrahepatic bile ducts on liver biopsy

2. Cardiovascular
- Peripheral pulmonary artery stenosis or hypoplasia, either isolated or associated with complex cardiovascular abnormalities

3. Musculoskeletal
- "Triangular" facies (broad overhanging forehead with deep-set eyes, flattened malar eminences, small, pointed mandible)
- Mid-arch deformities of thoracic vertebrae (particularly "butterfly" vertebrae)

- Short ulnae, short scaphoids, and short distal phalanges
- Sometimes growth retardation

4. Renal
- Congenital single kidney
- Renovascular hypertension

5. Endocrine
- Sometimes hypogonadism

6. Neurologic
- Sometimes areflexia
- Sometimes decreased intelligence

III. OCULAR MANIFESTATIONS

1. Cornea
- Posterior embryotoxin (prominent Schwalbe's line) (Fig. 22.1)
- Axenfeld's anomaly (iris strands to Schwalbe's line) (Fig. 22.2)
- Band keratopathy

2. Uvea
- Ectopic pupil (Fig. 22.3)
- Choroidal folds

3. Retina
- Pigmentary retinopathy
- Anomalous optic discs

4. Nonspecific
- Strabismus
- Infantile myopia

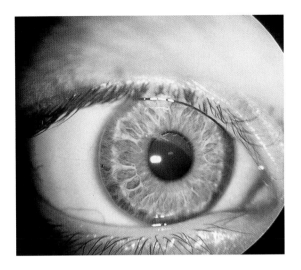

FIGURE 22.1. Prominent Schwalbe's line (posterior embryotoxin) is visible just inside temporal cornea of right eye.

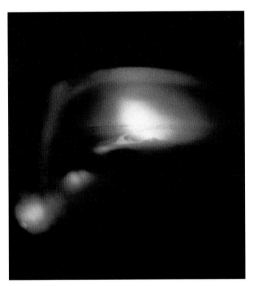

FIGURE 22.2. Gonioscope photograph of angle structure shows iris strands extending to Schwalbe's line (Axenfeld's anomaly).

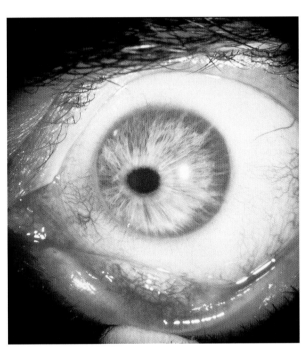

FIGURE 22.3. Ectopic pupil in left eye.

SUGGESTED READINGS

Hingorami M, Nischal KK, Davies A, et al. Ocular abnormalities in Alagille syndrome. *Ophthalmology* 1999;106:330–337.

Raymond WR, Kearney JJ, Parmley VC. Ocular findings in arteriohepatic dysplasia (Alagille's syndrome). *Arch Ophthalmol* 1989;107:1077.

Romanchuk KG, Judisch GF, LaBrecque DR. Ocular findings in arteriohepatic dysplasia (Alagille's syndrome). *Can J Ophthalmol* 1981;16:94–99.

Chapter 23

CROHN'S DISEASE
(INFLAMMATORY BOWEL DISEASE)

David L. Knox

I. SYSTEMIC MANIFESTATIONS

1. Arthritis
- Ankylosing spondylitis
- Monoarthropathy and stiffness
- HLA-B27 positive

2. Skin
- Erythema nodosum and multiforme

3. Eye
- See Ocular Manifestations

II. OCULAR MANIFESTATIONS: PRIMARY

1. Conjunctiva
- Repeated subconjunctival hemorrhage

2. Episclera
- Nongranulomatous focal or generalized episcleritis
- Granulomatous focal episcleritis (Fig. 23.1)

3. Cornea
- Anterior stromal, subepithelial opacification (Fig. 23.2)
- Limbal infiltrates

4. Sclera
- Scleritis

5. Uvea
- Chronic iridocyclitis
- Acute iritis
- Chronic pan-uveitis

6. Macula
- Edema, infiltrates, and exudative retinal detachments (Fig. 22.3)
- Central serous retinopathy

7. Orbit
- Proptosis and diplopia secondary to orbital myositis

8. Optic nerve
- Optic papillopathy
- Orbital optic neuritis
- Chiasmatic optic neuritis

III. MANIFESTATIONS: SECONDARY OCULAR

Definition: The ocular disorder is secondary to another complication of Crohn's disease

Ocular Disorder	Presumed Cause
Cataract	Systemic corticosteroids Chronic uveitis
Scleromalacia	Scleritis
Exudative retinal detachment	Psoas abscess Posterior scleritis
Decreased tear formation	Hypovitaminosis A, either low intake or poor absorption from absent or diseased gut
Night blindness	Hypovitaminosis A, see above
Candida endophthalmitis	Intravenous parenteral nutrition-induced candida sepsis

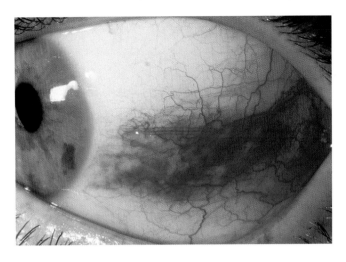

FIGURE 23.1. Episcleritis in a 33-year-old man.

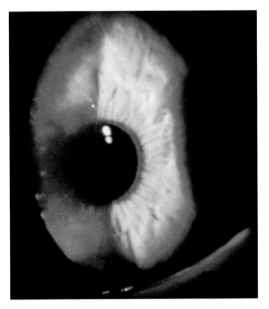

FIGURE 23.2. Keratopathy in a 50-year-old woman who also had dry eyes and night blindness.

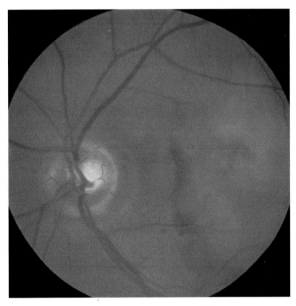

FIGURE 23.3. Retinopathy in a 30-year-old woman. Note mascular edema and subretinal hemorrhage.

SUGGESTED READINGS

Blase WP, Knox DL, Green WR. Granulomatous conjunctivitis in a patient with Crohn's disease. *Br J Ophthalmol* 1984;68:667–673.

Knox DL, Schachat AP, Mustonen E. Primary, secondary and coincidental ocular complications of Crohn's disease. *Ophthalmology* 1984;91:163–173.

Knox DL, Snip RC, Stark WJ. The keratopathy of Crohn's disease. *Am J Ophthalmol* 1980;90:862–865.

Chapter 24

PANCREATITIS

Erik F. Kruger
Joseph B. Walsh

I. GENERAL

1. May be acute or chronic
   - Acute form is usually self-limited.
   - Chronic form can result in endocrine and exocrine dysfunction.
2. Many possible etiologies
   - Alcoholism
   - Biliary tract disease
   - Trauma
   - Metabolic derangement
   - Drugs
3. The most common cause in the United States is alcohol followed by gallstones.
4. Pathogenic theory
   - Autodigestion of the pancreas by activated proteolytic enzymes

II. SYSTEMIC MANIFESTATIONS

1. Cardiovascular
   - Hypotension
     - Hypovolemia
     - Hypoalbuminemia
   - Sudden death
   - Nonspecific ST-T wave changes
   - Pericardial effusion
2. Pulmonary
   - Pleural effusion
   - Atelectasis
   - Mediastinal abscess
   - Pneumonitis
   - Adult respiratory distress syndrome
3. Gastrointestinal
   - Peptic ulcer disease
   - Gastritis
   - Hemorrhagic pancreatic necrosis
   - Portal vein thrombosis
   - Variceal hemorrhage
4. Hematologic
   - Disseminated intravascular coagulation (DIC)
5. Renal
   - Oliguria
   - Azotemia
   - Renal artery thrombosis
   - Renal vein thrombosis
6. Metabolic
   - Hyperglycemia
   - Hypertriglyceridemia
   - Hypocalcemia
   - Encephalopathy
7. Central nervous system
   - Psychosis
   - Fat emboli
8. Dermatologic
   - Subcutaneous nodules
9. Fat necrosis
   - Affecting bone
   - Affecting other tissues
10. Laboratory
    - Elevated serum amylase
    - Elevated serum lipase
    - Leukocytosis
    - Hyperbilirubinemia
    - Hypoxemia

III. OCULAR MANIFESTATIONS

1. Retina
   - Ischemic retinopathy
     - Only reported in acute pancreatitis related to alcohol
     - Similar in appearance to Purtscher's retinopathy
     - Findings predominantly in posterior pole
     - Multiple cotton-wool spots
       - May become confluent
     - Multiple nerve fiber layer hemorrhages
     - Diffuse retinal edema
     - Fluorescein angiography with typical findings
       - Obscuration of background fluorescence
       - Arteriolar and capillary nonperfusion
     - Indocyanine green angiography
       - Areas of persistent choroidal hypoperfusion
     - Etiology unclear
       - Fat emboli
       - Complement-induced leukocyte aggregation/embolization
       - Platelet aggregation/embolization
       - Fibrin embolization
     - No known treatment
2. Neuroophthalmologic
   - Related to ischemic retinopathy
     - Sudden visual loss
       - May be monocular or binocular
       - Recovery related to severity of initial visual deficit
     - Afferent pupillary defect
     - Visual field defects
       - Typically central scotomas

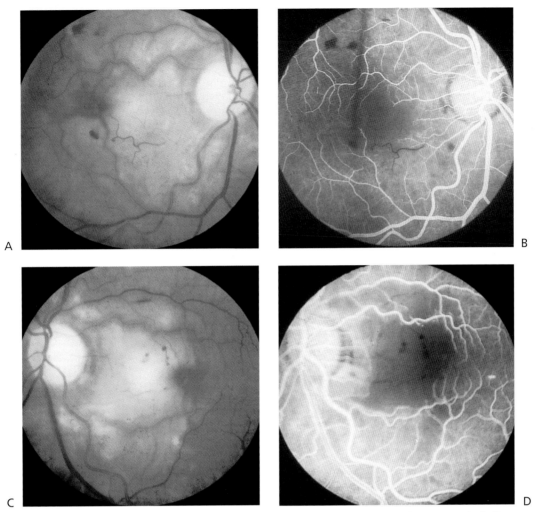

FIGURE 24.1. Man, aged 64, with acute loss of vision noted on recovering from acute alcoholic pancreatitis. Counting fingers vision in each eye. Both eyes revealed retinal infarction in the macula and nonperfusion of retinal vessels in posterior pole. (**A**) OD, (**B**) OD, (**C**) OS, (**D**) OS.

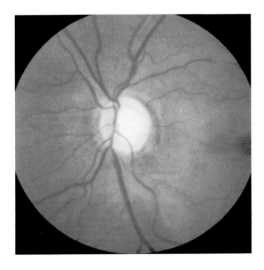

FIGURE 24.2. Follow-up shows optic nerve pallor OS at 3 months.

SUGGESTED READINGS

Behrens-Baumann W, Scheurer G, Schroer H. Pathogenesis of Purtscher's retinopathy. *Graefe's Arch Clin Exp Ophthalmol* 1992;230:286–291.

Greenberger NJ, Toskes PP, Isselbacher KJ. Acute and chronic pancreatitis. In: Isselbacher KJ, et al, eds. *Harrison's Principles of Internal Medicine,* 13th ed. New York: McGraw-Hill; 1994:1521–1530.

Inkeles DM, Walsh JB. Retinal fat emboli as a sequela to acute pancreatitis. *Am J Ophthalmol* 1975;80:935–938.

Sanders RJ, Brown GC, Brown A, et al. Purtscher's retinopathy preceding acute pancreatitis. *Ann Ophthalmol* 1992;24:19–21.

Williams JM, Gass JDM, O'Grady GE. Retinopathy of pancreatitis and the complement cascade. *Invest Ophthalmol Vis Sci* 1986;27(suppl):105.

Chapter 25

WHIPPLE'S DISEASE

Ann G. Neff
Guy W. Neff

I. GENERAL

1. Systemic bacterial infection caused by *Tropheryma whippeli*
2. More commonly affects middle-aged, white men
3. Multisystem disorder, but most common organs/systems affected are the intestinal tract, central nervous system (CNS), lymphatics, and heart; ocular manifestations may be due to CNS involvement, intraocular involvement, or both.
4. Common symptoms include fever, weight loss, diarrhea, arthralgias, and abdominal pain.
5. If untreated, or treatment delayed, may progress to significant neurologic sequelae or death.
6. Diagnosed by small-bowel biopsy, with identification of periodic acid-Schiff-positive inclusions within macrophages in the mucosa; electron microscopy and polymerase chain reaction techniques may also be used.
7. Treatment requires long-term antibiotic use, which should be coordinated by an infectious disease specialist.
8. Long-term follow-up necessary due to risk of relapse.

II. SYSTEMIC MANIFESTATIONS

1. Gastrointestinal
   - Abdominal pain
   - Diarrhea
   - Malabsorption
   - Ascites
   - Hepatomegaly
   - Splenomegaly
2. Neurologic
   - Confusion
   - Amnesia
   - Drowsiness
   - Personality changes
   - Ataxia
   - Seizures
3. Cardiac
   - Pericarditis
   - Endocarditis
   - Hypotension
   - Murmurs
4. Vascular
   - Aortic valvular lesions
5. Musculoskeletal
   - Migratory polyarthralgias
6. Pulmonary
   - Pleuritis
7. Hematologic
   - Anemia
8. Mucocutaneous
   - Skin hyperpigmentation
9. Ear/nose/throat
   - Hearing loss
   - Sore throat
10. Nonspecific
    - Fever
    - Weight loss
    - Lymphadenopathy

III. OCULAR MANIFESTATIONS

1. Neuroophthalmologic
   - Supranuclear ophthalmoplegia
   - Oculomasticatory myorhythmia
   - Gaze palsy
   - Nystagmus
   - Ptosis
2. Conjunctiva/sclera
   - Chemosis
3. Cornea
   - Keratitis
4. Uvea
   - Uveitis
5. Vitreous
   - Vitreous opacities
6. Retina
   - Retinal and choroidal inflammation
7. Optic nerve
   - Papilledema

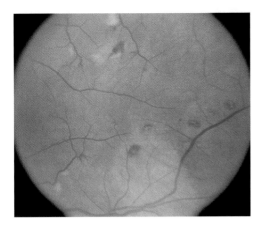

FIGURE 25.1. Left eye of a patient with Whipple's disease shows round, subretinal hemorrhages and small, round, grayish subretinal lesions temporal to macula.

SUGGESTED READINGS

Avila MP, Jalkh AE, Feldman E, et al. Manifestations of Whipple's disease in the posterior segment of the eye. *Arch Ophthalmol* 1984;102:384–390.

Hoeprich PD, Pittman FE. Whipple disease. In: Hoeprich PD, Jordan MC, Ronald AR, eds. *Infectious Diseases: A Treatise of Infectious Processes*. Philadelphia: JB Lipincott; 1994:1285–1291.

Trempe CL, Avila MP. Whipple's disease. In: Gold DH, Weingeist TA, eds. *The Eye in Systemic Disease*. Philadelphia: JB Lipincott; 1990:108–112.

PART 6. HEARING DISORDERS

Chapter 26

COGAN'S SYNDROME

John E. Sutphin

I. GENERAL

1. Typical Cogan's syndrome is interstitial keratitis and loss of hearing, vertigo, or tinnitus.
2. Atypical Cogan's syndrome consists of vestibuloauditory dysfunction and ocular inflammation other than keratitis.
3. Systemic steroids are needed to avoid permanent deafness.
4. Median age at onset is 25 years, ranging from 5 to 63 years.
5. Men equal women, and both eyes are typically involved.
6. Eyes or ears may be involved first, but both organs usually involved within 5 months.
7. The immune-mediated events of Cogan's syndrome may result from sensitization during an initial infectious episode. No infectious agent has yet been identified. Activated T cells and macrophages are found in the target tissues during the acute episodes.
8. Severe disease is related to vasculitis.

II. SYSTEMIC MANIFESTATIONS

1. Ear/nose/throat
   - Loss of hearing (60% permanent with no treatment, 80% reversible with systemic steroids)
   - Vertigo and tinnitus
   - Nausea and vomiting
   - Nystagmus
   - Ataxia
2. Nonspecific
   - Fever
   - Weight loss
   - Fatigue
   - Headache, discomfort, periorbital pain
   - Prodromal upper respiratory symptoms
3. Muscuolskeletal
   - Arthralgias and myalgias
   - Arthritis
4. Gastrointestinal
   - Abdominal discomfort
   - Hemorrhage
5. Vascular
   - Vasculitis
     - Multiple sites including femoral artery, central nervous system, skin, subcutaneous nodules, kidney, muscles, and coronary arteries
6. Cardiac
   - Aortic insufficiency
   - Systolic ejection murmur
   - Left ventricular hypertrophy
7. Pulmonary
   - Mild transient radiographic changes
   - Pleuritis
8. Genitourinary
   - Abnormal urinalysis
   - Testicular pain
9. Neurologic
   - Cranial neuropathy
   - Meningismus
   - Encephalitis
10. Lymphoreticular
    - Lymphadenopathy
    - Splenomegaly
    - Hepatomegaly
11. Mucocutaneous
    - Nodules
    - Nonspecific rash

III. OCULAR MANIFESTATIONS

1. Symptoms
   - Redness
   - Photophobia
   - Discomfort
   - Disurbances of visual acuity
2. Cornea
   - Interstitial keratitis
     - Patchy, stromal clouding of anterior and mid-stroma near the limbus
     - Vascularization and persistent haze may follow
   - Nummular anterior stromal keratitis
   - Both respond to topical corticosteroids
3. Conjunctivitis
4. Tearing
5. Ciliary flush
6. Uveitis
7. Episcleritis
8. Scleritis
9. Optic nerve
   - Papillitis
   - Papilledema
10. Retina
    - Chorioretinitis
    - Central retinal vein occlusion
11. Nonspecific
    - Pseudotumor
    - Glaucoma
    - Vitreous hemorrhage

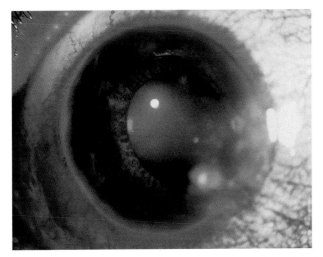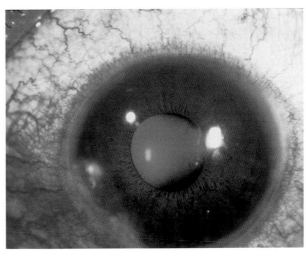

FIGURE 26.1. and FIGURE 26.2. Bilateral peripheral interstitial keratitis, diffuse anterior scleritis and mild iritis in a 36-year-old woman with Cogan's syndrome. Vertigo and deafness occurred 2 weeks later. Keratitis responded to topical corticosteroids, but deafness required high-dose oral steroids. Courtesy of James J. Reidy, MD, State University of New York at Buffalo.

SUGGESTED READINGS

Allen NB, Cox CC, Cobo M, et al. Use of immunosuppressive agents in the treatment of severe ocular and vascular manifestations of Cogan's syndrome. *Am J Med* 1990;88:296–301.

Cobo LM. Cogan's syndrome. In: Gold DH, Weingeist TA, eds. *The Eye in Systemic Disease.* Philadelphia: JB Lippincott; 1990:115–117.

Cogan DG. Syndrome of nonsyphilitic interstitial keratitis and vestibuloauditory symptoms. *Arch Ophthalmol* 1945;33:144–149. *Original report.*

Vollertsen RS, McDonald TJ, Younge BR, et al. Cogan's syndrome: 18 cases and a review of the literature. *Mayo Clin Proc* 1986;61:344–361. *A general review of ocular and systemic manifestations of Cogan's syndrome.*

Chapter 27

USHER SYNDROME

Brian E. Nichols
Richard J. H. Smith

I. GENERAL

1. Autosomal recessive inheritance
2. Present in 3% to 6% of deaf children
3. Most common cause of combined deafness and blindness in developed countries (16,000 deaf-blind persons in the United States; more than half have Usher type 1 (Ush1))
   - 4.4/100,000 in the United States (number underestimates incidence of Usher type 2 (Ush2))
   - 5/100,000 in Denmark (2:3, Ush1/Ush2)
   - 6.2/100,000 in England (2:3, Ush1/Ush2)
4. Earliest finding is sensorineural hearing loss (SNHL), profound in Ush1 and moderate to severe in Ush2 and Ush3.
5. Pigmentary retinopathy indistinguishable from retinitis pigmentosa
6. Visual field constriction with progressive retinal degeneration
7. Electroretinogram (ERG) attenuated or nonrecordable in the presence of pigmentary retinopathy
   - ERG can be markedly affected prior to pigmentary retinopathy in Ush1 (as young as 6 months of age)
   - Age at which ERG abnormalities can be expected in any type is unknown; therefore, a single normal ERG does not exclude Usher syndrome
8. Usher type 1
   - Characterized by profound congenital SNHL with retinitis pigmentosa (RP) prior to age 10 and vestibular areflexia (essential for the diagnosis)
   - Type 1A linked to chromosome 14q32 in French (Poitou-Charentes) families
   - Type 1B linked to chromosome 11q13.5 in British families
     - Responsible for 75% of type 1 Usher
     - Caused by mutations in *myosin VIIA* gene
     - Mutations in same gene also cause nonsyndromic hearing loss
   - Type 1C linked to chromosome 11p15.1 in Acadian families
   - Type 1D linked to chromosome 10q in Moroccan and Pakistani families
   - Type 1E linked to chromosome 21q21 in another subset of Moroccan families
   - Type 1F linked to chromosome 10q in Hutterite families
9. Usher type 2
   - Characterized by moderate-to-severe congenital down-sloping hearing loss with onset of RP in late teens, and intact vestibular function
   - Type 2A linked to chromosome 1q41
   - Type 2B includes families not linked to the 1q41 locus; accounts for 10% to 15% of Usher type 2
10. Usher type 3
    - Characterized by progressive SNHL, RP first noted at puberty, and vestibular hypoactivity
    - 2% of Usher overall, but highest in founder populations such as Finland (42%)
    - Clinically significant hypermetropia and astigmatism also felt to be characteristic
    - Linked to chromosome 3q21-q25 in French-Acadian and Finnish families
11. Pathophysiology
    - Vestibular and auditory hair cells, as well as photoreceptors, develop from ciliated progenitors
      - Usher syndrome may reflect an abnormality of axoneme structure
      - Type 1B is caused by mutations in the *myosin VIIA* gene, an unconventional myosin present in retinal pigment epithelium, the photoreceptor inner segments, and the cochlear and vestibular neuroepithelia.
      - Disease phenotype is dosage related. With no expression of the *myosin VIIA* gene, both auditory and visual impairment occur; with minimal expression, only auditory impairment occurs.
    - Histopathologic studies have documented severe loss of spiral ganglion cells, neural degeneration in the cochlea, and loss of supporting cells in the organ of Corti.
      - Pattern of neural degeneration is similar to that seen in the retina of patients with RP.

II. SYSTEMIC MANIFESTATIONS

1. Genitourinary
   - Decreased sperm motility in some men
2. Neurologic
   - Delayed developmental motor milestones (Ush1, due to vestibular dysfunction)
   - Paranoid psychosis, mental retardation, bipolar affective disorder, and major depressive disorder in up to 25% (may be a consequence of sensory deficits)
3. Hematologic
   - Possible decrease in plasma polyunsaturated fatty acids (docosahexaenoate and arachidonate)
4. Otolaryngologic
   - Congenital or progressive sensorineural hearing loss
     - Ush1 persons not aidable; use manual communication and, ultimately, Braille; some have received cochlear implants.
     - Ush2 and Ush3 aidable
   - Vestibular ataxia (Ush1)
   - Nasal cilia abnormalities (Ush1C)

1. Lens
   - Posterior subcapsular cataract (Fig. 27.1)
     - 50% of Usher patients older than 30
2. Vitreous
   - Posterior detachment of vitreous common
   - Vitreal cells
3. Retina
   - Depigmentation of retinal pigment epithelium with frequent bull's-eye lesions
   - Bone spicule pigmentation and perivascular intraretinal pigment migration varies widely and increases with time (Fig. 27.2)
   - Cystoid macular edema
   - Vascular attenuation (related to degree of retinal degeneration)
   - Loss of foveal reflex
   - Epiretinal membrane in virtually all eyes
   - Nonrecordable or depressed ERG
4. Optic nerve
   - Pallor
   - Optic nerve drusen (Fig. 27.3)
     - 20% Ush1; 8% Ush2

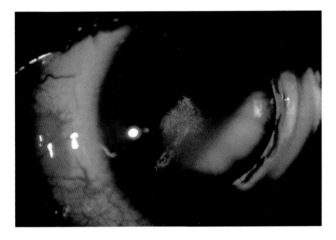

FIGURE 27.1. Posterior subcapsular cataract in a patient with Usher syndrome.

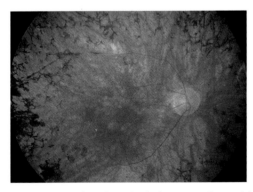

FIGURE 27.2. Peripheral retinal degeneration with bone spicule pigment in Usher type 2. This patient also demonstrates arteriolar attenuation and macular retinal pigment epithelium atrophic changes.

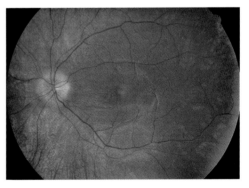

FIGURE 27.3. Virtually all patients with Usher syndrome have epiretinal membranes. This patient also has echographically diagnosed optic nerve drusen.

SUGGESTED READINGS

Boughman JA, Vernon M, Shaver KA. Usher's syndrome: Definition and estimate of prevalence from two high-risk populations. *J Chronic Dis* 1983;36:595–603. *Prevalence of Usher syndrome in the United States.*

Newsome DA. Usher's syndrome. In: Gold DH, Weingeist TA, eds. *The Eye in Systemic Disease.* Philadelphia: JB Lippincott; 1990:119–123. *A general review of the ocular manifestations of Usher syndrome.*

Online Mendelian Inheritance in Man, OMIM™. Center for Medical Genetics, Johns Hopkins University (Baltimore, MD) and National Center for Biotechnology Information, National Library of Medicine (Bethesda, MD), 1997. World Wide Web URL: http://www.ncbi.nlm.nih.gov/omim/. *A detailed review of the genetics of Usher syndrome.*

Shinkawa H, Nadol JB. Histopathology of the inner ear in Usher's syndrome as observed by light and electron microscopy. *Ann Otol Rhinol Laryngol* 1986;95:313–318.

Smith RJH, Berlin CI, Hejtmancik JF, et al. Clinical diagnosis of the Usher syndromes. *Am J Med Genet* 1994;50:32–38. *Diagnostic criteria as adopted by the Usher Syndrome Consortium.*

PART 7. HEMATOLOGIC DISORDERS

Chapter 28

ANEMIA

Helen K. Li
Ali M. Khorrami

I. GENERAL

1. Anemia results from a reduction in circulating red blood cells or hemoglobin.
2. Retinal hemorrhages are the most common ocular sign of anemia. Unless very severe (<8 g/100 mL), anemia does not result in ocular manifestations.
   - Thrombocytopenia (<50,000/mm^3), advanced age, and rapid development of anemia contribute to retinal manifestations.
   - Retinal hemorrhages occur in only 10% of patient with anemia.
   - However, 40% to 70% of patients with both anemia and thrombocytopenia develop retinal hemorrhages.
3. Pernicious anemia and anemia associated with primary disorders of bone marrow, for example, leukemia, are often accompanied by thrombocytopenia. Retinopathy of anemia is likely to be present in these two disorders.
4. The pathogenesis of retinopathy of anemia is thought to be related to hypoxic endothelial injury, with ensuing dilatation of the retinal venules, capillary leakage, intraretinal hemorrhages, and cotton-wool spots. White-centered retinal hemorrhages are due to an increased ratio of leukocytes to erythrocytes. Decreased platelet count also contributes to decompensation of the endothelial integrity.
5. Retinopathy of anemia is sometimes the first clinical manifestation of an underlying primary or secondary anemia with an associated systemic disease. Retinal hemorrhages resolve a few weeks after systemic treatment of the anemia and its precipitating cause.

II. SYSTEMIC MANIFESTATIONS

1. Cardiac
   - Tachycardia
   - Systolic ejection murmur
   - Cardiomegaly
2. Vascular
   - Orthostatic hypotension
   - Wide pulse pressure
   - Postural signs
3. Pulmonary
   - Dyspnea
4. Gastrointestinal
   - Anorexia
   - Indigestion
   - Nausea or bowel irregularity
   - Occult blood in stool
5. Neurologic
   - Dizziness
   - Headache
   - Syncope
   - Vertigo
   - Stupor
   - Coma
6. Hematologic
   - Abnormal red cell indexes
   - Reticulocyte count
   - Blood smear or bone marrow
7. Endocrine
   - Abnormal menstruation
   - Amenorrhea
   - Increased menstrual bleeding
   - Impotence
8. Musculoskeletal
   - Fatigue
   - Weakness
9. Mucocutaneous
   - Pallor of the skin
   - Palm crease
   - Nailbeds and oral mucous membranes cheilosis
   - Koilonychia
   - Icterus
   - Superficial skin ulceration
10. Ear/nose/throat
    - Tinnitis
11. Nonspecific
    - Irritable
    - Hypersensitive to cold
    - Palpitation
    - Diaphoretic
12. Other
    - Splenomegaly

1. Anterior segment
   - Palpebral conjunctival pallor
   - Subconjunctival hemorrhages
2. Retina
   - Flame-shaped hemorrhages
   - Dot and blot hemorrhages
   - White-centered hemorrhages (Roth's spot)
   - Subretinal or preretinal hemorrhages
   - Cotton-wool spots

   - Hard exudates
   - Dilated and tortuous retinal veins
   - Retinal vessels less red than normal
   - Retinal edema
   - Pale fundus
3. Neuroophthalmologic
   - Ischemic optic neuropathy
   - Cranial nerve palsies

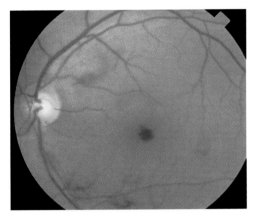

FIGURE 28.1. A 34-year-old female with history of alcohol abuse, folate deficiency, and hemoglobin of 4.6 g/dl.

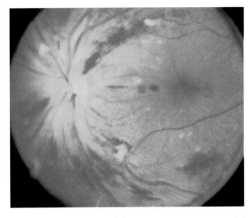

FIGURE 28.2. A 27-year-old pregnant woman with acute myeloblastic leukemia and associated pancytopenia. Hemoglobin = 2.5g/dl. Platelets = 12,000/ul. Patient and her fetus expired after hemorrhagic complications in the brain stem.

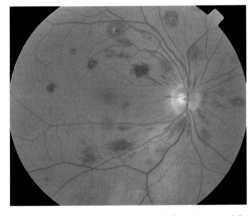

FIGURE 28.3. A 40-year-old male with HIV, on zidovudine. Hemoglobin/hematocrit = 3.1 g/dl/8.8%. Platelet = 125,000/ul.

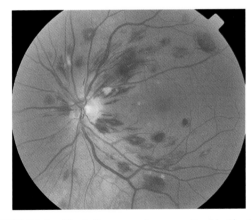

FIGURE 28.4. The fellow eye of same patient in Fig. 28.3.

SUGGESTED READINGS

Broan GC, Goldberg RE. Anemia. In: Gold DH, Weingeist TA, eds. *The Eye in Systemic Disease.* Philadelphia: JB Lippincott; 1990:127–129.

Bunn HF. Anemia. In: Isselbacher KJ, et al, eds. *Harrison's Principles of Internal Medicine,* 13th ed. New York: McGraw-Hill; 1994;313–317.

Lam S, Lam BL. Bilateral retinal hemorrhages from megaloblastic anemia: Case report and review of literature. *Ann Ophthalmol* 1992;24:86–90.

Rubenstein RA, Yanoff M, Albert DM. Thrombocytopenis, anemia, and retinal hemorrhage. *Am J Ophthalmol* 1968;65:435–439.

Chapter 29
COAGULATION DISORDERS

George A. Williams

I. GENERAL

1. Hemostasis is an intricately balanced system that precisely regulates formation and clearance of blood clots.
2. Coagulation is the formation of fibrin via the sequential activation of the intrinsic, extrinsic, and fibrinolytic pathways.
3. The interdependency of the intrinsic, extrinsic, and fibrinolytic pathways is demonstrated in coagulation disorders in which individual factors are lacking or dysfunctional due to hereditary or acquired disorders.
4. Hereditary disorders include deficiencies of factor VIII (hemophilia A), factor IX (hemophilia B), factor XI, antithrombin III, protein C, and protein S.
5. Acquired coagulation disorders are most commonly associated with anticoagulant medication.

II. SYSTEMIC MANIFESTATIONS

1. The systemic manifestations of coagulation disorders are characterized as joint, muscle, or intraperitoneal hemorrhage. The severity of the bleeding correlates with extent of the respective factor's deficiency.
2. Musculoskeletal
   - Hemarthrosis
   - Intramuscular hematomas
3. Neurologic
   - Central nervous system hemorrhage
4. Mucocutaneous
   - Ecchymosis
   - Purpura
5. Renal
   - Hematuria
6. Pulmonary
   - Hemoptysis
7. Genitourinary
   - Menorrhagia
   - Hematuria
8. Ear/nose/throat
   - Epistaxis
9. Nonspecific
   - Anemia

III. OCULAR MANIFESTATIONS

1. Retina
   - Central retinal vein occlusion
   - Central retinal artery occlusion
   - Retinal hemorrhages
   - Hemorrhagic retinal detachment
2. Vitreous
   - Vitreous hemorrhage
3. Uvea
   - Hemorrhagic choroidal detachment
4. Neuroophthalmologic
   - Cranial nerve palsies
   - Pupillary abnormalities
5. Optic nerve
   - Papilledema
6. Conjunctiva/sclera
   - Subconjunctival hemorrhage
7. Lids
   - Ecchymosis

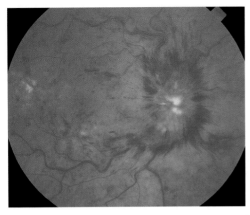

FIGURE 29.1 Central retinal vein occlusion in patient with anti-thrombin III deficiency.

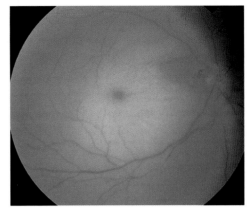

FIGURE 29.2 Central retinal artery occlusion in patient with protein S deficiency. Courtesy of John Hart, MD.

SUGGESTED READINGS

Williams GA. Coagulation disorders. In: Gold DH, Weingeist TA, eds. *The Eye in Systemic Disease.* Philadelphia: JB Lippincott; 1990:129–131.

Williams GA. Ocular manifestations of hematologic disease. In: Tasman W, Jaeger EA, eds. *Duane's Clinical Ophthalmology.* Philadelphia: JB Lippincott; 1991:1–12. *A comprehensive review of the ocular manifestations of coagulopathies.*

Chapter 30

DISSEMINATED INTRAVASCULAR COAGULATION

Helmut Buettner

I. GENERAL

1. Disseminated intravascular coagulation (DIC) is the clinical manifestation of a heterogenous group of consumptive thrombohemorrhagic disorders complicating a variety of primary disorders (infections, obstetric complications, hematopoietic and vascular disorders, neoplasms, advanced liver disease, massive tissue trauma, allergic reactions).
2. Fibrin thrombi form in small blood vessels, most frequently in the skin, brain, heart, lungs, kidneys, adrenal glands, spleen, and liver.
3. As intravascular thrombi form, platelets are consumed in large numbers, resulting in thrombocytopenia. Plasminogen, binding to fibrin, is converted to fibrinolytically active plasmin.
4. When plasmin formation exceeds the capacity of inhibitory factors, plasmin consumes certain clotting factors and in addition degrades fibrinogen and fibrin. The resulting fibrinogen–fibrin-split products inhibit fibrin thrombus formation.
5. Consumption of fibrinogen and platelets, the anticoagulative action of fibrinogen–fibrin-split products, and the fibrinolytic action of plasmin contribute to a hypocoagulative state, which severely deranges hemostasis.
6. There is no age, sex, or racial predilection for DIC, with the exception of cases associated with obstetric complications.

II. SYSTEMIC MANIFESTATIONS

1. Both thrombotic and hemorrhagic phenomena often occur simultaneously.
2. Skin
   - Patchy necrosis
   - Petechial and ecchymotic hemorrhages
3. Lungs
   - Acute respiratory distress
   - Pulmonary hemorrhages
4. Gastrointestinal tract
   - Submucosal necrosis
   - Acute ulceration
   - Massive bleeding
5. Kidneys
   - Cortical infarction
   - Hematuria
   - Oliguria/anuria
6. Adrenal glands
   - Hemorrhagic necrosis
   - Fulminant sepsis (Waterhouse-Friderichsen syndrome)
7. Central nervous system
   - Altered state of consciousness
   - Convulsions
   - Often bizarre neurologic symptoms

III. OCULAR MANIFESTATIONS

1. Anterior segment
   - Hemorrhages into conjunctiva, iris, and anterior chamber occur primarily in infants/children. When observed in adults, they are frequently a sign of terminal uremia or septicemia.
2. Posterior segment
   - Retinal and vitreous hemorrhages are primarily seen in infants/children.
   - Choroidal involvement in the form of vascular occlusion and hemorrhage is the most common manifestation of DIC in adults.
   - Associated serous retinal detachment in acute DIC.

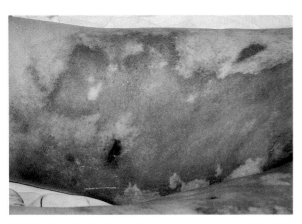

FIGURE 30.1. Patchy hemorrhages and necrosis of the skin of the thigh in a patient with fulminant DIC associated with multiple myeloma.

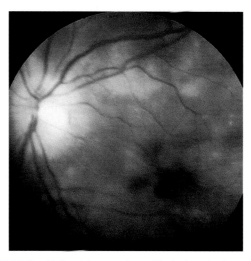

FIGURE 30.2. Yellowish gray plaquelike lesions in the posterior choroid of a patient with chronic DIC of unknown etiology. The retina is attached.

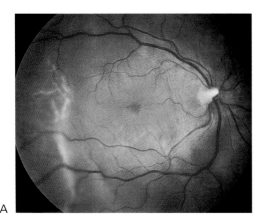

A

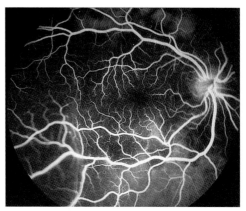

B

FIGURE 30.3. (**A**) Fundus photograph shows a serous retinal detachment in a pregnant woman presenting with abruptio placentae and a dead fetus. In the late venous phase of the fluorescein angiogram fluid leaks in a patchy fashion from the choroid into the subretinal space. (**B**) Leakage of fluorescein is also seen in the optic nerve head.

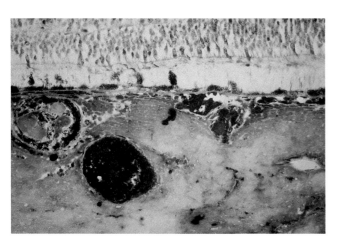

FIGURE 30.4. Photomicrograph of outer retina and choroid of the patient with chronic DIC whose fundus appearance is shown in Figure 30.2. Diffuse hemorrhage surrounds large choroidal vessels containing thrombi in varying stages of organization and recanalization (phosphotungstic acid hematoxylin; original magnification ×320).

SUGGESTED READINGS

Cogan DG. Ocular involvement in intravascular coagulopathy. *Arch Ophthalmol* 1975;93:1–8.

Marder VJ. Consumptive thrombohemorrhagic disorders. In: Williams WJ, et al, eds. *Hematology.* New York: McGraw-Hill; 1983:1433–1461.

Ortiz JM, Yanoff M, Cameron JD, Schaffer D. Disseminated intravascular coagulation in infancy and in the neonate; ocular findings. *Arch Ophthalmol* 1982;100:1413–1415.

Samples JR, Buettner H. Ocular involvement in disseminated intravascular coagulation (DIC). *Ophthalmology* 1983;90:914–916.

Chapter 31

DYSPROTEINEMIAS

Alan H. Friedman
Juan Orellana

I. GENERAL

1. Waldenström's macroglobulinemia, multiple myeloma, and benign monoclonal gammopathy
2. Excessive production of immunoglobulin or its derivative polypeptide
3. Hyperviscosity syndrome
4. Tumefactions in organs and bones

II. SYSTEMIC MANIFESTATIONS

1. Hematologic
   - Gamma globulin spike on immunoprotein electrophoresis
   - Hyperglobulinemia
   - Cryoglobulinemia
   - Pyroglobulinemia
   - Normocytic-normochromic anemia
   - Increased erythrocyte sedimentation rate
   - Hypercalcemia
   - Bence-Jones proteinuria
   - Amyloidosis
   - Purpura
2. Musculoskeletal
   - Punched-out lesions of the skull, vertebrae, and ribs
   - Carpal tunnel syndrome
3. Genitourinary
   - Uremia
4. Neurologic
   - Dizziness
   - Vertigo
   - Paresthesias
   - Headache
   - Nystagmus
   - Ataxia
   - Seizures
5. Cutaneous
   - Violaceous hue
   - Ecchymosis

III. OCULAR MANIFESTATIONS

1. Orbit
   - Proptosis
2. Lids
   - Violaceous hue
   - Tumors
3. Conjunctiva
   - Sludging of blood flow
   - Crystal deposition
4. Cornea
   - Crystal deposition
   - Copper deposition
5. Retina (Figure 31.1A)
   - Hyperviscosity
   - Hemorrhages
   - Exudates
   - Microaneurysms
   - Venous dilatation
   - Cotton-wool spots
   - Arteriolar dilatation
   - Arteriovenous crossing changes
   - Central retinal vein occlusion
6. Vitreous
   - Hemorrhage
7. Choroid
   - Tumors
   - Infiltrates
   - Infarction
8. Neuroophthalmic
   - Optic nerve infiltration
9. Lens
   - Copper deposition in lens capsule
10. Ophthalmic pathology
    - Macroglobulinemia
      - Cystoid spaces in retina containing immunoglobulin (Figure 31.1B and C)
      - Crystals
      - Microaneurysms
    - Multiple myeloma
      - Pars plana cysts containing immunoglobulin (Figure 31.2A and B)
    - Benign monoclonal gammopathy
      - Crystals (Figure 31.3A and B)
      - Crystals
      - Copper

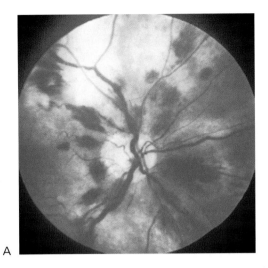

A

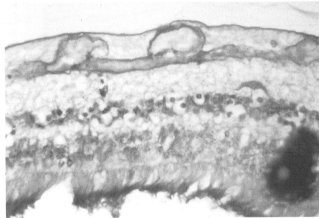

B

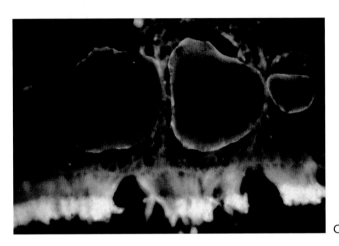

C

FIGURE 31.1. (**A**) Clinical photograph of a patient with Waldenström's macroglobulinemia shows congestion, hemorrhage, and leakage. Note the dilated vessels. (**B**) Photomicrograph of the retina of a patient who had Waldenström's macroglobulinemia. Note the microaneurysms in the superficial retina of the periphery. (**C**) Photomicrograph of the retina of a patient who had Waldenström's macroglobulinemia demonstrates IgM using fluorescein labeled antihuman IgM.

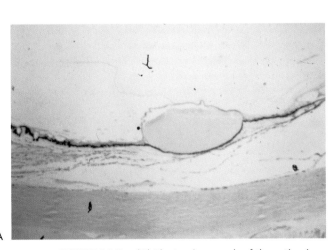

A

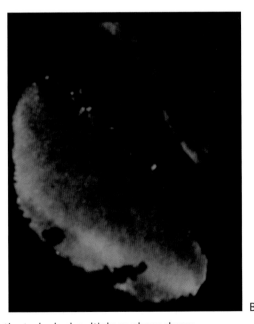

B

FIGURE 31.2. (**A**) Photomicrograph of the retina in a patient who had multiple myeloma shows the typical collection of immunoglobulin between the two epithelial layers of the pars plana. (**B**) Photomicrograph of the retina of a patient who had multiple myeloma demonstrates IgG using fluorescein-labeled antihuman IgG.

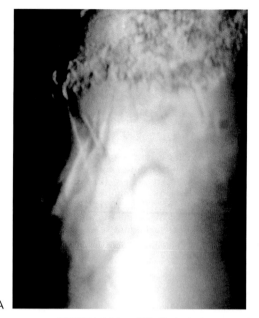
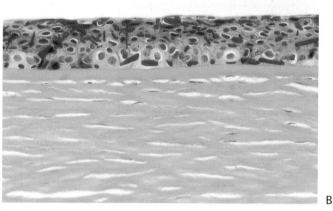

FIGURE 31.3. **(A)** Clinical photograph shows corneal deposits as viewed in the slit-lamp in a patient with benign monoclonal gammopathy. Courtesy of Merlyn Rodrigues, MD. **(B)** Photomicrograph of the trichrome-stained cornea of a patient with benign monoclonal gammopathy demonstrates the red crystals of immunoglobulin in the epithelium. Courtesy of Gordon Klintworth, MD.

SUGGESTED READINGS

Ackerman AL. The ocular manifestations of Waldenström's macroglobulinemia and its treatment. *Arch Ophthalmol* 1962;67:701–707.

Aronson SB, Shar R. Corneal crystals in multiple myeloma. *Arch Ophthalmol* 1959;61:541–546.

Efferman RA, Rodrigues MM. Unusual superficial stromal corneal deposits in benign monoclonal gammopathy. *Arch Ophthalmol* 1980;98:78–81.

Orellana J, Friedman AH. Ocular manifestations of multiple myeloma, Waldenström's macroglobulinemia and benign monoclonal gammopathy. *Surv Ophthalmol* 1981;26:157–169.

Rodrigues MM, Krachmer JH, Miller SD, et al. Posterior corneal crystalline deposits in benign monoclonal gammopathy. *Arch Ophthalmol* 1979;979:124–128.

Chapter 32

LEUKEMIA

Marilyn C. Kincaid

I. GENERAL

1. Nomenclature
   - Leukemia can be acute or chronic and can be from the myelogenous or lymphoid cell lines.
   - Leukemia is the result of clonal proliferation of cells.
   - Classification presently used is the FAB (French-American-British) to characterize the myeloid (M0 through M7) or lymphoid (L1 through L3) proliferation.
2. Predisposing factors
   - Myelodysplastic syndrome predisposes to acute myelocytic leukemia and can itself be primary or secondary.
   - Exposure to carcinogens
     - Chemical agents, including those used as chemotherapy for other malignancies
     - Ionizing radiation, including that used for other malignancies
   - Aneuploidy, such as Down syndrome (trisomy 21)
3. Pathophysiologic mechanisms
   - Oncogenes are promoters of tumorigenesis or loss of suppression.

II. SYSTEMIC MANIFESTATIONS

1. There may be no symptoms, particularly in older individuals, and particularly with chronic lymphocytic leukemia.
2. Signs and symptoms
   - Fatigue, weakness
   - Anemia from decreased red blood cell production
   - Easy bruisability from diminished platelets
   - Susceptibility to infection because of decreased normal white blood cells
   - Organomegaly from direct cellular invasion
   - Lymph node enlargement from accumulations of leukemic cells

III. OCULAR MANIFESTATIONS

1. Uveal tract
   - Most common site of direct cellular invasion; not always evident clinically
   - Infiltration may secondarily cause serous sensory retinal detachment or retinal pigment epithelial changes.
   - Infiltration may cause clinically evident change in iris color, with or without a pseudohypopyon.
2. Retina
   - Direct infiltration by leukemic cells
   - Vascular changes secondary to anemia, hyperviscosity, thrombocytopenia
     - Intraretinal, preretinal, and subretinal hemorrhages, which can be massive
     - Cotton-wool spots
     - Vascular occlusion
     - Neovascularization
3. Optic nerve
   - Papilledema secondary to central nervous system involvement with increased intracranial pressure
   - Direct infiltration by leukemic cells
     - Retrolaminar infiltration can be responsible for visual loss and is justification for emergency irradiation.
4. Cornea
   - Indirect involvement from altered limbal perfusion, leading to corneal ulcers
   - Peripheral corneal infiltrates
   - Corneal edema
5. Orbit and adnexa
   - Leukemic tumors creating a mass effect
     - Granulocytic sarcoma in acute myelogenous leukemia
     - Lymphocytic sarcoma in acute lymphocytic leukemia
     - Direct infiltration of eyelid
     - Lacrimal drainage involvement causing dacryocystitis
6. Other aspects
   - Infections, including endophthalmitis, because of immunocompromise
   - Effects of radiation, chemotherapy, and bone marrow transplant

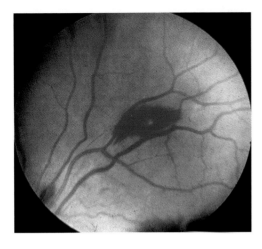

FIGURE 32.1. White-centered hemorrhage in patient with leukemia.

SUGGESTED READINGS

Britt JM, Karr DJ, Kalina RE. Leukemic iris infiltration in recurrent acute lymphocytic leukemia. *Arch Ophthalmol* 1991;109:1456–1457. *A brief case report with excellent color photographs.*

Kalina PH, Campbell RJ. *Aspergillus terreus* endophthalmitis in a patient with chronic lymphocytic leukemia. *Arch Ophthalmol* 1991;109:102–103. *A patient with fungal infection of the eye and the lung died of fungal sepsis.*

Kincaid MC. The eye in leukemia. In: Gold DH, Weingeist TA, eds. *The Eye in Systemic Disease.* Philadelphia: JB Lippincott; 1990;138–140. *A basic review of systemic and ocular manifestations of leukemia.*

Munro S, Brownstein S, Jordan DR, McLeish W. Nasolacrimal obstruction in two patients with chronic lymphocytic leukemia. *Can J Ophthalmol* 1994;29:137–140. *Two patients previously diagnosed with chronic lymphocytic leukemia developed obstructive symptoms, one bilaterally.*

Ohkoshi K, Tsiaras WG. Prognostic importance of ophthalmic manifestations in childhood leukaemia. *Br J Ophthalmol* 1992;76:651–655. *Children with leukemia were evaluated prospectively. Those with ocular manifestations had a lower 5-year survival (21.4%) than those who did not (45.7%). Ocular manifestations were associated with either bone marrow relapse or central nervous system leukemia.*

Wallace RT, Shields JA, Shields CL, et al. Leukemic infiltration of the optic nerve. *Arch Ophthalmol* 1991;109:1027. *A brief case report with excellent color photographs.*

Chapter 33

PERNICIOUS ANEMIA

Paul M. Tesser
Ronald M. Burde

I. GENERAL

1. Results from vitamin B_{12} deficiency secondary to decreased intrinsic factor production in the stomach
2. Results in deranged DNA synthesis causing megaloblastic hematopoietic cells and incorporation of abnormal fatty acids in myelin sheaths
3. The majority of cases occur in or beyond the fifth decade.
4. Usually high incidence in people of Scandinavian descent and in young African-American women
5. May be autoimmune in nature and is associated with Hashimoto's thyroiditis, vitiligo, rheumatoid arthritis, Sjögren's syndrome, and Graves' disease
6. Diagnosis is made by reversal of poor vitamin B_{12} absorption with exogenous intrinsic factor (*eg*, Shilling's test).

II. SYSTEMIC MANIFESTATIONS

1. Hematologic
   - Normochromic, macrocytic anemia
   - Hypersegmented neutrophils, macrocytes, and macroovalocytes
   - Hypercellular bone marrow
   - Megaloblastic changes in all cell lines

2. Nervous system
   - Symmetrical paresthesias in feet and fingers
   - Vibratory and proprioceptive disturbances
   - Spastic ataxia

III. OCULAR MANIFESTATIONS

1. Neuroophthalmologic
   - Optic neuropathy
   - Disc pallor
   - Central or cecocentral scotoma
   - Dyschromatopsia

2. Retina
   - Hemorrhages
   - Dilated veins
   - Retinal edema with exudate

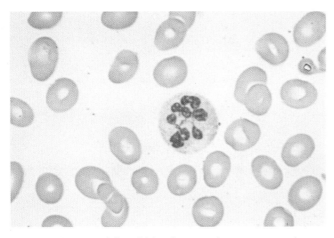

FIGURE 33.1. Peripheral blood smear demonstrates a hyper-segmented neutrophil, macrocytes, and macroovalocytes.

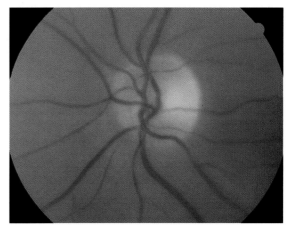

FIGURE 33.2. Optic nerve from the left eye of a patient with pernicious anemia demonstrates a wedge of temporal disc pallor.

SUGGESTED READINGS

Adams RD, Victor M. Diseases of the nervous system due to nutritional deficiency. In: Adams RD, Victor M, eds. *Principles of Neurology,* 5th ed. New York: McGraw-Hill; 1993:864–867.

Beck WS. Megaloblastic anemias. In: Wyngaarden JB, Smith LH Jr, eds. *Cecil Textbook of Medicine,* Part 1. Philadelphia: WB Saunders; 1982:853–860.

Cohen H. Optic atrophy as the presenting sign in pernicious anemia. *Lancet* 1936;2:1202–1203. *Cohen was the first to describe visual dysfunction due to optic atrophy in a patient with pernicious anemia. The ocular findings predated any other clinical manifestations.*

Rubin B, Munion L. Retinal findings in an adolescent with juvenile pernicious anemia. *N Y State J Med* 1982;82:1239–1241.

Stambolian D, Behrens M. Optic neuropathy associated with vitamin B_{12} deficiency. *Am J Ophthalmol* 1977;83:465–469.

Chapter 34
PLATELET DISORDERS
George A. Williams

I. GENERAL

1. Platelet disorders are best evaluated by the bleeding time and platelet count.
2. A prolonged bleeding time indicates a platelet disorder and the platelet count determines either thrombocytopenia or platelet dysfunction.
3. Thrombocytopenia may result from abnormal platelet production, platelet sequestration, or increased platelet destruction.
4. Platelet dysfunction syndromes are characterized by a prolonged bleeding time with a normal platelet count and may be inherited or acquired.

II. SYSTEMIC MANIFESTATIONS

1. Mucocutaneous
   - Petechiae
   - Purpura
   - Mucosal bleeding
   - Deep tissue bleeding
2. Neurologic—seen in thrombotic thrombocytopenic purpura (TTP)
   - Headache
   - Confusion
   - Aphasia
   - Transient paresis
   - Ataxia
   - Coma
3. Renal—seen in TTP
   - Hematuria
   - Proteinuria
   - Acute renal failure
4. Hematologic—seen in TTP
   - Microangiopathic hemolytic anemia
5. Ear/nose/throat
   - Epistaxis

III. OCULAR MANIFESTATIONS

1. Retina
   - Hemorrhages
   - Serous retinal detachment in TTP
   - Retinal pigment epithelial changes
   - Choroidal hemorrhage
2. Vitreous
   - Hemorrhage
3. Anterior chamber
   - Spontaneous or traumatic hyphema
4. Orbit
   - Idiopathic thrombocytopenic purpura associated with Graves' disease
5. Optic nerve
   - Optic neuritis
6. Nonspecific
   - Fever in TTP

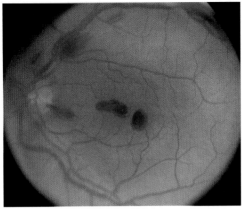

FIGURE 34.1. Preretinal and intraretinal hemorrhages in a patient with a platelet count of 10,000/mm³.

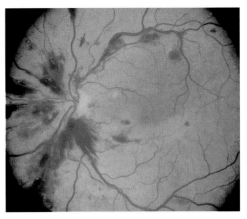

FIGURE 34.2. Retinal hemorrhages secondary to platelet dysfunction caused by Waldenström's macroglobulinemia. Courtesy of William F. Mieler, MD.

SUGGESTED READINGS

Handin RI. Hemorrhagic disorders II. Platelets and purpura. In: Beck WS, ed. *Hematology.* Cambridge, MA: MIT Press; 1985:433–456. *An excellent review of platelet biology and diseases.*

Lambert SR, High KA, Cotlier R, et al. Serous retinal detachments in thrombotic thrombocytopenic purpura. *Arch Ophthalmol* 1985;103:1172–1174.

Williams GA. Ocular manifestations of hematologic and oncologic disease. *Curr Opin Ophthalmol* 1990;1:181–186. *A review of ocular manifestations of platelet disorders with annotated references.*

Williams GA. Platelet disorders. In: Gold DH, Weingeist TA, eds. *The Eye in Systemic Disease.* Philadelphia: JB Lippincott; 1990:145–146.

Chapter 35
POLYCYTHEMIA

Kenneth G. Noble

I. GENERAL: ETIOLOGIES OF SECONDARY POLYCYTHEMIA

1. Hypoxia
   - High altitude
     - Acute mountain sickness
     - Chronic mountain sickness (Monge's disease)
   - Pulmonary disease
     - Chronic obstructive disease
     - Diffuse pulmonary infiltrates (fibrous, granulomatous)
     - Kyphoscoliosis
     - Multiple pulmonary emboli
     - Cor pulmonale (arterial desaturation, pulmonary artery hypertension)
     - Ayerza's syndrome (asthma, bronchitis, dyspnea, cyanosis, congestive failure, right ventricular hypertrophy due to pulmonary artery narrowing as a consequence of inflammation, *eg*, syphilis, arteriolar sclerosis, or congenital hypoplasia)
     - Cavernous hemangioma
     - Arteriovenous fistula
   - Congenital heart disease
     - Pulmonary stenosis (usually with patent foramen ovale, persistent patent ductus arteriosus, or defective ventricular or atrial septum)
     - Persistent truncus arteriosus
     - Complete transportation of the great vessels
     - Tetralogy of Fallot
   - Hypoventilation syndromes
     - Ondine's curse (idiopathic disease of the medullary respiratory center)
     - Secondary diseases of the respiratory center (bulbar poliomyelitis, vascular thrombosis, encephalitis)
     - Pickwickian syndrome (extreme obesity, somnolence, hypercapnia, cyanosis that may be reversed by weight loss)
   - Hemoglobin abnormalities
     - Inherited (many varieties)
     - Acquired
       - Drugs (nitrites, nitrates, sulfonamides, aniline and nitrobenzene compounds)
       - Chemicals (carboxyhemoglobin from heavy smoking, phosphorous)

2. Inappropriate Erythropoietin Production (in relative order of frequency)
   - Hypernephroma
   - Hepatocellular carcinoma
   - Cerebellar hemangioma
   - Cystic kidney disease
   - Leiomyosarcoma of uterus
   - Hydronephrosis
   - Rarely other renal tumors, pheochromocytoma, carcinomas

II. SYSTEMIC MANIFESTATIONS

1. General
   - Headache
   - Weakness
   - Dizziness
   - Sweating
   - Weight loss
2. Skin
   - Rubor (especially lips, cheeks, tip of nose)
   - Cyanosis (especially extremities)
   - Dry skin
   - Eczema
   - Acne
   - Urticaria
   - Intense itching after bathing (hot water results in vasodilation)
3. Mucous membranes
   - Intense redness
   - Easy bleeding of nose and gums
4. Central nervous system
   - Grand mal seizures
   - Paralysis
   - Myoclonus
   - Psychological disturbances
5. Other
   - Bleeding
     - Hemoptysis
     - Hemothorax
     - Gastrointestinal
     - Urogenital
   - Dyspnea
   - Abdominal fullness
     - Splenomegaly
     - Peptic ulcer
   - Gout (secondary to hyperuricemia)

1. Retina
- Plethoric fundus
  - Dark purple hue
  - Dark, dilated, tortuous veins
  - Hyperemic optic nerve
- Venous stasis retinopathy
  - Superficial and deep hemorrhages
  - Edema
- Papilledema
- Central retinal vein occlusion

2. Conjunctiva
- Congestion
- Mimics recalcitrant conjunctivitis

3. Visual symptoms secondary to cerebrovascular insufficiency
- Amaurosis
- Scotoma
- Blurred vision
- Visual hallucinations

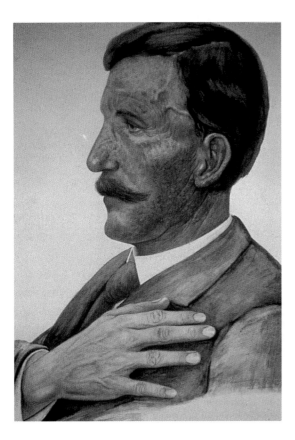

FIGURE 35.1. Painting of a patient of Dr. William Osler (1915) with polycythemia vera showing facial flushing and cyanosis of the extremities. Courtesy of C. Lockard Conley, MD.

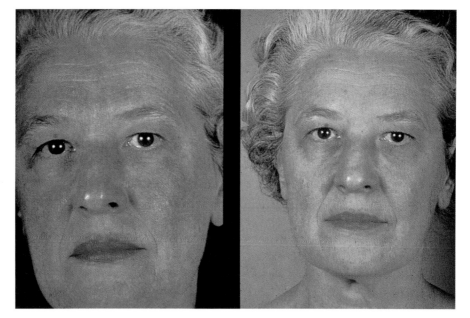

FIGURE 35.2. Adult woman with polycythemia vera showing marked reduction in facial rubor after phlebotomy. Courtesy of C. Lockard Conley, MD.

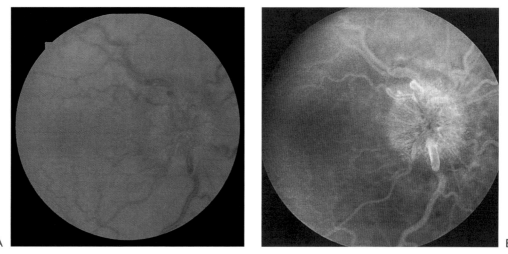

FIGURE 35.3. (**A**) Fundus of adult obese woman with chronic obstructive pulmonary disease showing secondary dilation, darkening, and tortuosity of the retinal veins in association with edema of the disc. (**B**) The fluorescein angiogram shows dilated capillaries on the optic disc.

SUGGESTED READINGS

Hoffman R, Wasserman LR. Natural history and management of polycythemia vera. *Adv Intern Med* 1979;24:255.

Kearns TP. Changes in the ocular fundus in blood diseases. *Med Clin North Am* 1956;40:1209.

Lindsey J, Insler MS. Polycythemia rubra vera and conjunctival vascular congestion. *Ann Ophthalmol* 1985;17:62.

Wagener HP, Rucker CW. Lesions of the retina and optic nerve in association with blood dyscrasias. In: Sorsby A, ed. *Modern Trends in Ophthalmology.* London: Butterworth; 1948:300.

Chapter 36

SICKLE CELL DISEASE

Aaron Perera Weingeist
Elaine L. Chuang

I. GENERAL

1. Autosomal recessive disease with codominant expression
2. Gene located 11p15 in the β-globin complex
3. 8% to 10% of African-Americans, and as many as 30% of blacks in some African nations, are heterozygous for the sickle cell gene.
4. Hemoglobin S (HbS)—single point mutation at codon β6 (valine for glutamic acid). Homozygotes have decreased life span.
5. Hemoglobin C (HbC)—single point mutation at codon β6 (lysine for glutamic acid)
6. AS—sickle cell trait (HbA is normal). Life expectancy and frequency of hospitalization are equal to those of normal individuals.
7. Double heterozygosity (HbS plus any of the other hemoglobin mutations) causes clinically significant sickle cell disease.
8. On deoxygenation, red blood cells containing HbS change from biconcave disks to "sickle" cells and occlude capillaries in a reversible fashion. Local ischemia causes further sickling and the initiation of a vicious cycle. The degree of sickling is greatly reduced by the presence of non-HbS (*ie*, A or F).
9. Heterozygotes have a decreased rate and severity of falciparum malaria infection.
10. Diagnosis is made by either the sickle test or the hemoglobin solubility test. Positive results are confirmed by hemoglobin electrophoresis.
11. Manifestations are due to microvascular infarction.

II. SYSTEMIC MANIFESTATIONS

Degree of systemic manifestations (SS > SC > AS). AS and AC rarely have systemic manifestations except under extreme hypoxia or acidosis. Either may have decreased ability to concentrate urine or hematuria.

1. Hematologic
   - Hemolytic anemia
2. Vascular
   - Arterial occlusion
3. Splenic/immunologic
   - Splenomegaly in infancy, then atrophy and autosplenectomy in childhood
   - Increased sepsis with encapsulated organisms (*Streptococcus pneumoniae, Haemophilus influenzae*)
4. Central nervous system
   - Cerebrovascular accident (ischemic in children, hemorrhagic in adults)
   - Cerebral atrophy
   - Aneurysms
5. Genitourinary
   - Priapism
   - Impotence
6. Musculoskeletal
   - Aseptic necrosis
   - Vertebral compression ("fish-mouth" vertebrae)
7. Cardiopulmonary
   - Acute chest syndrome
   - Generalized pulmonary fibrosis
   - Cor pulmonale
   - Pulmonary infarcts and dyspnea
   - Adult respiratory distress syndrome
   - Cardiomyopathy
   - Systolic heart murmur
   - Congestive heart failure
8. Mucocutaneous
   - Chronic lower extremity ulcerations
9. Renal
   - Inability to concentrate urine
   - Hematuria
   - Chronic renal failure secondary to obliterative glomerulosclerosis
10. Hepatobiliary
    - Hepatomegaly
    - Cirrhosis
    - Hyperbilirubinemia
    - Cholelithiasis
11. Nonspecific
    - Painful crises
    - Delayed growth and development

III. OCULAR MANIFESTATIONS

Frequency of ocular manifestations (SC > SS > AS)
1. Orbit
   - Proptosis
   - Pain
2. Lids
   - Edema
3. Conjunctiva
   - "Conjunctival sign" (comma-shaped vascular occlusions, usually inferior) telangiectasis
4. Sclera
   - Icterus

5. Anterior chamber
   - Hyphema (an ocular emergency)
6. Iris
   - Atrophy
   - Peripheral anterior synechia
   - Posterior synechia
   - Neovascularization and glaucoma
7. Fundus
   - Sickle cell "disk sign" (segmented blood in small vessels on the disk)
   - Increase in vessel tortuosity
   - Central retinal or branch retinal artery occlusions
   - Macular depression sign (concavity with a bright central reflection)
   - Mascular ischemia with enlargement of foveal avascular zone (rare)
   - "Salmon patch" hemorrhages
   - Retinoschisis cavities
   - Iridescent spots
   - "Black sunburst" chorioretinal scars
   - Sea fans (superotemporal quadrant most common)
   - Vitreous hemorrhage
   - Retinal detachment (tractional or rhegmatogenous)
   - Angioid streaks
   - Wedge-shaped choroidal infarcts

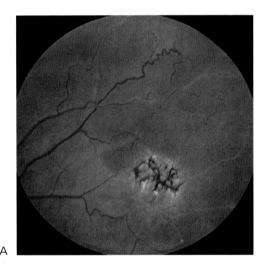
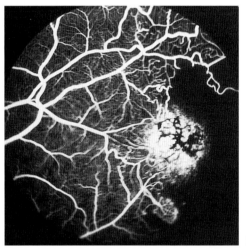

FIGURE 36.1. (**A**) Color fundus photograph and (**B**) corresponding fluorescein angiogram of black sunburst chorioretinal scar.

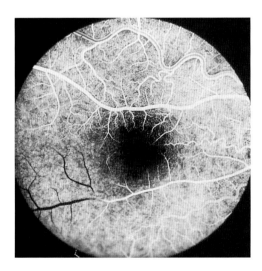

FIGURE 36.2. Fluorescein angiogram demonstrates macular arterial obstruction.

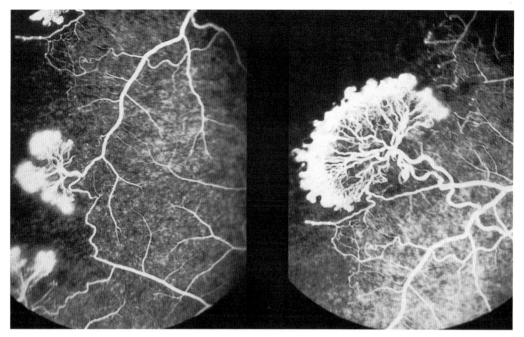

FIGURE 36.3. Fluorescein angiogram shows perfused sea fans and peripheral nonperfusion.

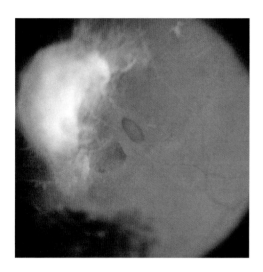

FIGURE 36.4. Color fundus photograph of elevated, autoinfarcted sea fan with atrophic retinal holes.

SUGGESTED READINGS

Clarkson JG. The ocular manifestations of sickle-cell disease: A prevalence and natural history study. *Trans Am Ophthalmol Soc* 1992;90:481–504.

Cohen SB, Ban Houten PA. Hemoglobinopathies. In: Ryan SJ, Schachat AP, Murphy RP, Patz A, eds. *Retina,* vol 2, *Medical Retinal,* 2nd ed. St. Louis: CV Mosby; 1994:1462–1472. *A detailed source on ocular manifestations with good photographs.*

Nagpal KC, Goldberg MF, Rabb MF. Ocular manifestations of sickle hemoglobinopathies. *Surv Ophthalmol* 1977;21:391–411. *Classic review article with good photos.*

Penman AD, Talbot JF, Chuang EL, et al. New classification of peripheral retinal vascular changes in sickle cell disease. *Br J Ophthalmol* 1994;78:681–689. *A new classification scheme of sickle cell associated vascular changes in the peripheral retina.*

Powars DR. Sickle cell anemia and major organ failure. *Hemoglobin* 1990;14:573–598. *A good review of the systemic manifestations of sickle cell disease.*

Serjeant GR. *Sickle Cell Disease.* Oxford, England: Oxford Medical Publications; 1985. *An excellent, detailed source covering all aspects of sickle cell disease.*

PART 8. INFECTIOUS DISEASES

Section A. Bacterial Diseases

Chapter 37

TULAREMIA

William G. Hodge
Gilbert Smolin
Robert Nozik

I. GENERAL

1. This very rare reportable infection is caused by *Francisella tularensis,* a small gram-negative nonmotile coccobacillus that is pleomophic in culture.
2. Culture requires cysteine-rich media such as thioglycolate at 37°C.
3. It is distributed throughout the northern hemisphere and has been recovered in more than 100 wild animals.
4. In North America, the most important reservoirs are rabbits, hares, muscrats, and ticks.
5. Humans acquire the infection after direct contact with a body fluid from an infected animal or via an animal bite.
6. Only 10 to 50 bacilli are needed to cause disease if inhaled or injected intradermally; the usual incubation period is 3 to 5 days.
7. The organism can survive for prolonged periods intracellularly. Early lesions are characterized by necrosis. Later, granuloma formation occurs.

II. SYSTEMIC MANIFESTATIONS

1. General
   - Fever, chills
   - Malaise and fatigue
2. Skin and lymphatics
   - Ulcerated skin lesions
   - Macular, maculopapular, or pustular rash
   - Erythema nodosum
   - Erythema multiforme
   - Painful regional lymphadenopathy
   - Lymphangitis rare
3. Respiratory
   - Asymptomatic but abnormal chest X ray
   - Lobar pneumonia
   - Pleural effusions
   - Adult respiratory distress syndrome rare
4. Other rare systemic manifestations
   - Hepatomegaly and abnormal liver function tests
   - Renal failure and rhabdomyolysis
   - Pericarditis
   - Peritonitis
   - Meningitis
   - Osteomyelitis

III. OCULAR MANIFESTATIONS

1. General
   - Usually unilateral
   - Pain, photophobia, and itching common
2. Lid
   - Eyelid ulceration
   - Lid and periorbital edema
   - Regional lymphadenopathy
3. Conjunctiva
   - Perinaud's oculoglandular syndrome
   - Conjunctival erythema, chemosis, and discharge
   - Conjunctival nodules 1 to 5 mm in size
   - Necrotic membranes
4. Cornea
   - Peripheral corneal infiltrates
   - Pannus
   - Limbal nodules
   - Cornea edema
   - Rarely, cornea ulceration and perforation
5. Lacrimal system
   - Dacryocystitis
6. Optic nerve
   - Bilateral optic neuritis

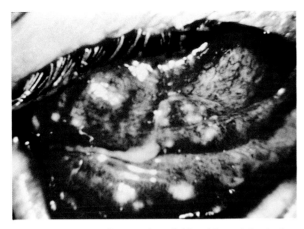

FIGURE 37.1. A purulent conjunctivitis with nodules is characteristic of this infection.

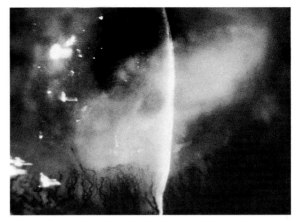

FIGURE 37.2. Cornea findings are rare but when they occur, large peripheral infiltrates can be seen.

SUGGESTED READINGS

Evans ME, Gregory DW, Schaffner W, et al. Tularemia: A 30-year experience with 88 cases. *Medicine* 1985;64:251–269. *An in depth review of the systemic clinical aspects of the disease.*

Ostler HB. *Diseases of the External Eye and Adnexa.* Philadelphia: Williams & Wilkins; 1993:431–434. *An excellent review of the ocular manifestations of this rare disorder.*

Provenza JM, Klotz SA, Penn RL. Isolation of *Francisella tularensis* from blood. *J Clin Microbiol* 1986;24:453–455.

Section B.   Helminthic Diseases

Chapter 38

CYSTICERCOSIS

Alex E. Jalkh
Arnaldo F. Bordon

I. GENERAL

1. Parasitic infestation by *Cysticercus cellulosae*
2. Worldwide disease, predominantly in Africa, Mexico, Southeast Asia, South America, and Eastern Europe
3. No sex or race predilections
4. Human acts as the intermediary host instead of definitive host as in *Taenia solium* life cycle.
5. Infestation occurs when food or water containing contaminated eggs is ingested. Autoinfestation may occur in individuals with poor hygiene or when eggs reflux from the intestine into the stomach.
6. *Cysticercus cellulosae* larvae perforate the gastrointestinal mucosae, gain access to the portal circulation, and locate mainly in the eye, brain, subcutaneous tissue, and skeletal muscles.

II. SYSTEMIC MANIFESTATIONS

1. The clinical presentation is determined by the location and size of the cysticercus.
2. Neurologic manifestations are the most common presentation.
   - Generalized, focal, or jacksonian seizures
   - Symptoms of increased intracranial pressure (nausea, vomiting, headache)
   - Ataxia
   - Confusion
   - Chronic meningitis or arachnoiditis (racemose form of cysticercosis)
3. Subcutaneous nodules (usually asymptomatic)
4. Skeletal muscle nodules (usually asymptomatic)
5. Other locations (tongue, visceral are rare)
6. Immunoblotting technique (enzyme-linked immunosorbent assay) has 98% specificity and 91% sensitivity. Other serologic tests show cross-reactivity with other tapeworm, filarial, and echinococcal infestation.
7. Cerebrospinal fluid analysis shows pleocytosis with mononuclear cell predominance, decreased glucose, and increased protein levels.
8. Computed tomography is helpful to identify calcified lesions and magnetic resonance imaging to detect cystic lesions in the brain.

III. OCULAR MANIFESTATIONS

1. Living parasite causes chronic uveitis that could lead to panophthalmitis if left untreated.
2. When the parasite dies toxins are released causing a severe inflammatory reaction.
3. Lids
   - Painless tumefaction, irritation
4. Anterior segment
   - Conjunctiva
     - Redness, irritation, tearing
     - Subconjunctival tumefaction
   - Anterior chamber
     - Pain, redness
     - Flare, cells, cysticercus floating in the anterior chamber
5. Posterior segment
   - Intravitreous
     - Decreased visual acuity, redness, or can be asymptomatic
     - Cysticercus floating freely in the vitreous cavity, vitreous cells, and intravitreous inflammatory opacities
     - Removal by pars plana vitrectomy is the treatment of choice.
   - Subretinal space
     - The most common posterior segment location, usually in the macular area
     - Decreased visual acuity
     - Vitreous cells and vitreous opacities
     - Subretinal lesion is seen ophthalmoscopically.
     - Treatment consists of cyst removal through a posterior sclerotomy.
6. Lacrimal system
   - Dacriops
7. Optic nerve
   - Unusual location and may mimic optic nerve glioma
   - Decreased vision
   - Retrobulbar neuritis can occur with orbital lesions.
8. Orbit
   - Unusual location
   - Asymptomatic or can be associated with considerable pain, redness, chemosis, exophthalmos, ptosis
   - Diplopia with restriction of extraocular movements
9. Neuroophthalmologic
   - Papilledema (associated with increased intracranial pressure)
   - Pupillary abnormalities, upward gaze paresis, skew deviation, nystagmus, eyelid retraction
   - Secondary optic atrophy
   - Abducens palsy
   - Homonymous hemianopia
   - Bitemporal hemianopia
   - Fourth nerve palsy (uncommon)

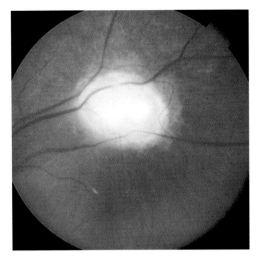

FIGURE 38.1. Subretinal cysticercus of the left eye showing fibrosis around the lesion. Courtesy of Pedro Paulo Bonomo, MD, São Paulo, Brazil.

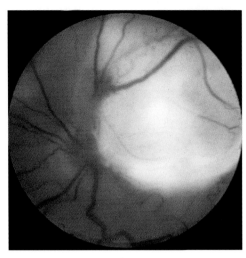

FIGURE 38.2. A large subretinal cysticercus is seen in the posterior pole of the left eye. Courtesy of Pedro Paulo Bonomo, MD, São Paulo, Brazil.

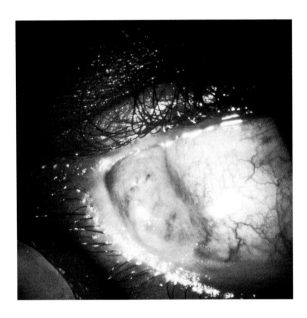

FIGURE 38.3. A case of subconjunctival cysticercus of the right eye. Courtesy of Élcio H. Sato, MD, São Paulo, Brazil.

SUGGESTED READINGS

Jalkh AE, Quiroz H. Cysticercosis. In: Gold DH, Weingeist TA, eds. *The Eye in Systemic Disease.* Philadelphia: JB Lippincott; 1990:175–178.

Keane JR. Neuro-ophthalmologic signs and symptoms of cysticercosis. *Arch Ophthalmol* 1982;100:1445–1448.

Kruger-Leite E, Jalkh AE, Quiroz H, Schepens CL. Intraocular cysticercosis. *Am J Ophthalmol* 1985;99:252–257.

Nutman TB, Weller PF. Cestodes. In: Isselbacher KJ, et al. *Harrison's Principles of Internal Medicine.* New York: McGraw-Hill; 1994:931–932.

Sen DK. Cysticercus cellulosae in the lacrimal gland, orbit, and the eyelid. *Acta Ophthalmol* 1980;58:144–147.

Chapter 39
ECHINOCOCCOSIS
J. Oscar Croxatto

I. GENERAL

1. Organisms
   - *Echinococcus granulosus* (hydatid cyst)
   - *Echinococcus multilocularis* (alveolar hydatid cyst)
   - *Echinococcus oligoarthrus*
   - *Echinococcus vogeli* (polycystic)
2. Endemic areas
   - Middle East
   - North Africa
   - South America
   - Central Europe and Mediterranean countries
   - Western United States
   - Alaska, Canada, and Siberia (northern strains)
3. Life cycle
   - Definitive hosts: dogs and wild carnivores
   - Intermediate host: sheep, pigs, domestic animals, and rodents
   - Humans, children and adults, act as accidental intermediate hosts.
4. Structure of the cyst
   - Inner germinative layer
     - Brood capsules
     - Protoscolices measuring 100 μm with hooklets
   - Outer "cuticular" laminated nonnucleated membrane
   - Adventitial layer (inflammatory reaction by the host)
5. Immunology
   - Antibody response limited by integrity of the cyst
   - Anaphylactic response after rupture
   - Serology: antigen 5 immunoelectrophoresis, enzyme-linked immunosorbent assay test to fertile bovine hydatid cyst fluid

II. SYSTEMIC MANIFESTATIONS

Location of the cysts
1. Cardiac
2. Pulmonary
   - Cough
   - Chest pain
   - Fever
   - Hemoptysis
   - Hydatid vomica after rupture
3. Renal
   - Pain
   - Hematuria
4. Gastrointestinal (liver)
   - Abdominal pain
   - Palpable mass in the liver
   - Jaundice
5. Neurologic (central nervous system)
   - Raised intracranial pressure
   - Epilepsy
6. Hematologic
   - Spleen involvement
7. Skeletal
   - Spontaneous fractures

III. OCULAR MANIFESTATIONS

1. Lids/conjunctiva
   - Chemosis
   - Lid edema
   - Pain
2. Ocular
   - Loss of vision
   - Papilledema
   - Vitritis
   - Subretinal mass
   - Vitreal cyst
   - Anterior chamber cyst
3. Orbit
   - Slowly progressive painless exophthalmos
   - Impaired extraocular motility
   - Palpable mass
   - Orbital cellulitis because secondary infection

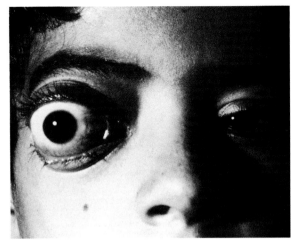

FIGURE 39.1. Axial proptosis in a 15-year-old boy from an endemic area.

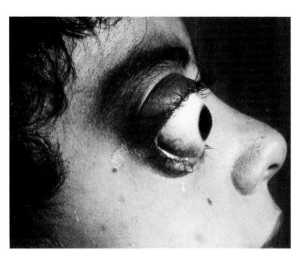

FIGURE 39.2. Lateral view of the patient depicted in Fig. 39.1.

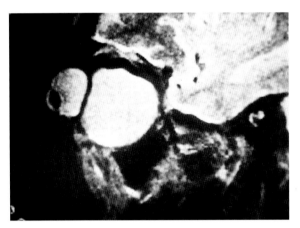

FIGURE 39.3. Nuclear magnetic resonance imaging (T_2-weighted) of a large watery orbital cyst.

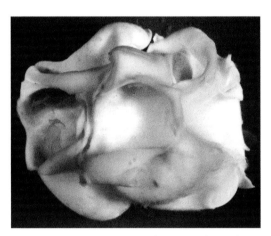

FIGURE 39.4. Gross appearance of an excised cyst showing the nonnucleated outer membrane.

SUGGESTED READINGS

Gomez Morales A, Croxatto JO. Echinococcosis. In: Gold DH, Weingeist TA, eds. *The Eye in Systemic Disease.* Philadelphia: JB Lippincott; 1990:178–180. *A short review of systemic and ocular manifestations, and therapy.*

Gomez Morales A, Croxatto JO, Crovetto L, Ebner R. Hydatid cyst of the orbit. A review of 35 cases. *Ophthalmology* 1988;95:1027–1032. *A review of a series of patients with orbital disease.*

Schantz PM. Echinococcosis. In: Steele JH. *CRC Handbook Series in Zoonoses. Section C: Parasitic Zoonoses,* vol 1. Boca Raton, FL: CRC Press; 1983:231–277. *A large review of parasitology and pathogenesis of echinococcosis.*

Williams DF, Williams GA, Caya JG, et al. Intraocular *Echinococcus multilocularis. Arch Ophthalmol* 1987;105:1106–1109.

Chapter 40

LOA LOA

David S. Gendelman

I. GENERAL

1. Uncommon outside of Africa
2. Most common west and central Africa in rain forests and swamplands
3. Parasitic nematode in adult stage occupying subcutaneous tissue
4. Adult released as microfilariae into host blood
5. Horsefly (*Chrysops*) ingests larvae from host's blood, the horsefly (acting as intermediate vector) injects microfilariae into blood
6. Worm matures over first year; may live as long as 15 years

II. SYSTEMIC MANIFESTATIONS

1. Cardiac
   - Endomyocardial fibrosis
2. Central nervous system
   - Meningoencephalitis
3. Musculoskeletal
   - Polyarticular arthritis
4. Mucocutaneous
   - Calabar swelling
5. Hematologic
   - Microfilaria in blood
   - Eosinophilia

III. OCULAR MANIFESTATIONS

1. Anterior segment
   - Subconjunctival worm
   - Conjunctivitis
   - Keratitis
   - Iridocyclitis
2. Retina
   - Loa loa retinopathy
     - Superficial hemorrhagic sheath
     - Yellow exudates on retina
3. Nonspecific
   - Eyelid subcutaneous worms
   - Worms in vitreous
   - Uveitis secondary to microfilaria

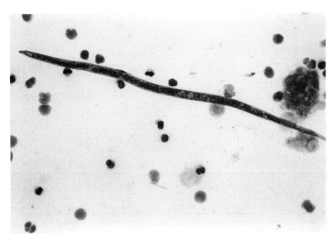

FIGURE 40.1. Peripheral blood smear showing microfilariae and eosinophils (hematoxylin-eosin; original magnification, ×40).

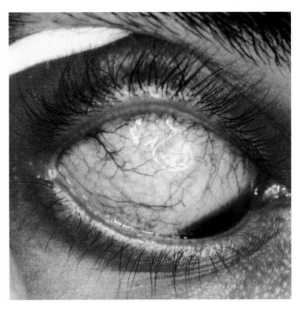

FIGURE 40.2. Subconjunctival worm in the superotemporal quadrant of the right eye.

SUGGESTED READINGS

Disease of the outer eye: conjunctiva. In: Duke-Elder W, ed. *System of Ophthalmology,* vol 8. St Louis: Mosby; 1965:403–405.

Gendelman D. Loa Loa. In: Gold D, Weingeist T, eds. *The Eye in Systemic Disease.* Philadelphia: JB Lippincott; 1990:180–182. *A general review of ocular Loa Loa.*

Gendelman D, Blumberg R, Sadun A. Ocular pathology for clinicians. Ocular loa-loa with cryoprobe extraction of subconjunctival worm. *Ophthalmology* 1984;91:300–303.

Manson-Bahr PEC, ed. *Manson's Tropical Diseases,* 18th ed. London: Balliere Tindall; 1982:161–174, 727–729.

Rogell G. Infectious and inflammatory diseases. In: Duane TD, ed. *Clinical Ophthalmology,* vol 5. Philadelphia: Harper & Row; 1982:19.

Toussaint D, Danis P. Retinopathy in generalized loa-loa filariasis: A clinicopathological study. *Arch Ophthalmol* 1965;74:470–476.

Chapter 41

SCHISTOSOMIASIS

Ernesto I. Segal
Rafael Cordero Moreno

I. GENERAL

1. Chronic infection by trematodes of the genus *Schistosoma*
2. Three major species infect humans: *S. haematobium* (Egypt, Africa, Middle East) causing urinary schistosomiasis, *S. japonicum* (Japan, Far East) causing the Katayama disease, and *S. mansoni* (Africa, southern North America, Central and South America) producing the intestinal schistosomiasis.
3. The life cycle has two sexual phases: sexual multiplication in adult stages in the definitive human host and an asexual phase during larval stages in the intermediate snail host.
4. Infected snails shed larval schistosomes in the water. The cercariae penetrates the human skin or mucous membranes and transform into schistosomules. These are carried through the venous circulation to the heart and lungs, from there proceeding to the liver. In the portal circulation they grow and copulate, and the *S. haematobium* migrate to the vesical veins, the *S. japonicum* to the inferior mesenteric veins and the *S. mansoni* to the superior mesenteric veins. At these locations, they lay eggs that can penetrate the vessel wall into the tissues of the bladder and the intestine, or the eggs can be excreted with the urine and feces. In the water the eggs hatch and liberate a larva called miriacidia, which can get into the snail host and restart the cycle.
5. Ocular and central nervous system involvement is unusual, seen mainly in children with severe hepatosplenic syndrome living in endemic areas. The mechanism is hematogenous spread, by embolism of eggs through the arterial system and local deposit in those tissues. There is a hypothetical immunologic mechanism causing ocular symptoms during the acute phase of the disease.
6. The immunologic mechanism involves both humoral and cellular responses that cause a dermatitis at the site of primary cercarial invasion of the skin. The live adult worms can acquire host antigens on their surface and evade the host immune response. The dead worms and eggs cause an active mixed response that results in production of antibodies and granulomatous reactions. An enzyme-linked immunosorbent assay with a sensitivity of 98% can help in the diagnosis.
7. The pathology shows granulomas with the calcified egg in the center, surrounded by layers of epithelioid cells, plasma, cells, lymphocytes, and eosinophils.
8. Treatment: oxamniquine and praziquantel

II. SYSTEMIC MANIFESTATIONS

1. Gastrointestinal
   - Hepatitis
   - Hepatic fibrosis
   - Portal hypertension
   - Hepatosplenomegaly
   - Esophageal varices
   - Ascites
   - Hematemesis
   - Intestinal mucous ulcers
   - Inflammatory polyps in the colon
   - Abdominal pain
   - Dysentery
2. Genitourinary
   - Cystitis
   - Hematuria
   - Dysuria
   - Urinary frequency
   - Calcified bladder
   - Hydroureters
   - Hydronephrosis
   - Pyelonephritis
   - Increased incidence of carcinoma of the bladder
3. Pulmonary
   - Cough
   - Hemoptysis
   - Pulmonary hypertension
4. Cardiac
   - Cor pulmonale
5. Neurologic
   - Seizures
   - Psychomotor epilepsy
   - Transverse myelitis
   - Spinal cord mass
6. Skin
   - Dermatitis at the site of primary penetration
   - Maculopapular pruritic rash
7. Hematologic
   - Eosinophilia
   - Elevated specific antibodies
8. Nonspecific
   - Katayama syndrome
   - Fever
   - Lymphadenopathies

III. OCULAR MANIFESTATIONS

1. Lids
   - Edema
   - Swelling
   - Urticaria
   - Mass
   - Ptosis

2. Conjunctiva/sclera
   - Granulomas
   - Yellowish white nodules
   - Polyps
3. Anterior chamber
   - Direct invasion by the worm
   - Hyphema
4. Retina and choroid
   - Yellowish white nodules near the blood vessels
   - Hyperfluroescent lesions on the fluorescein angiogram

5. Orbit and lacrimal system
   - Granuloma
   - Orbital pseudotumor
   - Direct invasion of orbital vessels by the worm
   - Dacryoadenitis
6. Nonspecific
   - Anterior nongranulomatous uveitis
   - Cataract

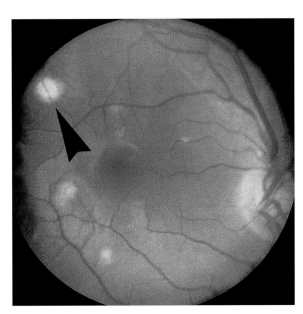

FIGURE 41.1. Fundus photo shows yellowish white lesions in the choroid, produced by the *S. mansoni* eggs. Reprinted from Orefice F, et al. *Br J Ophthalmol* 1985;69.

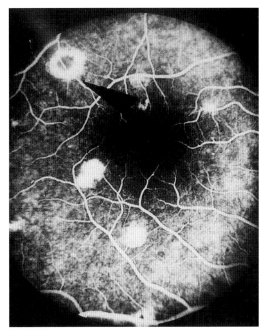

FIGURE 41.2. Early fundus fluorescein angiogram shows early hyperfluorescence of choroidal lesions produced by the *S. mansoni* eggs. Reprinted from Orefice F, et al. *Br J Ophthalmol* 1985;69.

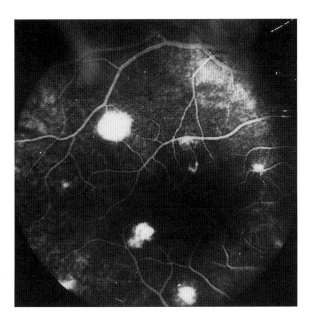

FIGURE 41.3. Late fundus fluorescein angiogram shows late hyperfluorescence of the same choroidal lesions. Reprinted from Orefice F, et al. *Br J Ophthalmol* 1985;69.

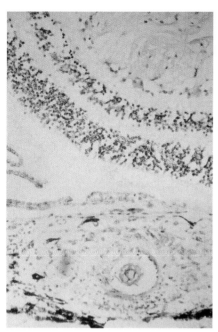

FIGURE 41.4. Pathology specimen shows choroidal granuloma containing in center the *S. mansoni* egg. Reprinted from Orefice F, et al. *Br J Ophthalmol* 1985;69.

SUGGESTED READINGS

Cordero-Moreno R. *Manifestaciones Oculares de Algunas Enfermedades Tropicales.* Caracas: Publicaciones de la Secretaria de la UCV; 1993:213–220

Elkhayat RA, Girgis M. Bilharzial granuloma of the conus: Case report. *Neurosurgery* 1993;32: 1022–1024.

Kabo AM, Warter A. Apropos of 1 case of ophthalmologic manifestation of bilharziasis. *Bull Soc Pathol Exot* 1993; 86:174–175.

Orefice F, Sinval LJR, Pitella JEH. Schistosomotic choroiditis. *Br J Ophthalmol* 1985;69:294–299.

Pitella JEH, Orefice F. Schistosomotic choroiditis: Report of the first case. *Br J Ophthalmol* 1985;69: 300–302.

Ramzy RM, Hillyer GV. Evaluation of an ELISA for the diagnosis of human infection with *S. haematobium. J Egypt Soc Parasitol* 1993;23:315–322.

Tabbara KF, Shoukrey N. Schistosomiasis. In: Gold DH, Weingeist T, eds. *The Eye in Systemic Disease.* Philadelphia: JB Lippincott; 1990:184–187.

Chapter 42
TOXOCARIASIS
Donald W. Park

I. GENERAL

1. Usually affects children
2. Boys are affected more than girls in ocular toxocariasis
3. Uniocular
4. Due to infection with *Toxocara canis* (dogs) and *Toxocara cati* (cats)
5. Ingestion of *Toxocara* ova from contaminated soil (*eg*, pica)
6. The ova develop into larvae in the gastrointestinal epithelium.
7. Larvae spread via blood vessels and lymphatics to multiple organs.
8. An eosinophilic zonal granulomatous inflammation develops around the *Toxocara* larvae.
9. Enzyme-linked immunosorbent assay (ELISA) can help confirm the diagnosis.
10. Humans are unnatural hosts and represent dead-end infections.

II. SYSTEMIC MANIFESTATIONS

1. Visceral larva migrans
   - General
     - Fever
     - Malaise
     - Weight loss
   - Hematologic
     - Blood eosinophilia
     - Anemia
     - Leukocytosis
   - Gastrointestinal
     - Hepatosplenomegaly
     - Diarrhea
   - Pulmonary
     - Cough and wheezes
     - Pulmonary infiltrates on chest X ray
   - Neurologic
     - Seizures
     - Meningitis
     - Encephalitis
   - Cardiac
     - Myocarditis
2. Ocular toxocariasis
   - Patients with ocular toxocariasis will usually have no evidence of the systemic visceral larval migrans.

III. OCULAR MANIFESTATIONS

1. Retina and choroid
   - White, granulomatous masses in the macula or peripheral retina
   - Retinal vascular distortion
   - Subretinal fluid
   - Subretinal hemorrhage
   - Retinal detachment
   - Vision variable depending on extent of macular involvement
2. Vitreous
   - Endophthalmitis form with dense vitritis and mild anterior chamber cells
   - Vitreous traction bands over granulomas may extend to macula.
3. Conjunctiva
   - Despite active uveitis, conjunctiva may look white and quiet.
4. Lens
   - Cataract
5. Ocular motility
   - Strabismus
6. Neuroophthalmologic
   - Neuroretinitis
7. Cornea
   - Keratitis
8. Nonspecific
   - Leukocoria

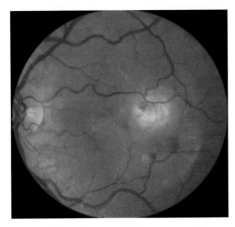

FIGURE 42.1. This is a 12-year-old boy who noted poor vision in the left eye over the preceding 2 months. His visual acuity measured 20/20 RE and 20/100 LE. Toxocara serum titer (ELISA) was positive at 1:4. Ophthalmoscopic photograph, left eye. Note the deep, subretinal white mass with surrounding hemorrhage, lipid, and retinal edema.

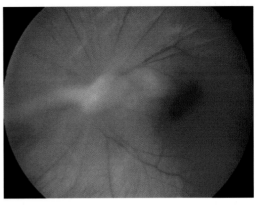

FIGURE 42.2. This is an 8-year-old girl with a *Toxocara* lesion by the optic nerve and vitreal inflammation. Visual acuity measured 20/25 RE and 20/100 LE. Ophthalmoscopic photograph, left eye. There is a white mass over the optic nerve head. Also, note the significant vitritis associated with the mass. White, fingerlike projections from the white mass extend into the peripheral retina.

SUGGESTED READINGS

Schantz PM, Glickman LT. Toxocaral visceral larva migrans. *N Engl J Med* 1978;298:436–439.

Shields JA. Ocular toxocariasis: A review. *Surv Ophthalmol* 1984;28:361–381. *A thorough review of ocular toxocariasis and the differential diagnosis.*

Smith RE, Nozik R. Ocular toxocariasis. In: *Uveitis. A Clinical Approach to the Diagnosis and Management,* 2nd ed. Baltimore: Williams & Wilkins; 1989:135–140. *A well-written source on ocular toxocariasis.*

Wehrle PF, Top FH. Visceral larva migrans. In: *Communicable and Infectious Diseases,* 9th ed. St. Louis: CV Mosby; 1981: 358–362.

Chapter 43

TRICHINOSIS

Ernesto I. Segal
Rafael Cordero Moreno

I. GENERAL

1. Human infection by roundworms of species *Trichinella spiralis*
2. Mainly a zoonosis, common in rodents and pigs, man is an incidental host, who becomes infected by eating undercooked or raw pork or other meat with encysted larvae.
3. During the life cycle, the ingested cyst wall is digested in the stomach and the infective larvae are released. They migrate to the duodenal and jejunal mucosa, where they grow into adult worms. These copulate and some of the larvae are excreted with the feces; other new larvae migrate by hematogenous and lymphatic spread to the striated muscle tissue, mainly to the skeletal muscles of the limbs, diaphragm, masseters, tongue, extraocular muscles, and others. At these locations, they coil up, become encapsulated, and transform into third-stage larvae.
4. The immunologic response involves the role of cell-mediated immunity at the intestinal mucosa. During the migration phase there is an antibody response, in combination with a cellular response that involves a typical hypereosinophilia.
5. The pathology specimens show encysted larvae within striated muscle fibers with variable inflammatory response.
6. Treatment consists of the use of different antiparasitics: diethylcarbamizine, thiobendazol, mebendazol, and flubendazol, as well as analgesics and systemic steroids.

II. SYSTEMIC MANIFESTATIONS

1. Gastrointestinal
   - Gastroenteritis
   - Anorexia
   - Nausea and vomiting
   - Abdominal cramps
   - Diarrhea
   - Constipation
   - Peritonitis
2. Musculoskeletal
   - Myositis
   - Severe myalgias
   - Decreased muscle strength
   - Elevation of serum muscle enzymes
   - Difficulty in mastication, breathing, and swallowing
3. Neurologic
   - Meningoencephalitis
   - Cortical infarcts
4. Cardiac
   - Myocarditis
5. Pulmonary
   - Bronchitis
   - Pneumonia
6. Renal
   - Nephritis
7. Nonspecific
   - High fever
   - Weakness
   - Headaches
   - Hypereosinophilia
   - Edema
   - Dehydration
   - Toxic syndrome

III. OCULAR MANIFESTATIONS

1. Lids
   - Bilateral edema
   - Ptosis (levator invasion)
   - Decreased palpebral fissure (orbicularis invasion)
2. Conjunctiva/sclera
   - Chemosis
   - Subconjunctival hemorrhage
   - Angular conjunctivitis
3. Iris and lens
   - Mydriasis
   - Accommodation paresis
4. Vitreous
   - Vitreitis
   - Hemorrhage
5. Retina
   - Hemorrhage
   - Edema
6. Optic nerve
   - Disc edema
7. Orbit
   - Retroorbital pain (with eye movements)
   - Bilateral periorbital edema ("classic" triad with fever and hypereosinophilia)
   - Proptosis
8. Neuroophthalmologic
   - Extraocular muscle palsies or restriction
   - Ophthalmoplegia
   - Diplopia
   - Facial palsy and diplegia

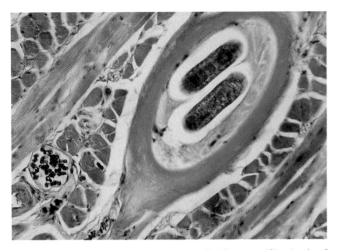

FIGURE 43.1. Pathology specimen (high magnification) of *Trichinella spiralis* encysted within human striated muscle. Reprinted from Cordero-Moreno R. *Manifestaciones Oculares de algunas Enfermedades Tropicales.* Caracas: Publicaciones de la Secretaria de la UCV, 1993.

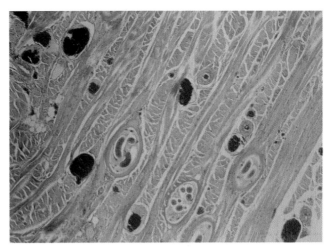

FIGURE 43.2. Pathology specimen (low magnification) of *Trichinella spiralis* encysted within human striated muscle.

SUGGESTED READINGS

Cordero-Moreno R. *Manifestaciones Oculares de Algunas Enfermedades Tropicales.* Caracas: Publicaciones de la Secretaria de la UCV; 1993:179–185.

Feydy A, Touze E, Miaux Y, et al. MRI findings in a case of neurotrichinosis. *Neuroradiology* 1996;38(Suppl 1):S80–S82.

Harms G, Binz P, Feldmeier H, et al. Trichinosis: A prospective controlled study of patients ten years after acute infection. *Clin Infect Dis* 1993;17:637–643.

Lopez-Lozano JJ, Garcia Merino JA, Liano H. Bilateral facial paralysis secondary to trichinosis. *Acta Neurol Scand* 1988;78:194–197.

Tabbara KF, Shoukrey N. Trichinosis. In: Gold DH, Weingeist T, eds. *The Eye in the Systemic Disease.* Philadelphia: JB Lippincott; 1990:191–192.

Section C.   Mycobacterial Diseases

Chapter 44

LEPROSY

Timothy J. ffytche

I. GENERAL

1. Leprosy is widely distributed in the developing world with an estimated 5 to 10 million people affected.
2. Leprosy is caused by *Mycobacterium leprae* and probably spread by droplet infection.
3. The organism affects nerves in the cooler parts of the body—skin, hands, feet, nose, eyes, and testis.
4. Two basic forms occur, depending on the immune response of the affected individual: paucibacillary, where there is a high degree of immunity, and multibacillary, where immunity is low.
5. The disease is chronic and slowly progressive, but acute reactions in nerves and various organs can occur when the immunity alters.
6. The disease manifestations vary according to the patient's immunity and many other factors.
7. Multidrug therapy (dapsone, rifampicin, and clofazimine) should be effective in preventing major disabilities if commenced early in the disease, but the continuing stigma of leprosy often stops patients from presenting for treatment.

II. SYSTEMIC MANIFESTATIONS

1. Mucocutaneous
   - Skin patches, plaques, and nodules
   - Loss of skin sensation: pain, temperature, touch
   - Thickened nerves
   - Plantar ulcers
   - Nasal destruction
2. Musculoskeletal
   - Paralysis
   - Dactylitis
   - Contractures
   - Limb deformities
3. Systemic reactions
   - Fever, malaise
   - Erythema nodosum leprosum
   - Acute neuritis
   - Myositis
   - Tenosynovitis
   - Nephritis
   - Orchitis

III. OCULAR MANIFESTATIONS

1. Lids
   - Madarosis
   - Blepharochalasis
   - Nodules
   - Entropion
   - Ectropion
   - Lagophthalmos
2. Lacrimal system
   - Dacryocystitis
3. Cornea
   - Reduced or absent sensation
   - Thickened corneal nerves
   - Superficial stromal keratitis
   - Corneal opacities
   - Exposure keratopathy
4. Sclera
   - Episcleritis
   - Scleritis
   - Scleral nodules
   - Staphyloma
5. Uveal tract (multibacillary disease)
   - Acute iridocyclitis and sequelae
   - Chronic iridocyclitis
   - Miosis
   - Iris atrophy
   - Iris pearls
   - Corectopia
   - Ocular hypotension
6. Lens
   - Secondary cataract

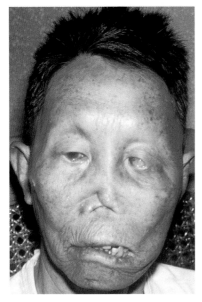

FIGURE 44.1. Facial deformities in a Korean leprosy patient. Madarosis, bilateral lagophthalmos with lateral tarsorrhaphies, total corneal opacity from exposure, nasal destruction.

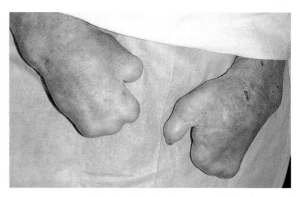

FIGURE 44.2. Hands of patient in Fig. 44.1, which show deformities.

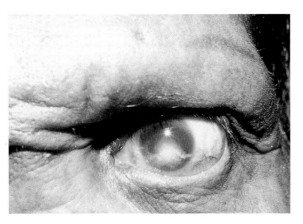

FIGURE 44.3. Corneal scarring with secondary cataract.

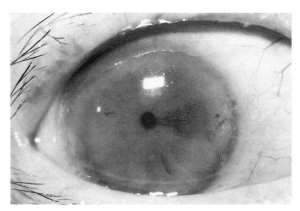

FIGURE 44.4. Chronic iridocyclitis in patient with multibacillary disease showing iris atrophy and miosis. Ciliary body failure had reduced the intraocular pressure to less than 10 mm Hg.

SUGGESTED READINGS

Brand MB. *The Care of the Eye in Hansen's Disease,* 2nd ed. Gillis W, ed. Carville: Long Hansen's Disease Center; 1987. *An excellent manual on the prevention and management of the eye complications of leprosy.*

Brand MB, ffytche TJ. Ocular complications of leprosy. In: Hastings RC, ed. *Leprosy.* New York: Churchill-Livingstone; 1985.

Courtright P, Johnson GJ. *Prevention of Blindness in Leprosy,* revised ed. London: International Centre for Eye Health; 1991.

ffytche TJ. Leprosy or Hansen's disease. In: Gold DH, Weingeist TA, eds. *The Eye in Systemic Disease.* Philadelphia: JB Lippincott; 1990.

Chapter 45

TUBERCULOSIS

Craig J. Helm
Gary N. Holland

I. GENERAL

1. Infection with *Mycobacterium tuberculosis* occurs by inhalation of airborne droplets containing organisms.
2. Bacilli are engulfed by macrophages and spread through lymphatics, eventually entering the bloodstream to seed distant organs.
3. Tuberculosis (the disease state caused by *M. tuberculosis*) develops in approximately 10% of all infected persons.
4. The prevalence of tuberculosis in patients with acquired immunodeficiency syndrome (AIDS) is almost 500 times that in the general population.
5. Intravenous drug users, prison inmates, and the homeless are among groups with a high rate of human immunodeficiency virus (HIV) and *M. tuberculosis* infection.
6. Resistance to development of tuberculosis may be lowered by diseases or conditions that alter immunity, such as diabetes mellitus, malignancy, malnutrition, alcoholism, old age, and immunosuppressive drug therapy.
7. Resistance to development of tuberculosis may also be lower during the first 2 years of life, during puberty and adolescence, and in the postpartum period.

II. SYSTEMIC MANIFESTATIONS

1. Pulmonary
   - Hilar lymphadenopathy
   - Infiltrates (predilection for apical posterior segments of upper lobes)
   - Cavitary lesions
   - Calcification
2. Serosal surfaces
   - Pleurisy with effusion
   - Pericarditis
   - Peritonitis
3. Gastrointestinal
   - Ileitis
4. Central nervous system
   - Meningitis
5. Renal
   - Pyuria
   - Hematuria
6. Endocrine
   - Adrenal tuberculosis
7. Musculoskeletal
   - Skeletal tuberculosis (Pott's disease)
8. Cutaneous
   - Lupus vulgaris
9. Ear/nose/throat
   - Adenitis
10. Nonspecific
   - Fever
   - Chills
   - Night sweats
   - Hemoptysis
   - Malaise
   - Weight loss

III. OCULAR MANIFESTATIONS

1. Conjunctiva
   - Conjunctivitis
     - Chronic
     - Unilateral
     - Ulcer or mass lesion
     - Associated regional lymphadenopathy
   - Phlyctenulosis
2. Sclera
   - Scleritis (unilateral, ulcerative, or nodular)
3. Cornea
   - Interstitial keratitis
   - Ulcerative keratitis
   - Phlyctenules
4. Uvea
   - Iritis (chronic, usually granulomatous)
   - Ciliary body tuberculoma
   - Multifocal choroiditis (usually unilateral)
   - Choroidal tuberculoma (usually unilateral)
   - Panuveitis
5. Retina
   - Retinal vasculitis
   - Retinal tuberculoma (exceptionally rare)
6. Orbit
   - Orbital tuberculoma (unilateral, bony erosion common)
7. Lids
   - Abscess
8. Neuroophthalmologic
   - Papillitis

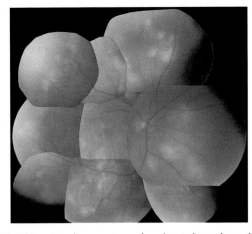

FIGURE 45.1. Fundus montage showing tuberculous chorioretinitis in a 56-year-old patient with normal chest x-ray. Diagnosis was confirmed by chorioretinal endobiopsy. Reprinted from Barondes MJ, Sponsel WE, Stevens TS, Plotnik RD. Tuberculosis choroiditis diagnosed by chorioretinal endobiopsy. *Am J Ophthalmol* 1991;112:460–461, with permission from *The American Journal of Ophthalmology.* Copyright by the Ophthalmic Publishing Company.

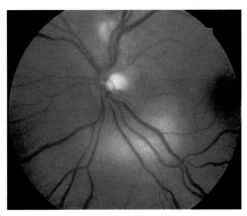

FIGURE 45.2. Choroidal tuberculoma in a 43-year-old HIV-infected male patient with pulmonary tuberculosis. Courtesy of Ronald N. Brown, Jr, MD.

SUGGESTED READINGS

American Thoracic Society. Diagnostic standards and classification of tuberculosis. *Am Rev Respir Dis* 1990;142:725–735.

Barnes PF, Block AB, Davidson PT, Snider DE Jr. Tuberculosis in patients with human immunodeficiency virus infection. *N Engl J Med* 1991;324:1644–1650.

Helm CJ, Holland GN. Ocular tuberculosis. *Surv Ophthalmol* 1993;38:229–256. *A detailed review of the manifestations, diagnosis, and treatment of ocular tuberculosis.*

Section D.   Mycotic Diseases

Chapter 46

HISTOPLASMOSIS

David M. Brown
Ronald E. Smith
Thomas A. Weingeist

I. GENERAL

1. Presumed ocular histoplasmosis syndrome (POHS) common in Mississippi and Ohio river valleys (5–10% of asymptomatic individuals)
2. Exposure to soil and airborne vectors with self-limited nonspecific upper respiratory tract infection
3. Fungemia spreads *Histoplasma capsulatum* organisms throughout the body including the choroid.
4. Presumably, immunologic reaction results in formation of "histo spots"—one-third disc area hypo- and hyperpigmented lesions of the fundus.
5. 5% to 10% of these individuals are at risk for choroidal neovascular membrane formation and subsequent visual loss.
6. Rarely immunocompromised individuals may develop endogenous endophthalmitis or subretinal abscesses at the time of initial infection.

II. SYSTEMIC MANIFESTATIONS

1. Pulmonary
   - Bronchopneumonia
   - Tuberculosis-like granulomatous infection
   - Pulmonary fibrosis
2. Hepatic
   - Calcific foci
   - Rare abscesses
3. Spleen
   - Calcific foci
4. Nonspecific
   - Fever
   - Chills
   - Malaise
   - Upper respiratory infectionlike symptoms

III. OCULAR MANIFESTATIONS

1. Retina (histoplasmosis systemic infection)
   - "Granulomatous disease" of vitreous/choroid
   - Acute endophthalmitis in immunosuppressed persons (acquired immunodeficiency syndrome)
2. Nonspecific (systemic disease)
   - Anterior uveitis (not seen in POHS)
3. Retina (POHS)
   - "Histo spots" (one-third disc area hypo- and hyperpigmented lesions)
   - Peripapillary atrophy
   - Peripheral linear streaks
   - No vitreous inflammation
   - Choroidal neovascular membrane formation

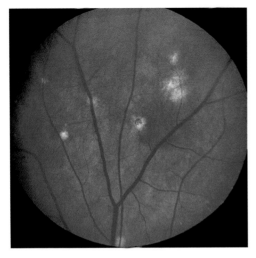

FIGURE 46.1. Peripheral hypopigmented histo spots.

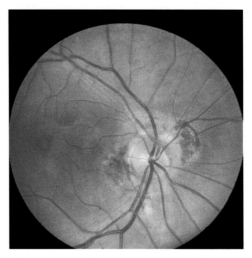

FIGURE 46.2. Peripapillary scarring in ocular histoplamosis syndrome.

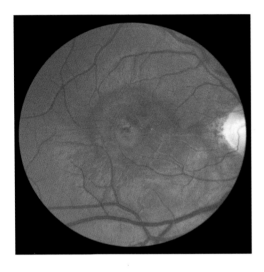

FIGURE 46.3. Choroidal neovascular membrane in the macula of a patient with the ocular histoplasmosis syndrome.

SUGGESTED READINGS

Brown DM, Smith RE, Weingeist TA. Ocular histoplasmosis. In: Prepose JS, Holland GN, Wilhelmus KR, eds. *Ocular Infection and Immunity.* St. Louis: Mosby-Year Book; 1994: *Reference and bibliography of ocular histoplasmosis.*

Macular Photocoagulation Study Group. Persistent and recurrent neovascularization after krypton laser photocoagulation for neovascular lesions of ocular histoplasmosis. *Arch Ophthalmol* 1989;107: 344–352. *Treatment recommendations for POHS-related choroidal neovascular membranes.*

Watzke RC. Mycotic diseases. In: Gold DH, Weingeist TA, eds. *The Eye and Systemic Disease.* Philadelphia: JB Lippincott; 1990:200–205. *Reviews endogenous fungal endophthalmitis and POHS.*

Chapter 47

METASTATIC FUNGAL ENDOPHTHALMITIS

Gholam A. Peyman
Aref Rifai

I. GENERAL

1. Pathogens
   - *Candida albicans* most common
   - *C. tropicalis, C. stelattoidea, C. parapsilosis*
   - *Aspergillus fumigatus*
   - *Blastomyces dermatitidis*
   - *Histoplasma capsulatum*
   - *Cryptococcus neoformans*
   - *Coccidioides immitis*
   - *Sporothrix schenckii*
2. Source of infection with predisposing conditions
   - Exogenous
     - After ophthalmic surgery
     - Penetrating injury
     - Extension of a mycotic corneal ulcer
   - Endogenous
     - Intravenous hyperalimentation
     - Prolonged antibiotics therapy
   - Systemic corticosteroids
   - Immunosuppressive therapy
   - Abdominal surgery
   - Hemodialysis
   - Intravenous drug abuse
   - Acquired immunodeficiency syndrome
   - Malignancy
   - Massive trauma
   - Alcoholism
   - Hepatic insufficiency
   - Postpartum
   - Prematurity
   - Genitourinary manipulation

II. SYSTEMIC MANIFESTATIONS

1. Symptoms
   - Blurred vision
   - Red eyes
   - Pain
   - Floaters
   - Photophobia
   - Cobwebs
   - Veil across the vision
   - May also be asymptomatic
2. Findings
   - Anterior segment
     - Conjunctival injection and ciliary flush
     - Anterior chamber reaction with or without hypopyon
     - Episcleritis
     - Scleritis
     - Pupillary membranes
     - Mycotic corneal infiltrate
   - Posterior segment
     - Creamy, white, well-circumscribed lesion involving the retina and choroid of the posterior pole
     - Intraretinal hemorrhages
     - Roth's spots (white-centered hemorrhages)
     - Vitreous opacities with strands, a "string of pearls" appearance
     - Epiretinal membrane formation, vitreoretinal traction, and retinal detachment occurring late
     - Chorioretinal scarring, with choroidal neovascular membrane rarely

III. OCULAR MANIFESTATIONS

1. Differential diagnosis may include
   - Toxoplasmic retinochoroiditis
   - Viral retinitis
   - Nematode endophthalmitis
   - Phacoanaphylactic reactions
   - Large-cell lymphoma of the eye
   - Uveitis due to sarcoidosis
   - Familial amyloidosis
2. Diagnosis
   - Clinical presentation
   - Cultures: blood, urine, sputum, indwelling catheter
   - Diagnostic vitreous tap
   - Anterior chamber paracentesis
3. Treatment options
   - Intravitreal injection of amphotericin
   - Systemic antifungal medications
     - Amphotericin
     - Ketoconazole
     - 5-Fluorocytosine
   - Vitrectomy

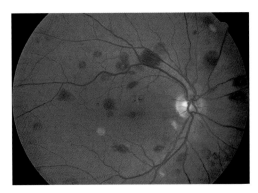

FIGURE 47.1. Multiple Roth's spots seen along the arcades with nerve fiber layer hemorrhages and few cotton-wool spots.

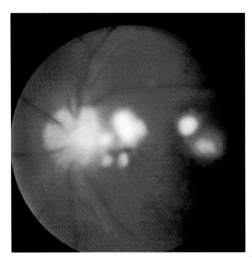

FIGURE 47.2. White opacities in the vitreous with an intraretinal yellowish lesion involving the macula.

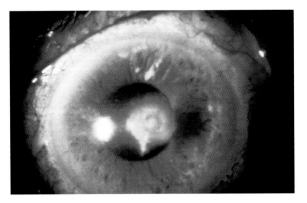

FIGURE 47.3. Mycotic corneal infiltrate.

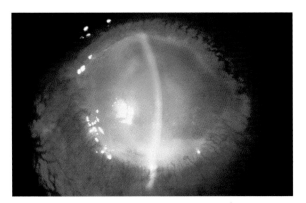

FIGURE 47.4. Acute fungal endophthalmitis with hypopyon.

SUGGESTED READINGS

Brod RD, Clarkson JG, Flynn HW Jr, Green WR. Endogenous fungal endophthalmitis. In: Tasman W, Jaeger EA, eds. *Duane's Clinical Ophthalmology,* vol 3, ch 11. Philadelphia: JB Lippincott; 1993: *A good review of the different mycotic pathogens found in endogenous fungal endophthalmitis.*

Getnick RA, Rodrigues MM. Endogenous fungal endophthalmitis in a drug addict. *Am J Ophthalmol* 1974;77:680–683. *A general review of the etiologies, presentation, and treatment of metastatic fungal endophthalmitis.*

Peyman GA, Schulmann JA. *Intravitreal Surgery: Principles and Practice,* 2nd ed. Norwalk, CT: Appleton & Lange; 1994:851–922. *A general review of endophthalmitis.*

Schulman JA, Peyman GA. Metastatic fungal endophthalmitis. In: Gold DH, Weingeist TA, eds. *The Eye in Systemic Disease.* Philadelphia: JB Lippincott; 1990:203–205.

Chapter 48
MUCORMYCOSIS

Roger Kohn

I. GENERAL

1. Fungal infection of class *Phycomycetes* and order *Mucorales*
2. Ubiquitous fungi occurring in soil, air, skin, and food
3. Inoculation by inhalation into nasopharynx and oropharynx
4. Spreads to paranasal sinuses, subsequently to orbits, meninges, and brain by direct extension
5. Opportunistic infection
6. Predisposed in diabetic ketoacidosis and immunocompromised hosts
7. Exceptionally high morbidity and mortality
8. Early recognition and treatment improve prognosis.

II. SYSTEMIC MANIFESTATIONS

1. Vascular
   - Invades walls of blood vessels, resulting in vascular occlusion, thrombosis, and infarction.
   - Vision loss from ophthalmic artery compromise or involvement of cavernous sinus or internal carotid artery
2. Hematologic
   - Predisposed in leukemia, lymphoma, multiple myeloma, anemia, patients treated with chemotherapeutic agents, folic acid antagonists, ionizing radiation, or corticosteroids
3. Infectious disease
   - Predisposed in septicemia, tuberculosis, fluid–electrolyte imbalance
   - Characteristic large, branching, nonseptate hyphae
4. Gastrointestinal
   - Predisposed in enteritis, hepatitis, cirrhosis
5. Renal
   - Predisposed in glomerulonephritis, acute tubular necrosis, uremia
6. Pulmonary
   - Predisposed in alveolar proteinosis
7. Cardiovascular
   - Predisposed in congenital heart disease
8. Neurologic
   - Suggestive symptoms include multiple cranial nerve palsies
9. Endochrine
   - Predisposed in diabetic ketoacidosis
10. Mucocutaneous
    - Black eschar on palate or within nose

III. OCULAR MANIFESTATIONS

1. Orbital and periorbital
   - Unilateral periorbital pain
   - Orbital inflammation
   - Eyelid edema
   - Acquired blepharoptosis
   - Proptosis
2. Neuroophthalmologic
   - Acute motility changes
   - Internal or external ophthalmoplegia
   - Headache
   - Acute loss of vision
3. Evaluation
   - Computed tomography (CT) of paranasal sinuses, orbit, and anterior cranial areas
   - Prompt biopsy for microscopic examination (frozen sections), histopathologic examination (paraffin sections), and fungal stains and cultures
4. Treatment
   - Early definitive diagnosis
   - Correction of diabetic ketoacidosis or other concomitant metabolic derangement
   - Wide local excision and debridement of all involved and devitalized oral, nasal, sinus, and orbital tissue
   - Establishing adequate sinus and orbital drainage
   - Daily irrigation and packing of involved orbital and paranasal areas with amphotericin B
   - IV amphotericin B
   - Extent of surgical excision should balance the degree of morbidity and mutilation against the life-threatening risk this organism may present.

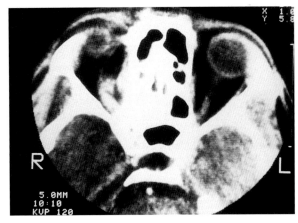

FIGURE 48.1. CT scan of a patient with rhinoorbital mucormycosis demonstrates a right ethmoidal sinusitis and subperiosteal abscess extending into the right medial orbit.

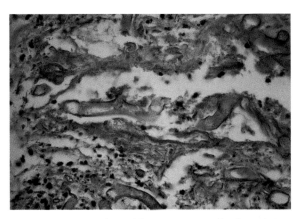

FIGURE 48.2. Large, branching, nonseptate hyphae characteristic of mucormycosis (hematoxylin-eosin; original magnification, ×40).

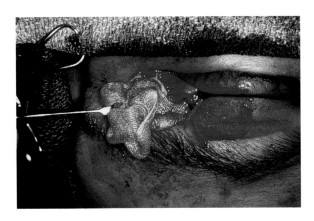

FIGURE 48.3. A patient with rhinoorbital mucormycosis demonstrates amphotericin B packing placed in the ethmoidal sinus and superior medial orbit.

SUGGESTED READINGS

Baum J. Rhino-orbital mucormycosis occurring in an otherwise healthy individual. *Am J Ophthalmol* 1967;63:335–339.

Ferry A, Abedi S. Diagnosis and management of rhinoorbitocerebral mucormycosis (phycomycosis). *Ophthalmology* 1983;90:1096–1104.

Fleckner R, Goldstein J. Mucormycosis. *Br J Ophthalmol* 1969;53:542–548.

Kohn R, Hepler R. Management of limited rhino-orbital mucormycosis without exenteration. *Ophthalmology* 1985;92:1440–1444.

Straatsma B, Zimmerman L, Gass J. Phycomycosis. A clinopathologic study of 51 cases. *Lab Invest* 1962;11:963.

Section E. Protozoan Diseases

Chapter 49

ACANTHAMEOBA INFECTION

Kenneth C. Chern
David M. Meisler

I. GENERAL

1. The free-living ameba, *Acanthamoeba,* is ubiquitous in nature and may be found in the soil, contaminated and stagnant water, tap water, swimming pools, and hot tubs.
2. *Acanthamoeba* exists in two forms: a motile trophozoite and a protected cyst, more resistant to treatment.
3. *Acanthamoeba* is visible histologically with many common stains (Gram, Giemsa, hematoxylin-eosin). The chemofluorescent stain, calcofluor white, binds to the cell wall highlighting the organisms. On transmission electron microscopy, locomotive pseudopodia, distinctive acanthapodia, bull's-eye nucleus, and osmotic vacuoles can be identified.
4. *Acanthamoeba* cultured on nonnutrient agar with a bacterial overlay (*Escherichia coli* or *Klebsiella*) will create tracks along the agar surface as it phagocytoses bacteria. *Acanthamoeba* may also be grown axenically in proteose peptone-yeast extract-glucose (PYG) media.
5. Confocal microscopy may be a helpful adjunct in the diagnosis of *Acanthamoeba. Acanthamoeba* organisms may appear as reflective, ovoid bodies in the epithelium or anterior stroma.
6. Acanthamoebic keratitis is associated with corneal trauma, contact lens wear (especially soft contact lens wear with use of homemade saline or tap water), and exposure to soil or contaminated water (swimming pools, hot tubs).
7. Patients with *Acanthamoeba* keratitis may have severe pain despite a relative paucity of clinical findings.
8. The chronic, indolent keratitis caused by *Acanthamoeba* may mimic corneal infection by herpes simplex virus or fungi.
9. *Acanthamoeba* is variably sensitive to many drugs making medical treatment prolonged and difficult.
10. Surgical treatments include epithelial scraping for superficial infection confined to the epithelium and penetrating keratoplasty for deeper infection unresponsive to antimicrobial agents. Recurrence of *Acanthamoeba* in grafts is particularly problematic.

II. SYSTEMIC MANIFESTATIONS

1. Systemic *Acanthamoebic* infection not usually associated with ocular disease
2. Pulmonary
   - Pneumonitis
3. Neurologic
   - Granulomatous amoebic encephalitis (immunosuppressed individuals)
4. Mucocutaneous
   - Amebic skin lesions
5. Ear/nose/throat
   - Sinusitis

III. OCULAR MANIFESTATIONS

1. Cornea
   - Epithelial cysts
   - Elevated epithelial lines
   - Dendriform keratitis
   - Subepithelial infiltrates
   - Radial keratoneuritis
   - Ring-shaped stromal infiltrate
   - Interstitial keratitis
2. Conjunctiva/sclera
   - Sclerokeratitis
3. Iris
   - Unilateral nongranulomatous uveitis (one case report)

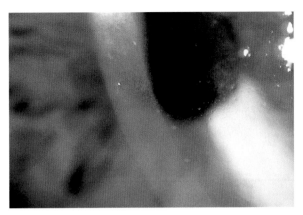

FIGURE 49.1. Among the early signs of *Acanthamoebic* infection are epithelial cysts.

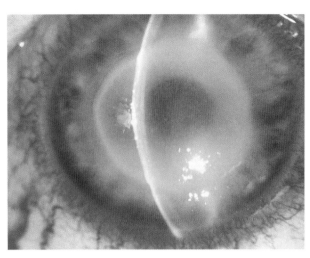

FIGURE 49.2. The characteristic ring-shaped stromal infiltrate.

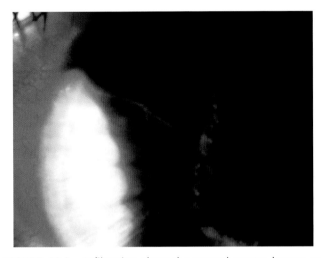

FIGURE 49.3. Infiltration along the corneal nerves, known as radial keratoneuritis.

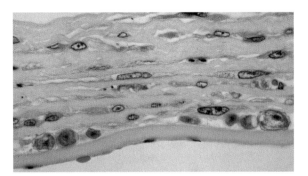

FIGURE 49.4. Histologic section of the cornea demonstrating *Acanthamoeba* organisms abutting Descemet's membrane (hematoxylin-eosin; original magnification, ×200).

SUGGESTED READINGS

Cohen EJ, Parlato CJ, Arentsen JJ, et al. Medical and surgical treatment of *Acanthamoeba* keratitis. *Am J Ophthalmol* 1987;103:615. *Multidrug therapy may be effective in treating* Acanthamoeba *keratitis; however, advanced cases require penetrating keratoplasty.*

Elder MJ, Kilvington S, Dart JKG. A clinicopathologic study of in vitro sensitivity testing and *Acanthamoeba* keratitis. *Invest Ophthalmol Vis Sci* 1994;35:1059. *Polyhexamethylene biguanide and chlorhexidine have the highest in vitro activity against* Acanthamoeba *cysts. In vitro sensitivity testing does not always correlate with clinical response.*

Ficker LA, Kirkness C, Wright P. Prognosis for keratoplasty in *Acanthamoeba* keratitis. *Ophthalmology* 1993;100:105. *Penetrating keratoplasty in cases of active* Acanthamoeba *infection and inflammation has a poor prognosis with a high incidence of graft failure and recurrent disease.*

Moore MB, McCulley JP, Newton C, et al. *Acanthamoeba* keratitis: a growing problem in soft and hard contact lens wearers. *Ophthalmology* 1987;94:1654. *The use of contact lenses and improper lens care are significant risk factors for the development of* Acanthamoeba *keratitis.*

Theodore FH, Jakobiec FA, Juechter KB. The diagnostic value of a ring infiltrate in *Acanthamoeba* keratitis. *Ophthalmology* 1985;92:1471. *Excellent review of the clinical, microbiologic, and pathologic features of* Acanthamoeba *keratitis.*

Chapter 50

LEISHMANIASIS

Merlyn M. Rodrigues
Hyong S. Choe

I. GENERAL

1. Leishmaniasis, an endemic disease in Asia, Africa, Mediterranean, and the Americas, is caused by the protozoan *Leishmania.* It is transmitted to human by the bite of the sandfly vector.
2. The skin is usually the primary portal of entry of the parasites (promastigote), which activate the host's complement system, attracting macrophages and lymphocytes.
3. The organisms can be destroyed by an oxidative burst in macrophages, killing the phagocytized parasites or by lymphocyte-mediated cytotoxicity.
4. Systemic disease occurs if the parasites overcome the host defense mechanisms with involvement of the reticuloendothelial system, bone marrow, liver, and spleen.
5. Diagnosis is by Giemsa, reticulin stain, monoclonal antibody, culture, or polymerase chain reaction.

II. SYSTEMIC MANIFESTATIONS

1. Cutaneous (Oriental sore)
   - Caused by *L. tropica, L. major,* or *L. mexicana*
2. Mucocutaneous
   - Caused by *L. braziliensis*
   - Facial skin
   - Mucous membrane
   - Soft and cartilaginous tissue of the nose and oropharynx
   - Epistaxis
   - Respiratory problems
3. Visceral disease (Kala azar)
   - Caused by *L. donovani*
   - Fever
   - Hepatosplenomegaly
   - Weakness and weight loss
   - Pancytopenia
   - Ascites

III. OCULAR MANIFESTATIONS

1. Lids (most common)
   - Nodules
   - Ulcers
   - Scarring and cicatrization
2. Conjunctiva (limbus)
   - Nodules
3. Keratitis
4. Miscellaneous
   - Uveitis
   - Retinitis
   - Central retinal vein thrombosis
   - Papillitis

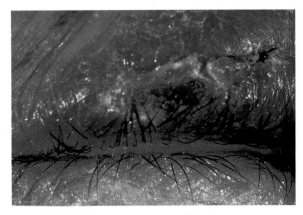

FIGURE 50.1. Upper lid ulcer.

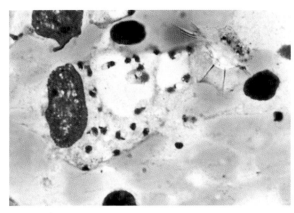

FIGURE 50.2. Impression Giemsa smear of a biopsy shows organisms with a prominent nucleus and dotlike kinetoplast, within a macrophage.

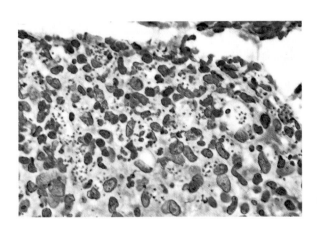

FIGURE 50.3. Lid tissue shows myriad dotlike organisms, some within macrophages (reticulin stain).

SUGGESTED READINGS

Chu FC, Rodrigues MM, Cogan DG, et al. Leishmaniasis affecting the eyelids. *Arch Ophthalmol* 1983;101:84–91.

de Brujin MH, Labrada LA, Smyth AJ, et al. A comparative study of diagnosis by the polymerase chain reaction and by current clinical methods using biopsies from Colombian patients with suspected leishmaniasis. *Trop Med Parasitol* 1993;44:201–207.

Ferry AP. Cutaneous leishmaniasis (oriental sore) of the eyelid. *Am J Ophthalmol* 1977;84:349–354.

Moss JT, Wilson JP. Current treatment recommendations for leishmaniasis. *Ann Pharmacother* 1992;26:1452–1455.

Sodaify M, Aminlari A, Resaer H. Ophthalmic leishmaniasis. *Clin Exp Dermatol* 1981;6:485–488.

Chapter 51

MALARIA

Sornchai Looareesuwan

1. Human malaria is caused by protozoa of the genus *Plasmodium*. Of the four species infecting humans (*P. vivax, P. malariae, P. ovale, P. falciparum*) only, *P. falciparum* produces severe complications and death.
2. Malaria is usually associated initially with nonspecific flulike systemic symptoms.
3. Cytokines resulting from the rupture of infected red blood cells trigger symptoms such as fever, chills, and rigors.
4. Massive destruction of infected and uninfected red blood cells may lead to anemia, jaundice, and hemoglobinuria.
5. Sequestration of parasitized red blood cells in deep vascular spaces of internal organs is the main pathophysiologic phenomenon of severe malaria.
6. Retinal hemorrhage is a poor prognostic sign and occurs in 10% to 15% of patients with cerebral malaria.

II. SYSTEMIC MANIFESTATIONS

1. Cardiac
   - Tachycardia associated with high fever
   - High-output cardiac failure associated with severe anemia (usually young children)
2. Vascular
   - Postural hypotension
3. Pulmonary
   - Acute respiratory distress syndrome carries a high mortality rate of 20% to 50%.
4. Renal
   - Acute renal failure caused by acute tubular necrosis
5. Gastrointestinal
   - Anorexia
   - Nausea
   - Vomiting
   - Diarrhea
   - Jaundice
   - Hepatosplenomegaly
6. Genitourinary
   - Hemoglobinuria (dark urine)
7. Central nervous system
   - Confusion
   - Delirium
   - Coma
   - Convulsions
8. Hematologic
   - Anemia
   - Thrombocytopenia
   - Leukocytosis associated with severe disease
9. Endocrine and metabolic
   - Hypoglycemia
   - Hyponatremia
10. Mucocutaneous
    - Pallor
11. Nonspecific
    - Fever
    - Chills
    - Malaise

III. OCULAR MANIFESTATIONS

1. Conjunctiva/sclera
   - Pallor
   - Jaundice
   - Hemorrhages
2. Retina
   - Hemorrhages (deep and superficial)
   - Roth's spots
   - Cotton-wool spots
   - Macular and extramacular edema
   - Papilledema (rare)
3. Neuroophthalmologic
   - Dysconjugate gaze
   - Nystagmus
   - Cranial nerve palsy (rare)

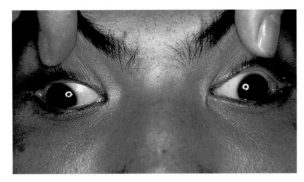

FIGURE 51.1. A comatose cerebral malaria patient with dysconjugate gaze.

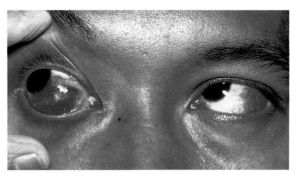

FIGURE 51.2. Bilateral subconjunctival hemorrhages in a patient with uncomplicated falciparum malaria.

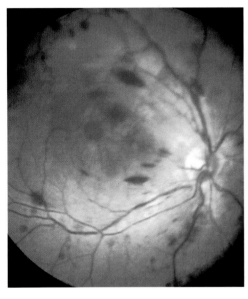

FIGURE 51.3. Multiple retinal hemorrhages in the right eye of a cerebral malaria patient. Courtesy of Prof. N. J. White.

SUGGESTED READINGS

David MW, Vaterlaws AL, Simes J, Torzillo P. Retinopathy in malaria. *P N G Med J* 1982;25:19–22.

Davis TME, Suputtamongkol Y, Spencer JL, et al. Measures of capillary permeability in acute falciparum malaria. Relation to severity of infection and treatment. *Clin Infect Dis* 1992;15:256–266.

Grant WM. Ocular complications of malaria. *Ophthalmol Rev* 1946;35:48–54.

Looareesuwan S, Warrell DA, White NJ, et al. Retinal hemorrhage, a common sign of prognostic significance in cerebral malaria. *Am J Trop Med Hyg* 1983;32:911–915.

Warrell DA, Molyneux ME, Beales PF. Severe and complicated malaria. *Trans R Soc Trop Med Hyg* 1990;84 (suppl):1–65.

Chapter 52

TOXOPLASMOSIS

Maria H. Berrocal
Jose A. Berrocal

I. GENERAL

1. Caused by the intracellular protozoan *Toxoplasma gondii*
2. Worldwide in distribution
3. About 50% of adults in the United States are seropositive for toxoplasmosis.
4. Cysts and trophozoites of toxoplasma are found in humans.
5. Oocysts in the intestines are shed by the cat, spread by many vectors, injested directly or by contaminated meat.
6. Common disease in mammals and birds, but the cat is the definite host.
7. Systemic toxoplasmosis can be acquired or congenital.
8. The congenital form is due to transplacental passage during the primary infection of a pregnant woman.
9. The acquired infection causes lymphadenopathy, is usually asymptomatic, but may be life-threatening in the immunosupressed person.
10. Recrudescence of the disease can occur when dormant cysts rupture, releasing organisms and causing inflammation.
11. The organism has a preference for muscle, neural tissue, and the retina.

II. SYSTEMIC MANIFESTATIONS

1. Central nervous system
   - Cerebral calcifications
   - Seizures
   - Encephalitis
   - Meningoencephalitis
   - Hydrocephalus
   - Microcephaly
   - Psychomotor retardation
   - Cranial nerve palsies
   - Headache
2. Cardiovascular
   - Myocarditis
   - Pericarditis
   - Polymyositis
   - Focal necrosis
3. Pulmonary
   - Pneumonitis
4. Gastrointestinal
   - Hepatosplenomegaly
   - Pancreatic necrosis
   - Abdominal pain
5. Mucocutaneous
   - Maculopapular rash
   - Jaundice
6. Hematologic
   - Lymphadenopathy
7. Other
   - Malaise
   - Fever
   - Fatigue
   - Myalgia
   - Abortion

III. OCULAR MANIFESTATIONS

1. Retina/vitreous
   - Retinochoroiditis
   - Cystoid macular edema
   - Retinal detachment
   - Vasculitis
   - Vein and artery occlusions
   - Neovascularization
   - Vitritis
2. Neuroophthalmologic
   - Papillitis
   - Papilledema
   - Nystagmus
   - Neuroretinitis
   - Visual field defects
   - Strabismus
3. Uvea
   - Granulomatous iridocyclitis
4. Other
   - Microphthalmia
   - Cataracts
   - Glaucoma
   - Photophobia
   - Pain
   - Scleritis

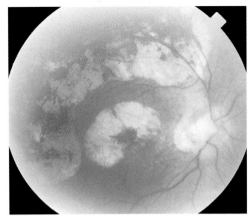

FIGURE 52.1. Multiple chorioretinal scars in a patient with a history of congenital toxoplasmosis.

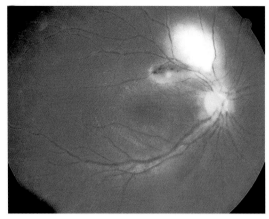

FIGURE 52.2. An area of active retinochoroiditis (white) next to a pigmented toxoplasmosis scar. Vasculitis and vitritis are also present.

SUGGESTED READINGS

Berrocal J. Toxoplasmosis. In: Gold DH, Weingeist TA, eds. *The Eye in Systemic Disease.* Philadelphia: JB Lippincott; 1990:217–219.

Fish RH, Hoskins JC, Kline LB. Toxoplasmosis neuroretinitis. *Ophthalmology* 1993;100:1177–1182.

Morgan CM, Gragoudas ES. Branch retinal artery occlusion associated with recurrent toxoplasmic retinochoroiditis. *Arch Ophthalmol* 1987;105:130–131.

Nussenblatt RB, Palestine AG. *Uveitis—Fundamentals and Clinical Practice.* Chicago: Year Book Medical Publishers; 1989:336–354. *A good review of the ocular disease with sample cases.*

Section F.   Rickettsial Diseases

Chapter 53

RICKETTSIAL INFECTIONS

Joseph B. Michelson

I. GENERAL

1. Usually disease of young or middle-aged patient
2. *Rickettsia rickettsii*
3. Gram-negative coccobacilli
4. Like viruses: obligate intracellular parasite
5. Most active in spring/summer
6. Eastern United States, especially south, but ubiquitous in continental United States
7. Infect endothelial cells of capillaries/venules
8. Mortality rate is 3% to 8%.
9. Focal or proliferative vasculitis

II. SYSTEMIC MANIFESTATIONS

Focal damage
1. Liver thrombosis/infarction
2. Ocular
3. Heart
4. Central nervous system

III. OCULAR MANIFESTATIONS

1. Conjunctivitis
2. Petechiae or conjunctiva
3. Subconjunctival hemorrhage
4. Corneal ulcer
5. Iritis
6. Endophthalmitis
7. Neuroretinitis
8. Optic nerve inflammation
9. Optic nerve pallor
10. Retinal hemorrhage/exudates
11. Panuveitis

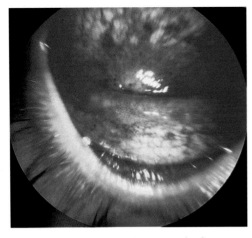

FIGURE 53.1. A 31-year-old white man had severe myalgia, arthralgia, headache, chills, and fever, and a sore, red eye, with conjunctival papillae, chemosis, and petechiae on both the bulbar and palpebral conjunctiva. Note prominent petechiae on the bulbar conjunctiva. Visual acuity was 10/10. The patient's history revealed tick exposure 7 days earlier. Courtesy of David A. Snyder, MD.

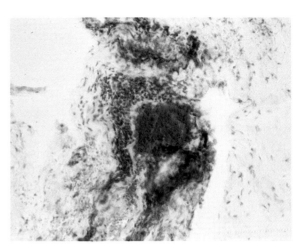

FIGURE 53.2. Histopathology of conjunctival biopsy demonstrates a mononuclear cell infiltration with perivasculitis. (Giemsa stain; original magnification, ×150). Courtesy of David A. Snyder, MD.

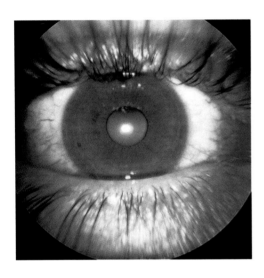

FIGURE 53.3. External photograph of same patient shows conjunctival erythema.

SUGGESTED READINGS

Alio S, Ruiz-Beltra JR, Herrera I. Rickettsial keratitis in a case of Mediterranean spotted fever. *Eur J Ophthalmol* 1992;2:41–43. *This is the first documented case of infectious keratitis ascribed to* Rickettsia conorii *in a patient with systemic dissemination from a region where Mediterranean spotted fever is endemic.*

Duffey RJ, Haming ME. The ocular manifestations of Rocky Mountain spotted fever. *Ann Ophthalmol* 1987;19:301–306.

Kelsey DS. Rocky Mountain spotted fever. *Pediatr Clin North Am* 1979;26:367–376.

Kuhne F, Morlat P, Riss I, et al. Is A29, B12 vasculitis caused by the Q fever agent? *J Fr Ophthalmol* 1992;15:315–321. *A recent report of two cases of retinal vasculitis associated with Q fever.*

Sulenski ME, Green WR. Ocular histopathologic features of a presumed case of Rocky Mountain spotted fever. *Retina* 1986;6:128–130.

Section G. Spirochetal Diseases

Chapter 54

LEPTOSPIROSIS

Susan Barkay
Hanna Garzozi

I. GENERAL

1. Spirochetal epidemic or endemic disease primarily in young men
2. Organisms are harbored by animal hosts, with long-lasting leptospiruria. Human infection is by contact with infected urine or direct contact with infected dead animals.
3. Pathogenic leptospiras belong to *Leptospira interrogans*.
4. Rapid invasion into bloodstream, after 24 hours virtually into all organs, cerebrospinal fluid (CSF), brain, and anterior chamber of the eyes. Virulence seems to depend on toxin production.
5. Biphasic illness, after incubation period of 3 to 26 days
6. First leptospiremic phase, acute febrile illness with circulating leptospiras until the ninth day; homogenous clinical picture; culture of leptospiras from blood or CSF with semisolid medium (Fletcher or Stuart)
7. Short asymptomatic interval (1–3 days) after 10 days leptospiruria, 1 to 11 months.
8. Second, immune phase, appearance of leptospira antibodies in blood, reaching peak in third or fourth week. Individual variation in clinical picture, some patients are almost symptomless, about 50% have high fever and are severely ill. Serologic tests are based on immune reactions.
9. Prognosis is mostly good. In patients with jaundice, Weil's syndrome, if untreated have a 25% to 40% mortality rate.
10. Late uveitis cases, even years after general illness subsided, no clear pathogenesis.
11. Ecchymoses and petechiae in striated muscles, kidneys, adrenals, liver, lungs, spleen, stomach, skeletal muscles, changes from vacuoles to necrosis

II. SYSTEMIC MANIFESTATIONS: FIRST, LEPTOSPIREMIC PHASE

1. Nonspecific
   - High fever
   - Chills
   - Malaise
   - Severe headaches
   - Sensory disturbances
2. Respiratory
   - Pharyngeal injection
   - Coughing
3. Gastrointestinal
   - Nausea
   - Vomiting
   - Diarrhea
4. Musculoskeletal
   - Myalgias
5. Mucocutaneous
   - Skin rash
   - Hemorrhage

II. SYSTEMIC MANIFESTATIONS: SECOND, IMMUNE PHASE

1. Persistent, high fever
2. Central nervous system
   - Meningismus
   - High protein in CSF
   - Pleocytosis
   - Encephalitis
   - Guillain-Barré
   - Cranial nerve involvement
   - Peripheral nerve lesions
3. Renal
   - Hematuria
   - Pyuria
   - Uremia
   - Acute tubular necrosis
4. Gastrointestinal
   - Hepatomegaly
   - Jaundice
5. Hemorrhagic
   - Hemoptysis
   - Epistaxis
   - Gastrointestinal bleeding
   - Subarachnoidal hemorrhage

III. OCULAR MANIFESTATIONS

1. Lids
   - Palpebral herpes
2. Conjunctiva
   - Engorged vessels
   - Leptospiras in conjunctival discharge
3. Uvea
   - Iridocyclitis in immune phase
   - Late uveitis (after long interval, even years)
     - Mild to severe exudative inflammation
     - Mutton fat precipitates
     - Hypopyon
   - Pupillary occlusion
   - Secondary glaucoma
   - Choroiditis
4. Vitreous
   - Membranes
5. Retina
   - Exudates
   - Hemorrhages
6. Neuroophthalmologic
   - Optic neuritis
   - Cranial nerve palsies

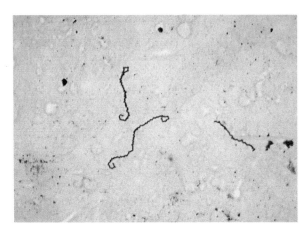

FIGURE 54.1. Smear from culture of leptospira using silver impregnation stain.

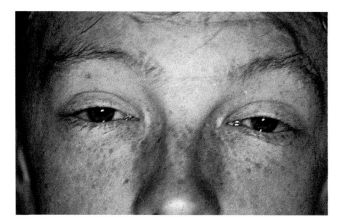

FIGURE 54.2. Suffusion of conjunctiva in leptospirosis.

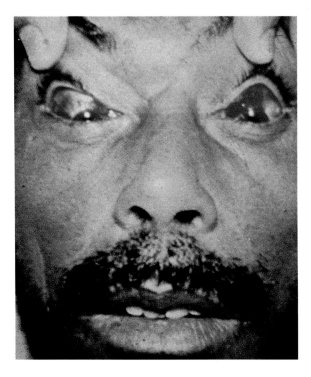

FIGURE 54.3. Face of patient with Weil's syndrome.

SUGGESTED READINGS

Barkay S, Garzozi H. Leptospirosis and uveitis. *Ann Ophthalmol* 1984;16:164–168.

Duke-Elder S. *System of Ophthalmology,* vol 9. *Diseases of the Uveal Tract.* London: Henry Kimpton; 1966:322–325.

Fraunfelder FT, Hampton Roy F. *Current Ocular Therapy,* 14th ed. Philadelphia: WB Saunders; 1995:30–32.

Javetz E, Melnik JL, Adelberg EA. *Review of Medical Microbiology,* 14th ed. Los Altos CA: Lange Medical Publications; 1980:259–260.

Chapter 55

SYPHILIS

William J. Wirostko
Jose S. Pulido

I. GENERAL

1. Syphilis is a sexually transmitted disease caused by the spirochete *Treponema pallidum*.
2. Since the early 1980s, the incidence of acquired and congenital syphilis has been rapidly increasing, especially among illicit drug users, teenagers, and individuals with human immunodeficiency virus (HIV). The concurrent HIV epidemic makes this statistic especially concerning.
3. *T. pallidum* inoculation occurs through physical contact with an infectious chancre. The presence of a chancre also increases the risk of HIV acquisition and HIV transmission during sexual contact. Congenital syphilis is produced by the transplacental passage of the spirochete from the mother to the fetus.
4. Primary syphilis is characterized by the development of a chancre at the inoculation site. From this lesion, *T. pallidum* disseminates throughout the body to produce the dermatologic, ocular, and constitutional manifestations of secondary (disseminated) syphilis. Although neurologic symptoms are uncommon in secondary syphilis, individuals with HIV can develop an early and aggressive form of neurosyphilis during this time.
5. Eventually, the symptoms of secondary syphilis abate and the latent stage is entered. This occurs despite the continued presence of *T. pallidum* throughout the body. Rarely, patients may reactivate back to the secondary stage from latency.
6. After a variable latency period, tertiary syphilis develops in about one third of untreated individuals. Manifestations include neurosyphilis, aortitis, and gummata. Uveitis, retinitis, and optic neuritis are also possible. Histologically, an obliterative endarteritis is seen.
7. The diagnosis of syphilis is based on clinical findings and serologic testing. Patients who test positive for syphilis should be tested for other sexually transmitted diseases and patients infected with other sexually transmitted diseases should be tested for syphilis. Reagin-based tests may be nonreactive during early disease, latency, and in HIV-infected individuals.
8. Although penicillin remains the preferred antibiotic therapy for syphilis, benzathine penicillin should not be used for the treatment of tertiary syphilis and luetic uveitis. Benzathine penicillin does not obtain an adequate concentration in the eye or in the central nervous system to completely eradicate *T. pallidum*. Individuals with concomitant HIV disease respond slower and require longer therapeutic courses of penicillin with doses similar to those used for neurosyphilis.

II. SYSTEMIC MANIFESTATIONS*

1. Dermatologic
   - Chancre
   - Maculopapular rash involving the palms of the hands and the soles of the feet
   - Alopecia
   - Mucous patches
   - Condyloma lata
   - Gummata
   - Desquamative skin rash (C)
   - Jaundice (C)
2. Neurological
   - Meningitis
   - Altered mental status
   - Cranial neuropathies
   - Cerebrovascular accidents
   - Radiculopathies
   - Tabes
   - Paresis
   - Gummata
3. Cardiovascular
   - Ascending aortic aneurysm
   - Aortic insufficiency
   - Left ventricular hypertrophy
   - Congestive heart failure
   - Angina
4. Musculoskeletal
   - Gummata
   - Periostitis (C)
   - Clutton's joints (C)
   - Sabre shins (C)
5. Gastrointestinal
   - Hepatosplenomegaly (C)
   - Abdominal distention (C)
   - Gummata
6. Ear/nose/mouth
   - Deafness (C)
   - Hutchinson's teeth (C)
   - Snuffles (C)
   - Saddle-nose deformity (C)
   - Frontal bossing (C)
   - Mulberry molars (C)
   - Rhagades (C)
   - Gummata
7. Nonspecific
   - Headache
   - Fever
   - Malaise
   - Lymphadenopathy

* (C) indicates manifestations appearing primarily in congenital syphilis.

1. Conjunctiva
   - Chancre
   - Mucous patches
2. Sclera
   - Scleritis (anterior, posterior, diffuse, or nodular)
   - Episcleritis
3. Cornea
   - Interstitial keratitis
4. Iris
   - Iritis
   - Iris roseata
   - Papulata/nodules
5. Retinal vessels
   - Perivasculitis
   - Vascular occlusions
   - Neovascularization

6. Retina and choroid
   - Chorioretinitis (diffuse or placoid)
   - Neuroretinitis
   - Retinitis
   - Vitritis
   - Cystoid macular edema
   - Exudative retinal detachment
   - Salt-and-pepper retinopathy
   - Hypo- and hyperpigmentation of the retinal pigment epithelium
7. Neuroophthalmologic
   - Optic neuritis
   - Optic atrophy
   - Papillitis
   - Cranial mononeuropathies
   - Argyll-Robertson pupils

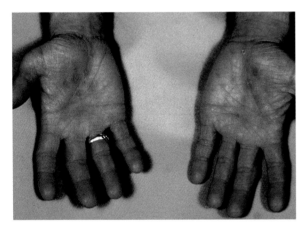

FIGURE 55.1. Typical maculopapular skin rash of secondary syphilis.

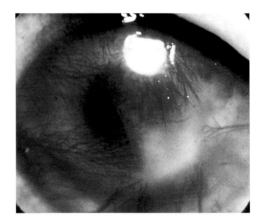

FIGURE 55.2. Active interstitial keratitis. Courtesy of Robert A. Hyndiuk, MD.

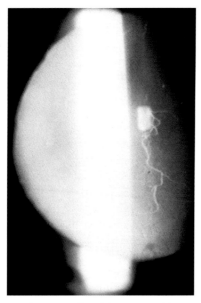

FIGURE 55.3. Ghost vessels. Old interstitial keratitis. Courtesy of Robert A. Hyndiuk, MD.

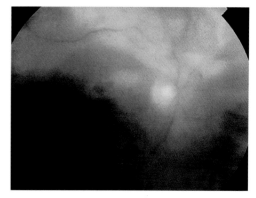

FIGURE 55.4. Active retinitis in a patient whose rapid plasma reagin titer was 1:4096 and fluorescent treponemal antibody absorption was positive. Courtesy of James F. Vander, MD.

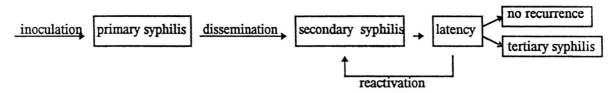

FIGURE 55.5. Clinical course of untreated syphilis.

SUGGESTED READINGS

Evans HE, Frenkel LD. Congenital syphilis. *Clin Perinatol* 1994;21:149–162.

Hook EW, Marra CM. Acquired syphilis in adults. *N Engl J Med* 1992;326:1060–1069.

Musher DM: Syphilis. In: Gorbach SL, Bartlett JG, Blacklow NR, eds. *Infectious Diseases*. Philadelphia: WB Saunders; 1992:822–828. *A general review of syphilis.*

Musher DM, Hamill RJ, Baughn RE. Effects of human immunodeficiency virus (HIV) infection on the course of syphilis and on the response to treatment. *Ann Intern Med* 1990;113:872–881.

Pulido JS, Corbett JJ, McLeish WM. Syphilis. In: Gold DH, Weingeist TA, eds. *The Eye in Systemic Disease*. Philadelphia: JB Lippincott; 1990:233–239. *A review of the ocular manifestations of syphilis.*

Section H. Viral Diseases

Chapter 56

ACQUIRED IMMUNODEFICIENCY SYNDROME

Baruch D. Kuppermann
Gary N. Holland

I. GENERAL

1. Acquired immunodeficiency syndrome (AIDS) is a late manifestation of infection with human immunodeficiency virus (HIV), type 1, an RNA retrovirus. Also caused by HIV, type 2 in Africa.
2. HIV transmission
   - Sexual
     - Anal intercourse (major mode of transmission among homosexual/bisexual men)
     - Vaginal intercourse (major mode of transmission worldwide)
   - Intravenous drug use
   - Receipt of contaminated blood or blood products (now uncommon in Western countries due to screening)
   - Transplacental infection of fetus (30–50% of HIV-infected mothers; reduced by maternal antiviral drug use)
3. No known racial or other predispositions; certain genes (*CKR-5*) may be protective against HIV infection.
4. Pathogenesis
   - Immediately after infection, virus actively replicates, producing 10 billion virions per day, even if no symptoms.
   - The immune system initially is capable of clearing most newly produced virions.
   - Over prolonged periods, immune system fails and virus burden increases.
   - Infection is initially localized to lymph nodes; over time spreads hematogenously.
   - Decrease in the number of CD4+ T lymphocytes
   - Development of "opportunistic" infections
     - Exogenous pathogens that would normally be cleared by an intact immune system
     - Reactivation of latent infections
   - Development of clinical disease frequently delayed 10 years or more; progression from diagnosis of AIDS to death typically less than 5 years. Intervals may increase because of antiretroviral therapy.
5. Diagnosis of AIDS
   - Centers for Disease Control and Prevention (CDC) system for classification of HIV infection and AIDS
     - Uses both clinical conditions as "AIDS-indicator diseases" (see Systemic Manifestations) and absolute CD4+ T-lymphocyte count (≤200 cells/μL in peripheral blood; the best marker of deterioration of immune function) as definition of AIDS.
6. Treatment
   - Use of various antiviral agents in combination reduces HIV load and inhibits or delays progression of disease.

II. SYSTEMIC MANIFESTATIONS

1. HIV seroconversion illness
   - Flulike syndrome
   - 40% to 60% of individuals
   - Occurs within 1 to 3 weeks of infection
   - Symptoms last 1 to 3 weeks in most cases
   - Possible disorders associated with early HIV disease
     - General
       - Headache
       - Retrobulbar pain
       - Myalgias
       - Sore throat
       - Fever
       - Lymphadenopathy
       - Lethargy
       - Malaise
     - Cutaneous
       - Nonpruritic macular erythematous rash
     - Mucosal
       - Oral candidiasis with or without anal or esophageal ulcerations
     - Central nervous system
       - Meningitis
       - Encephalitis
     - Pulmonary
       - Pneumonitis
     - Gastrointestinal
       - Distress symptoms
       - Diarrhea
2. Chronic disorders
   - Lymphadenopathy, lethargy, malaise
   - Persistant for months
3. Following resolution of early HIV-related disorders, individuals are usually clinically asymptomatic for months to years
4. AIDS
   - Classification system for HIV infection and expanded AIDS surveillance case definition for adolescents and adults (1993).

CLINICAL CATEGORIES

CD4+ T-lymphocyte Categories[a]	(A) Asymptomatic, Acute (Primary) HIV or PGL[b]	(B) Symptomatic, Not (A) or (C) Conditions	(C) AIDS-Indicator Conditions
(1) ≥500/μL	A1	B1	C1[c]
(2) 200–499/μL	A2	B2	C2[c]
(3) <200/μL	A3[c]	B3[c]	C3[c]

[a] The lowest, but not necessarily the most recent, CD4+ T-lymphocyte count should be used for classification purposes.
[b] PGL, persistent generalized lymphadenopathy.
[c] Categories A3, B3, C1–3 constitute a diagnosis of AIDS.

5. Description of categories
- Category A: one or more of the conditions listed below in an individual at least 13 years of age with documented HIV infection, in the absence of conditions listed in categories B and C.
  - Asymptomatic HIV infection
  - Persistent generalized lymphadenopathy
  - Acute (primary) HIV infection with accompanying illness or history of acute HIV infection
- Category B: symptomatic conditions in an HIV-infected individual at least 13 years of age that are not included in the conditions listed in category C and that meet at least one of the following criteria: (a) the conditions are attributed to HIV infection or are indicative of a defect in cell-mediated immunity; or (b) the conditions are considered by physicians to have a clinical course or to require management that is complicated by HIV infection. Examples include (list is not exhaustive)
  - Bacillary angiomatosis
  - Candidiasis, oropharyngeal (thrush)
  - Candidiasis, vulvovaginal; persistent, frequent, or poorly responsive to therapy
  - Cervical dysplasia (moderate or severe)/cervical carcinoma in situ
  - Constitutional symptoms such as fever or diarrhea last more than 1 month
  - Hairy leukoplakia, oral
  - Herpes zoster (shingles) involving at least two distinct episodes or more than one dermatome
  - Idiopathic thrombocytopenic purpura
  - Listeriosis
  - Pelvic inflammatory disease, particularly if complicated by tuboovarian abscess
  - Peripheral neuropathy

- Category C: AIDS-defining illnesses, when occurring in association with HIV infection. Once a category C condition has occurred, the person will remain in category C.
  - Candidiasis of bronchi, trachea, or lungs
  - Candidiasis, esophageal
  - Cervical cancer, invasive
  - Coccidioidomycosis, disseminated or extrapulmonary
  - Cryptococcosis, extrapulmonary
  - Cryptosporidiosis, chronic intestinal (>1 month)
  - Cytomegalovirus (CMV) disease (other than liver, spleen, or nodes)
  - CMV retinitis
  - Encephalopathy, HIV-related
  - Herpes simplex virus: chronic ulcer(s) (>1 month duration); or bronchitis, pneumonitis, or esophagitis
  - Histoplasmosis, disseminated or extrapulmonary
  - Isosporiasis (>1 month duration)
  - Kaposi's sarcoma
  - Lymphoma, Burkitt's (or equivalent term)
  - Lymphoma, immunoblastic (or equivalent term)
  - Lymphoma, primary, of brain
  - *Mycobacterium avium* complex or *Mycobacterium kansasii,* disseminated or extrapulmonary
  - *Mycobacterium tuberculosis,* any site (pulmonary or extrapulmonary)
  - *Mycobacterium,* other species or unidentified species, disseminated or extrapulmonary
  - *Pneumocystis carinii* pneumonia
  - Pneumonia, recurrent
  - Progressive multifocal leukoencephalopathy
  - *Salmonella* septicemia, recurrent
  - Wasting syndrome due to HIV

1. A variety of ophthalmic disorders are associated with HIV infection and AIDS. The majority of HIV-infected individuals will develop one or more ophthalmic disorders during the course of their HIV disease.

2. Ophthalmic disorders associated with HIV infection and AIDS fall into four major categories.

- HIV-related vasculopathy
  - Most common intraocular disorder associated with AIDS
  - Not caused by direct HIV infection
  - Microvasculopathy characterized by swollen endothelial cells, loss of pericytes, thickened basal laminae, and narrowed capillary lumens.
  - Clinical findings include conjunctival vascular sludging, cotton-wool spots (Fig. 56.1), intraretinal hemorrhages, and retinal microaneurysms.
- Opportunistic infections
  - CMV retinitis (Fig. 56.2)
    - Affects up to 30% to 40% of people with AIDS
    - Usually occurs with absolute CD4+ counts T lymphocyte less 50/μL
    - Accounts for over 90% of all AIDS-related ocular infections
    - Full-thickness retinal necrosis
    - Lesions characterized clinically by granular, yellow-white opacification with irregular granular borders
    - Associated hemorrhage may or may not be present
  - Varicella-zoster virus retinitis
    - Progressive outer retinal necrosis syndrome variant (Fig. 56.3)
      - Outer retinal infection, which leads to full thickness necrosis
      - Lesions are multifocal, involving the periphery and posterior pole.
      - Minimal or no vitreous inflammatory reaction
      - Progression is hyperfulminant with most cases leading to blindness.
    - Can also present as acute retinal necrosis syndrome
  - Toxoplasmic retinochoroiditis (Fig. 56.4)
    - More common in countries with high rates of *Toxoplasma gondii* infection
    - Dense retinal opacity
    - Scant hemorrhage
    - May have minimal overlying vitreous inflammatory reaction
    - Responds well to therapy
    - Without treatment, lesions continue to enlarge.
  - Other opportunistic infections
    - *P. carinii* choroiditis
    - Cryptococcal chorioretinitis and papillitis
    - Syphilitic chorioretinitis and papillitis
    - Histoplasmic chorioretinitis
    - *Aspergillus* species chorioretinitis
    - Herpes zoster ophthalmicus
    - Herpes simplex virus retinitis (rare) and keratitis
- Neoplasms
  - Kaposi's sarcoma (Fig. 56.5)
    - Involves eyelid, conjunctiva (palpebral or bulbar), caruncle, or orbit (rare)
    - Does not involve intraocular tissues
    - Spreads slowly
  - Lymphoma
    - B-lymphocyte origin
    - Occurs with central nervous system (CNS) disease, visceral disease, or as isolated ocular disorder
    - With CNS disease, more likely to involve the retina
    - With visceral disease, more likely to involve uveal tissues
    - Appearance frequently confused with other diseases; may require chorioretinal biopsy
- Neuroophthalmic manifestations
  - Manifestations of orbital or intracranial neoplasms (lymphoma) or infections
    - Papilledema
    - Visual field defects
    - Optic atrophy
    - Cranial nerve palsies
    - Eye movement disorders
    - Cortical blindness
  - Cryptococcal meningitis
    - The most common cause of papilledema
    - Ophthalmic disorders seen in greater than 50% of cases
  - Other infectious causes of intracranial disease
    - Toxoplasmosis
    - Varicella-zoster virus encephalitis/cerebritis
    - CMV encephalitis
    - Progressive multifocal leukoencephalopathy

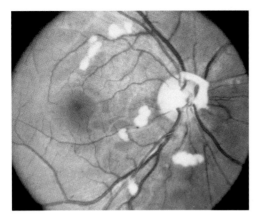

FIGURE 56.1. Cotton-wool spots, which are lesions related to HIV-associated, noninfectious retinal microvasculopathy, commonly known as "HIV retinopathy." Other manifestations can include intraretinal hemorrhages, microaneurysms, and Roth's spots.

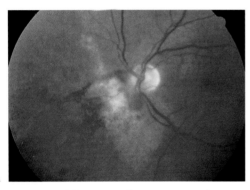

A

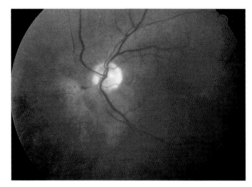

B

FIGURE 56.2. **(A)** Untreated CMV retinitis, demonstrating the irregular granular borders characteristic of this infection. **(B)** The same lesion 4 weeks after initiating therapy; retinal opacification has decreased and there has been no enlargment of the area of infection.

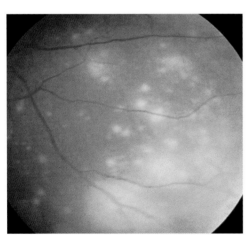

FIGURE 56.3. The progressive outer retinal necrosis syndrome variant of varicella-zoster virus retinitis in a person with advanced AIDS. Lesions are multifocal, associated with little or no vitreous inflammatory reaction, and spread rapidly to confluence. Occlusive vasculopathy is not a primary feature of the syndrome.

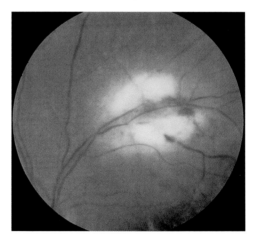

FIGURE 56.4. Toxoplasmic retinochoroiditis demonstrating the dense opacity and scant hemorrhage that is characteristic of this infection in patients with AIDS. Often, there is much less vitreous inflammatory reaction than would be seen in immunocompetent hosts.

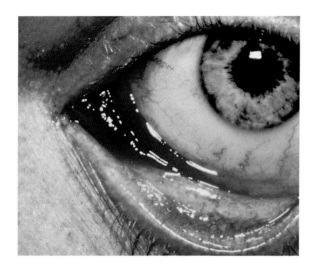

FIGURE 56.5. Kaposi's sarcoma lesion of the conjunctiva. This neoplasm can occur on the conjunctiva (most commonly in the inferior fornices, but can also develop initially on the bulbar or palpebral surface), eyelid, caruncle, or (less commonly) the orbit. It does not invade the globe.

SUGGESTED READINGS

Kuppermann BD. Non cytomegalovirus-related chorio-retinal manifestations of the acquired immuno-deficiency syndrome. *Semin Ophthalmol* 1995;10:125–141.

Levy JA. *HIV and the Pathogenesis of AIDS.* Washington DC: ASM Press; 1994.

Pepose JS, Holland GN, Nestor MS, et al. Acquired immunodeficiency syndrome: Pathogenic mechanisms of ocular disease. *Ophthalmology* 1985;92:472–484. *This paper describes the histopathologic characteristics of the most common ocular manifestations of AIDS with clinicopathologic correlations.*

Pepose JS, Holland GN, Wilhelmus KR, eds. *Ocular Infection & Immunity.* St. Louis: CV Mosby; 1996. *Many of the chapters in this textbook deal with ophthalmic infections that can occur in patients with AIDS; in addition, there is an overview of HIV disease and its relationship to the eye.*

1993 revised classification system for HIV infection and expanded surveillance case definition for AIDS among adolescents and adults. *MMWR* 1992;41 (RR-17):1–19.

Chapter 57

CYTOMEGALOVIRUS INFECTION

Peter L. Sonkin

1. Cytomegalovirus (CMV) is a DNA virus in the herpes family, capable of producing severe disease in the developing fetus, newborn, and immunocompromised patient.
2. In healthy children and adults, CMV infection is more often asymptomatic or produces only mild mononucleosis-like symptoms (fever, lymphadenopathy, and hepatitis).
3. Up to 80% of adults have serologic evidence of prior exposure.
4. Approximately 1% to 2% of newborns in the United States are seropositive at birth.
5. Modes of infection
   - Infection in infants and children usually occurs transplacentally, during birth, from breast milk, and from other infected infants and children (*eg*, in day care programs). Prolonged asymptomatic viral shedding in young children serves as a reservoir and likely plays a role in transmission of disease in this age group.
   - Primary infection is often a result of respiratory droplet spread. Viral shedding occurs for up to 2 to 3 years in the urine and other body secretions after primary infection.
   - Infection may also result from reactivation of latent virus. Mononuclear leukocytes are the likely reservoir for latent infection.
   - CMV can also be acquired via transplacental spread, blood transfusions, and organ transplantation.
   - Sexual contact may also be a means of spread, likely resulting from viral shedding from the cervix or semen.
   - Congenital infection in newborns can occur in seronegative women infected during pregnancy.
   - Incidence of infection is greater in lower socioeconomic groups.
6. Systemic illness can occur with both exogenous and latent reactivation mechanisms, with the former usually more serious. It occurs secondary to hematogenous viral spread.
7. CMV isolated from retinal tissue reveals necrosis of the involved retina with normal adjacent tissue. Inflammation in the form of a mild mononuclear infiltration is often seen in the choroid and overlying vitreous. Histopathology reveals large intracytoplasmic and intranuclear inclusions. The classic owl's-eye cell has a large basophilic nuclear inclusion adjacent to a clear rim of nucleoplasm.
8. Timing of maternal infection likely is important in the pathogenesis of CMV-induced central nervous system lesions.
9. Primary infection does not provide immunity, and maternal antibodies do not protect the fetus from intrauterine infection.
10. Risk of fetal infection is estimated to be 30% to 40% with primary maternal infection during pregnancy.

1. Clinical manifestations can range from no symptoms to fatal pneumonia.
2. Severity varies with patient age and immune status.
3. Tissues most commonly infected include lung, liver, spleen, intestine, adrenal gland, kidney, eye, and the central nervous system.
4. Approximately 7% to 10% of infected newborns have evidence of clinical cytomegalic disease and are symptomatic.
5. Nonocular manifestations of congenital CMV infection
   - Spontaneous abortion
   - Stillbirth
   - Intrauterine growth retardation
   - Premature birth
   - Periventricular calcifications on skull x-ray
   - Psychomotor retardation
   - Neuromuscular problems
   - Seizures
   - Microcephaly
   - Hydrocephalus
   - Hepatomegaly and jaundice
   - Splenomegaly, thrombocytopenia, purpura, and petechial rash
   - Hearing loss (sensorineural)
   - Dental abnormalities
   - Pneumonitis (particularly with infection acquired during birth)
   - Mild mental retardation
6. Of these symptomatic infants, approximately 80% to 90% will eventually have problems with hearing, motor function, cognitive function, or vision. In one study by Bale and colleagues, neonates with microcephaly, seizures, and abnormal imaging studies of the central nervous system (eg, periventricular calcifications) were at higher risk for severe developmental sequelae. Other complications of congenital CMV (birth weight, jaundice, hepatosplenomegaly, petechiae, or chorioretinitis) were not associated with developmental problems in this study.
7. The asymptomatic infants have a better prognosis, but 15% will still have sequelae, usually involving a hearing deficit.
8. Clinical disease in older children includes mild mental retardation, seizures, sensorineural hearing loss, and psychomotor retardation.
9. Primary infection in immunocompetent patients is usually asymptomatic or with a mononucleosislike syndrome. Laboratory findings include a lymphocytosis with atypical lymphocytes and a mild elevation in liver transaminase levels.
10. Immunosuppressed patients are prone to develop serious illness.
    - Fever, myalgias, anemia, pneumonia, hepatitis, gastritis, enterocolitis, and chorioretinitis
    - There is a high rate of CMV viremia and viruria in heart, kidney, and bone marrow transplant patients.
    - In transplant patients, infection of the transplanted organ can cause graft rejection.
    - Disseminated disease can result in death.
    - Patients with acquired immunodeficiency syndrome (AIDS) have a high incidence of CMV infection and often develop symptomatic disease.
    - Pneumonia is common in bone marrow trans-plant patients, and retinitis predominates in AIDS patients.
11. CMV in the immunocompromised patient can represent primary infection, reactivation, or superinfection.

1. Ocular manifestations (and associations) of congenital CMV infection
   - Chorioretinitis
     - Approximate 15% incidence
     - Characterized by chorioretinal scarring and inflammation; can be diffuse or localized
   - Pigmentary retinopathy
   - Optic atrophy
   - Optic neuritis
   - Strabismus
   - Nystagmus
   - Miscellaneous: retinal detachment, optic nerve hypoplasia, coloboma, microphthalmia, glaucoma, cataracts, iritis
   - Evaluation: ocular examination within the first few months of life is recommended for infants diagnosed with congenital CMV infection, with annual follow-ups.
   - Treatment: usually no therapy indicated for ocular sequelae (most retinal lesions are inactive at time of diagnosis); when active chorioretinitis is detected, intravenous ganciclovir can be considered; referral to audiologist is also recommended.
2. Ocular sequelae are more common among children who were
   - Symptomatic at birth in comparison to those that had mild or no symptoms
   - Born after a primary maternal infection in comparison to those born after recurrent maternal infection
3. Retinal disease is much less severe in congenital CMV infection (including those with progressive retinal changes) in comparison to CMV infection in the immunosuppressed patient.
4. Chorioretinitis
   - Symptoms
     - Can present with asymptomatic disease of the retinal periphery
     - More commonly present with complaints of blurred vision, floaters, and visual field loss
   - Examination
     - In infants and asymptomatic children and adults, often find old atrophic pigmentary changes diffusely involving the retina and choroid
     - Active disease
       - Necrotizing retinitis with associated retinal hemorrhages and vasculitis
       - Often multifocal in origin and bilateral

- Initially presents as white infiltration often with hemorrhages; ultimately becomes granular and necrotic with variable retinal pigment epithelium stippling and atrophy
- Vascular attenuation and optic atrophy can develop.
  - In immunocompromised patients, margins and borders of inactive areas often remain smoldering with active necrotizing retinitis.
- Diagnosis is based predominantly on the examination findings in consideration of the clinical setting.
- Approximately 2% to 5% of heart and kidney transplant patients develop CMV retinitis (less common in patients with bone marrow transplants).
- Patients with AIDS have a high incidence of CMV infection, with CMV retinitis being the most common opportunistic ocular infection.
- Differential diagnosis
  - Immunocompetent patients
    - Branch retinal vein occlusion
    - Diabetic retinopathy
    - Anemic retinopathy
    - Acute retinal necrosis
  - Immunocompromised patients
    - HIV retinopathy
    - Ocular toxoplasmosis
    - Cryptococcal retinitis
    - Candida chorioretinitis
    - Endogenous bacterial infections
    - Ocular herpes virus infections
    - Acute retinal necrosis
- Treatment
  - For active disease, IV ganciclovir is often initial therapy. It is selectively phosphorylated in CMV-infected cells by cellular enzymes. The triphosphate form of the drug acts by competitively inhibiting viral DNA polymerase and preventing viral replication. Ganciclovir is virostatic and requires long-term maintenance dosing, often complicated by myelosuppression. Foscarnet and cidofovir are often second choices. Route of therapy is predominantly IV with intravitreal injections and intraocular implants as alternatives (particularly in adult immunocompromised patients).
5. Ocular manifestations (and associations) of CMV infection in the immunosuppressed patient (see Chapter 56).

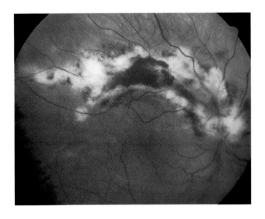

FIGURE 57.1. Cytomegalovirus retinopathy with granular patches of retinal whitening with associated hemorrhage. Note optic disc swelling.

SUGGESTED READINGS

Anderson KS, Amos CA, Boppana S, et al. Ocular abnormalities in congenital cytomegalovirus infection. *J Am Optom Assoc* 1996;67:273–278.

Bale JR Jr, Blackman JA, Sato Y. Outcome in children with symptomatic congenital cytomegalovirus infection. *J Child Neurol* 1990;5:131–136.

Cantril HL. Cytomegalovirus infection. In: Gold DH, Weingeist TA, eds. *The Eye in Systemic Disease.* Philadelphia: JB Lippincott; 1990:243–246.

Johnson RP, Baker AS. Cytomegalovirus (CMV). In: Albert DM, Jakobiec FA, eds. *Principles and Practices of Opthamology.* Philadelphia: WB Saunders; 1994, vol. 5:3024.

Kieval SJ. Cytomegalovirus. In: Albert DM, Jakobiec FA, eds. *Principles and Practice of Ophthalmology.* Philadelphia: WB Saunders; 1994; vol 2:963–964.

Kieval SJ. Cytomegalovirus infection. In: Isselbacher KI, Bruanwald E, Wilson JD, et al. *Harrison's Principles of Internal Medicine,* 13th ed. New York: McGraw-Hill; 1994:794–797.

Stagno S, Pass RF, Cloud G, et al. Primary cytomegalovirus infection in pregnancy: Incidence, transmission to fetus, and clinical outcome. *JAMA* 1986;256:1904–1908.

Chapter 58

HERPES SIMPLEX VIRUS

Thomas J. Liesegang

I. GENERAL

1. Herpes simplex virus (HSV) is a ubiquitous alpha herpesvirus that causes symptomatic and asymptomatic disease in multiple organs, especially skin and mucous membranes; enhanced and more frequent disease occurs in immunocompromised individuals.

2. HSV type I usually involved in ocular and oropharyngeal region (recurrent in 20–40% of population); HSV-II usually involved in genital region (recurrent in 5% of population); some overlap

3. HSV causes severe primary disease in children and neonates and can cause encephalitis, meningitis, erythema multiforme, hepatitis, and dissemination.

4. HSV-I and HSV-II have similar DNA homology; less homology with other herpes viruses (Epstein-Barr virus, varicella-zoster, cytomegalovirus, human herpers virus [HHV]-6, HHV-7, HHV-8).

5. Spread by personal contact with receptor specificity and host cell factors determining ability of particular viruses to infect a cell type; clinical disease depends on the virus strain and host immune response. Pathophysiology is related to infection and the inflammatory or immune response initiated.

6. Virion enters neurons, travels to nucleus, and becomes latent in the nucleus; capable of reactivating in response to stimuli or spontaneously.

7. The oral mucous membrane route provides access to trigeminal nerve and subsequently to the eye.

8. Humans are the only natural host; many experimental animal models.

9. Asymptomatic shedding (especially labial, oral, and genital) is an important source of transmission.

10. Ocular disease affects males and females equally; 400,000 patients with ocular HSV in the United States.

11. Initial ocular episode involves eyelid or conjunctiva in 54%, superficial cornea in 63%, corneal stroma in 6%, and uvea in 4%; recurrence rates of 10% at 1 year, 23% at 2 years, and 63% at 20 years. Bilateral disease in 12% of patients. Approximately 20% ultimately have stromal disease; 92% of patents maintain 20/40 or better vision.

II. SYSTEMIC MANIFESTATIONS

1. Congenital HSV infection
   - Skin vesicles
   - Jaundice
   - Hepatosplenomegaly
   - Bleeding diathesis
   - Intrauterine growth retardation
   - Microcephaly
   - Encephalitis, seizures, irritability
   - Psychomotor retardation
   - Cortical blindness
   - Hypopigmented skin lesions

2. Neonatal HSV infection
   - Skin vesicles
   - Seizures
   - Cranial nerve palsies
   - Lethargy, coma, seizures, irritability, shock
   - Encephalitis
   - Intravascular coagulation
   - Disseminated disease with liver and adrenal involvement
   - Multiple internal organs involved

3. Primary HSV ifection
   - Cutaneous vesicles localized and, rarely, disseminated
   - Disseminated can lead to visceral disease
   - Gingivostomatitis, pharyngitis, rhinitis, tonsillitis, myalgias, fever, chills
   - Regional lymphadenopathy
   - Genital herpes (penis, vulva, perineum, buttocks, cervix, vagina, anus)
   - Encephalitis
   - Meningoencephalitis
   - Radiculomyelitis, Bell's palsy
   - Finger herpetic whitlows
   - Eczema herpeticum in patients with atopic dermatitis

4. Recurrent HSV infection
   - Recurrent herpes labialis
   - Recurrent genital and anal lesions
   - Aseptic meningitis
   - Encephalitis
   - Tracheobronchitis
   - Interstitial pneumonia
   - Esophagitis
   - Hepatitis
   - Leukopenia, thrombocytopenia, disseminated intravascular coagulation
   - Disseminated disease
   - Adrenal necrosis, cystitis, arthritis
   - Erythema multiforme
   - Cofactor in cervical cancer
   - Idiopathic Bell's palsy
   - Multiple sclerosis, Mollaret syndrome, ascending myelitis, trigeminal neuralgia, temporal lobe epilepsy

1. Congenital HSV infection
   - Posterior lenticular opacification
   - Microphthalmia, microcornea
   - Iridocyclitis
   - Iris atrophy
   - Nystagmus
   - Posterior synechiae
   - Optic neuritis and atrophy
   - Retinitis
   - Chorioretinitis
   - Macular scars
   - Vitreous masses
2. Neonatal HSV infection
   - Periocular skin disease
   - Conjunctivitis
   - Epithelial keratitis
   - Stromal keratitis
   - Retinal exudate, perivasculitis
   - Vitreous inflammatory reaction
   - Superficial and deep retinal hemorrhages
   - Later, optic atrophy
   - Hypopigmented and hyperpigmented chorioretinal changes
   - Neovascularization and detachment of the retina
   - Attenuated retinal vasculature
3. Primary ocular HSV infection
   - Acute follicular conjunctivitis
   - Conjunctival dendrites
   - Corneal dendrites
   - Preauricular lymph nodes
   - Periocular and eyelid skin vesicles
4. Recurrent ocular HSV disease
   - Lid
     - Lid and lid margin vesicles
   - Conjunctiva
     - Conjunctival follicles
     - Conjunctival dendrites
     - Pseudomembranes
   - Cornea
     - Dendritic epithelial keratitis
     - Geographic epithelial keratitis
     - Marginal ulcerations
     - Stromal keratitis
       - Necrotizing stromal keratitis
       - Interstitial keratitis
     - Endotheliitis
       - Disciform
       - Diffuse
       - Linear
     - Metaherpetic disease
       - Granular epithelial lesions
       - Neurotrophic corneal disease
       - Indolent corneal ulceration
   - Uvea
     - Iridocyclitis
     - Trabeculitis
   - Retina
     - Necrotizing retinitis (retinal whitening, vasculitis, papilledema, nerve fiber hemorrhage, anterior chamber, and vitreous reaction); late retinal detachment, vitreous clouding
     - Acute retinal necrosis (retinal whitening with confluent necrosis, vitritis, retinal vasculitis)
     - HSV retinitis in immunocompromised patients
       - Variable retinal necrosis

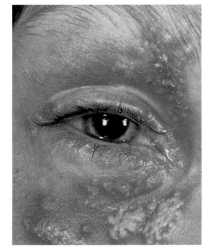

FIGURE 58.1. Recurrent HSV infection of the eyelid skin, eyelid margin, and conjunctiva in an otherwise healthy child.

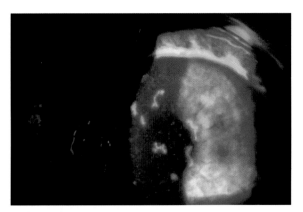

FIGURE 58.2. Multiple HSV corneal dendritic lesions demonstrated by fluorescein and cobalt blue filter at a different recurrent episode in the same child as shown in Figure 58.1.

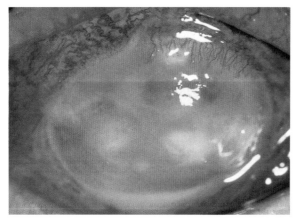

FIGURE 58.3. Marked HSV necrotizing stromal keratitis with multiple corneal abscesses, an epithelial defect, and hypopyon in a patient following recurrent and severe bouts of stromal keratitis.

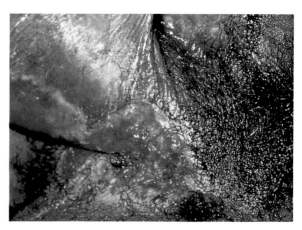

FIGURE 58.4. Severe HSV infection of the perineal region in an HIV-positive male patient.

SUGGESTED READINGS

Liesegang TJ. Biology and molecular aspects of herpes simplex and varicella-zoster virus infections. *Ophthalmology* 1992;99:781–799.

Margolis TP, Atherton SA. Herpes simplex virus diseases: Posterior segment of the eye. In: Pepose JS, Holland GN, Wilhelmus KR, eds. *Ocular Infections and Immunity*. St. Louis: CV Mosby; 1996:1155–1167.

Pepose JS. Herpes simplex keratitis: Role of viral infection versus immune response. *Surv Ophthalmol* 1991;35:345–352.

Pepose JS, Leib DA, Stuart PM, Easty DL. Herpes simplex virus diseases: Anterior segment of the eye. In: Pepose JS, Holland GN, Wilhelmus KR, eds. *Ocular Infections and Immunity*. St. Louis: CV Mosby; 1996:905–932.

Roizman B, Sears AE. Herpes simplex viruses and their replication. In: Fields BN, Knipe DM, Chanock RM, et al, eds. *Field's Virology*. New York: Raven Press; 1996:2231–2295.

Whitley RJ. Herpes simplex virus. In: Fields BN, Knipe DM, Chanock RM, et al, eds. *Field's Virology*. New York: Raven Press; 1996:2297–2342.

Chapter 59

HERPES ZOSTER

Thomas J. Liesegang

I. GENERAL

1. The identical varicella virus that causes chickenpox becomes latent in sensory ganglia and recurs as herpes zoster.
2. Almost all adults have clinical or serologic evidence of prior chickenpox; approximately 10% to 20% develop herpes zoster.
3. A pain prodrome frequently precedes the appearance of the zoster rash.
4. Silent reactivation of herpes zoster (without skin lesions) may occur periodically with cellular immune containment.
5. A viremia with a few disseminated vesicles frequently occurs.
6. Herpes zoster occurs most commonly in areas of the body most heavily involved with varicella; about 15% of herpes zoster involve the trigeminal nerve.
7. The incidence of herpes zoster is associated with increased age and immune suppression, especially in association with acquired immunodeficiency syndrome.
8. Herpes zoster is more severe, more prolonged, and more likely to be associated with dissemination, visceral, and neurologic complications in patients with immune suppression.

II. SYSTEMIC MANIFESTATIONS

1. Cutaneous
   - Dissemination (micro or diffuse)
   - Dermal scarring
   - Bacterial superinfection
   - Herpes gangrenosum
2. Visceral
   - Pneumonitis
   - Esophagitis
   - Enterocolitis
   - Myocarditis
   - Pancreatitis
3. Neurologic
   - Acute neuralgia
   - Postherpetic neuralgia
   - Encephalitis
   - Meningoencephalitis
   - Central nervous system granulomatous angiitis with hemiplegia
   - Myelitis
   - Guillain-Barré syndrome
   - Motor neuropathies
     - Cranial
       - Ophthalmoplegia (III, IV, VI)
       - Ramsay Hunt syndrome (VII, VIII)
       - Other cranial nerves
     - Peripheral
       - Diaphragmatic paralysis
       - Neurogenic bladder
4. Psychiatric
   - Depression

1. Skin/lids
   - Vesicular rash
   - Bacterial superinfection
   - Dermal contracture
   - Ptosis
   - Lid retraction
   - Trichiasis
   - Cicatricial ectropion
   - Ischemic lid necrosis
2. Conjunctiva
   - Follicular conjunctivitis
   - Vesicular eruption
   - Pseudomembrane
   - Punctal stenosis
3. Episclera/sclera
   - Anterior or posterior scleritis
   - Nodular episcleritis
   - Scleral thinning
   - Sclerokeratitis
4. Cornea
   - Punctate epithelial keratitis
   - Pseudodendritic keratitis
   - Nummular keratitis
   - Keratouveitis/endotheliitis
   - Disciform keratitis
   - Neurotrophic keratitis
   - Exposure keratitis
   - Mucous plaque keratitis
   - Lipid keratopathy
   - Interstitial keratitis
   - Secondary band keratopathy
5. Uveal tract
   - Anterior uveitis
   - Keratic precipitates
   - Iris hyperemia or hemorrhage
   - Anterior and posterior synechia
   - Iris atrophy
   - Anterior segment ischemia
   - Phthisis bulbi
6. Glaucoma
   - Trabeculitis
   - Rubeosis
   - Synechial angle closure
7. Cataract
8. Retina/optic nerve
   - Retinal vasculitis
   - Ischemic optic neuritis
   - Acute retinal necrosis
9. Extraocular muscles
   - Paresis, paralysis

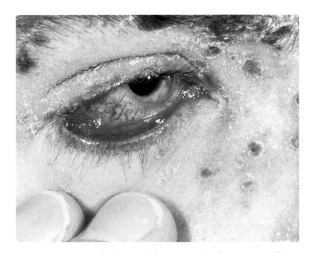

FIGURE 59.1. Dried skin vesicles 1 week after onset of herpes zoster ophthalmicus. There is a conjunctival vesicle, mild conjunctival injection, and a ciliary flush.

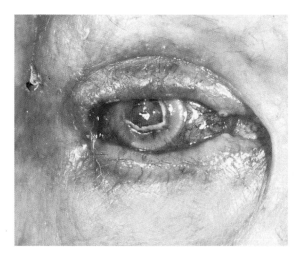

FIGURE 59.2. Deep dermal scarring from herpes zoster ophthalmicus resulting in dermal contracture of the upper lid, shiny skin, inability to close the lid, and a secondary calcific band keratopathy.

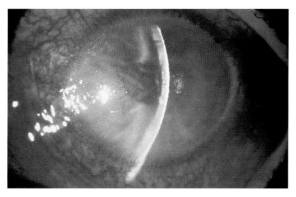

FIGURE 59.3. Severe keratouveitis secondary to herpes zoster ophthalmicus with conjunctival injection, ciliary flush, corneal stria, and keratic precipitates.

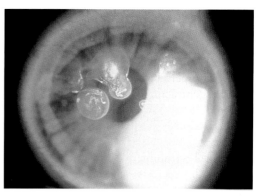

FIGURE 59.4. Lipid keratopathy scars from chronic herpes zoster keratitis.

SUGGESTED READINGS

Cobo M, Foulks GN, Liesegang T, et al. Observations on the natural history of herpes zoster ophthalmicus. *Curr Eye Res* 1987;6:195–199.

Karbassi M, Raizman MB, Schuman JS. Herpes zoster ophthalmicus. *Surv Ophthalmol* 1992;36: 395–410.

Liesegang TJ. Biology and molecular aspects of herpes simplex and varicella-zoster virus infections. *Ophthalmology* 1992;99:781–799.

Liesegang TJ. Diagnosis and therapy of herpes zoster ophthalmicus. *Ophthalmology* 1991;98:1216–1229.

Liesegang TJ. Corneal complications from herpes zoster ophthalmicus. *Ophthalmology* 1985;92: 316–324.

Marsh RJ, Cooper M. Ophthalmic herpes zoster. *Eye* 1993;7:350–370.

Chapter 60
MOLLUSCUM CONTAGIOSUM

Curtis E. Margo

I. GENERAL

1. Cutaneous infection occurs worldwide. DNA virus, genus *Molluscipoxvirus;* humans are only known reservoir.
2. Virus is transmitted by direct contact, both person to person and via fomites. Autoinnoculation probably is important in personal spread. Sexual transmission can occur. Localized epidemics are traced to swimming pools, gymnasiums, and public baths.
3. Incidence highest in childhood. Because serologic tests are not well standardized, epidemiology not fully characterized.
4. Incubation period ranges from 7 days to 6 months based on clinical reports. In experimental innoculation studies, incubation period was 20 to 50 days.
5. Can occur at any age. Infection is more common and more severe in immunocompromised patients. Severe dissemination can occur in acquired immunodeficiency syndrome (AIDS).
6. Infection can be prevented by avoiding direct contact with lesions and potential fomites. Isolation of infected children is not recommended, but infected persons should avoid activities that are associated with person-to-person contact.
7. Disease is self-limited in immunocompetent persons. Involution usually occurs within 2 to 8 months without scarring. Involution can be hastened by a variety of methods including cryotherapy or curettage. Treatment usually is not effective in patients with underlying immunodeficiency disease.

II. SYSTEMIC MANIFESTATION

1. Skin
   - Smooth-surfaced papule, 2 to 7 mm diameter
   - Umbilication of vertex
   - Flesh color, yellowish, or off white
   - Isolated papule or pupules in clusters
   - Painless, may itch
   - Secondary infection with scratching
   - Face, trunk, and proximal extemities most often involved in children
   - Lower abdominal skin, pubis, and thighs most often involved in adults

III. OCULAR MANIFESTATIONS

1. Lids
   - Isolated papule or papules in clusters
   - Can occur on lid margin, pretarsal skin, or periocular skin
   - Same clinical characteristics as cutaneous lesion elsewhere
   - Exuberant nodule formation can occur in patients with AIDS

2. Conjunctiva
   - Secondary toxic keratoconjunctivitis
   - Follicular conjunctival reaction
   - Usually associated with lesion on lid margin
   - Keratoconjunctivitis resolves with involution or successful treatment of lid lesion
   - Conjunctival infection rare; usually in patients with severe immunodeficiency condition

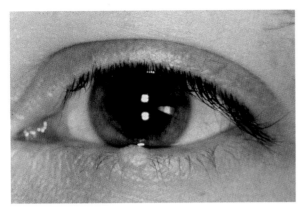

FIGURE 60.1. Solitary nodule of molluscum contagiosum in the middle of the left lower lid. The vertex is crusted but not yet umbilicated. There are no signs of secondary conjunctivitis.

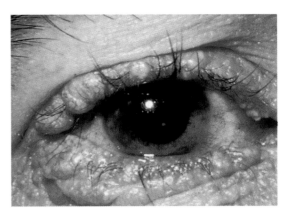

FIGURE 60.2. Confluent nodules of molluscum contagiosum on both upper and lower lids in a patient with AIDS. Courtesy of Henry Perry, MD.

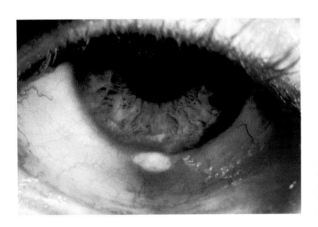

FIGURE 60.3. Limbal papule of molluscum contagiosum in a patient with AIDS. The patient also had cutaneous lesions of the eyelid. From Charles NC, Freidburg DN. Epibulbar molluscum contagiosum in a patient with acquired immune deficiency syndrome. *Ophthalmology* 1992; 99:1123–1126.

SUGGESTED READINGS

Charles NC, Friedburg DN. Epibulbar molluscum contagiosum in acquired immune deficiency syndrome. *Ophthalmology* 1992;99:1123–1126.

Margo C, Katz NNK. Management of periocular molluscum cantagiosum in children. *J Pediatr Ophthalmol Strab* 1983;20:19–21.

Postlethwaite R. Molluscum contagiosum. A review. *Arch Environ Health* 1970;21:432–452.

Redfield RR, James WD, Wright DC, et al. Severe molluscum contagiosum infection in a patient with human T cell lymphotropic (HTLV-III) disease. *J Am Acad Dermatol* 1985;13:821–824.

Robinson MR, Udell IJ, Garber PF, et al. Molluscum contagiosum of the eyelid in patients with acquired immune deficiency syndrome. *Ophthalmology* 1992;99:1745–1747.

Chapter 61

MUMPS

Kirk R. Wilhelmus

I. GENERAL

1. Mumps virus is spread by airborne respiratory droplets. Infected persons are contagious for about 1 week after onset of parotid gland swelling.
2. Mumps is a systemic disease, and virus can be cultured from saliva, urine, and other sites. Rapid diagnostic tests include immunofluorescence for mumps antigen and polymerase chain reaction for viral RNA.
3. Antibody responses are detected by serologic testing using complement fixation and enzyme immunoassay. Immune-mediated responses may account for postviral neurologic complications.
4. Mumps is being eradicated through vaccination programs with live attenuated virus strains.

II. SYSTEMIC MANIFESTATIONS

1. Mucocutaneous
   - Parotitis
   - Submaxillary sialadenitis
2. Central nervous system
   - Meningitis
   - Postviral encephalitis and encephalomyelitis
   - Hearing loss
   - Cranial nerve palsy
   - Guillain-Barré syndrome
3. Genitourinary
   - Orchitis
   - Epididymitis
   - Prostatitis
   - Oophoritis
   - Nephritis
4. Endocrine
   - Pancreatitis
   - Thyroiditis
5. Pulmonary
   - Bronchitis
6. Gastrointestinal
   - Splenomegaly
   - Hepatitis
7. Hematologic
   - Thrombocytopenia
   - Hemolytic anemia
8. Musculoskeletal
   - Mastitis
   - Arthritis
   - Myositis
9. Cardiac
   - Myocarditis

III. OCULAR MANIFESTATIONS

1. Lacrimal system
   - Acute dacryoadenitis
2. Conjunctiva/sclera
   - Conjunctivitis
   - Episcleritis
   - Scleritis
3. Cornea
   - Disciform stromal keratitis
4. Uvea
   - Iridocyclitis
   - Choroiditis
5. Retina/RPE
   - Acute posterior multifocal placoid pigment epitheliopathy
6. Optic nerve
   - Optic neuritis and neuroretinitis

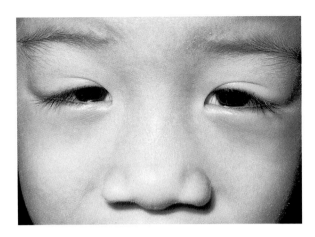

FIGURE 61.1. Acute bilateral dacryoadenitis in mumps.

SUGGESTED READINGS

Al-Rashid RA, Cress C. Mumps uveitis complicating the course of acute leukemia. *J Pediatr Ophthalmol* 1977;14:100–102. *Case report of iritis occurring during mumps parotitis.*

Meyer RF, Sullivan JH, Oh JO. Mumps conjunctivitis. *Am J Ophthalmol* 1974;78:1022–1024. *Culture-proven acute follicular conjunctivitis during mumps parotitis.*

Sugita K, Ando M, Minamitani K, et al. Magnetic resonance imaging in a case of mumps postinfectious encephalitis with asymptomatic optic neuritis. *Eur J Pediatr* 1991;150:773–775. *Neuroanatomy of postviral optic neuritis with demyelination.*

Sutphin JE. Mumps keratitis. *Ophthalmol Clin North Am* 1994;7:557–566. *Literature review of corneal inflammation due to mumps.*

Chapter 62
CONGENITAL RUBELLA SYNDROME
Timothy D. Polk

I. GENERAL

1. Rubella is an RNA virus in the togavirus group and causes German measles.
2. Postnatal infection is usually mild and self-limited.
3. Pregnant women who contract rubella during the first or second trimester may transmit the infection to their fetuses with severe consequences (congenital rubella syndrome).
4. 10% to 20% of women of child-bearing age have not been exposed to rubella and thus are susceptible.
5. Chronic contagious infection. Virus may be isolated years after birth.
6. Infection causes a widespread slowing of cell growth in the fetus.
7. Vaccination, available since 1969, has dramatically reduced the incidence of the congenital rubella syndrome.

II. SYSTEMIC MANIFESTATIONS

1. Central nervous system
   - Bilateral sensorineural hearing loss
   - Mental retardation
   - Psychomotor retardation
   - Microcephaly
   - Progressive panencephalitis
   - Meningitis
   - Cerebral vasculitis
2. Cardiac
   - Patent ductus arteriosus
   - Pulmonary artery stenosis
   - Ventricular septal defect
   - Atrial septal defect
   - Valvular stenosis
   - Coarctation of the aorta
   - Congestive heart failure
3. Dental
   - Dental hypoplasia
   - Micrognathia
   - Cleft lip
4. Endocrine
   - Diabetes mellitus
   - Hypothyroidism
   - Hyperthyroidism
   - Thyroiditis
   - Growth hormone deficiency
   - Hypoadrenalism
5. Hematologic
   - Thrombocytopenia with purpura
   - Hemolytic anemia
6. Nonspecific
   - Growth retardation
   - Failure to thrive
   - Low birth weight
7. Musculoskeletal
   - Longitudinal areas of radiolucency in long bones
   - Large anterior fontanelle
   - Scoliosis
   - Syndactyly
8. Visceral
   - Hepatitis
   - Hepatosplenomegaly
9. Pulmonary
   - Interstitial pneumonitis
10. Genitourinary
    - Undescended testes
    - Inguinal hernia
    - Recurrent urinary tract infections

III. OCULAR MANIFESTATIONS

1. Retina
- "Salt and pepper" mottling of retinal pigment epithelium
- Choroidal neovascularization
- Absent foveal reflex
- Retinal detachment

2. Lens
- Nuclear or total cataract
- Spontaneous lens absorption
- Retained cell nuclei in central lens
- Spherophakia

3. Intraocular pressure
- Glaucoma

4. Nonspecific
- Microphthalmia
- Myopia or hyperopia

5. Uvea
- Iris hypoplasia
- Angle dysgenesis
- Nongranulomatous iridocyclitis
- Pupillary membrane
- Poor pupil dilatation

6. Ocular motility
- Strabismus
- Nystagmus

7. Cornea
- Corneal clouding
- Punctate epithelial keratitis
- Keratic precipitates
- Keratoconus
- Microcornea
- Corneal hydrops

8. Optic nerve
- Optic neuritis
- Optic atrophy

9. Conjunctiva
- Conjunctivitis

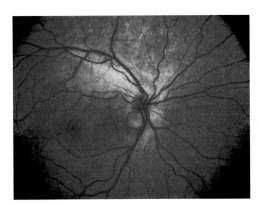 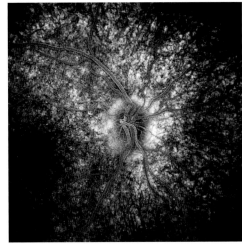

FIGURE 62.1. "Salt and pepper" retinopathy of congenital rubella syndrome. Color fundus photograph (left). Fluorescein angiogram (right).

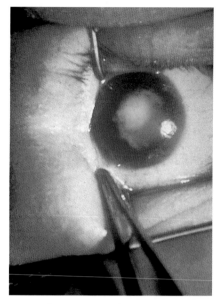

FIGURE 62.2. Nuclear cataract of congenital rubella syndrome. Courtesy of G. Frank Judisch, MD.

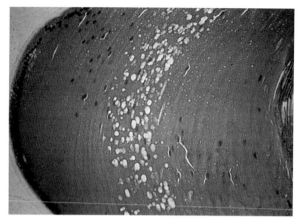

FIGURE 62.3. Retained cell nuclei in nucleus of rubella cataract.

SUGGESTED READINGS

Givens KT, Lee DA, Jones T, Ilstrup DM. Congenital rubella syndrome: Ophthalmic manifestations and associated systemic disorders. *Br J Ophthalmol* 1993;77:358–363. *A 20-year follow-up study of 125 patients with congenital rubella syndrome.*

O'Neill JF, Drack AV. Rubella: German measles. In: Gold DH, Weingeist TA, eds. *The Eye in Systemic Disease.* Philadelphia: JB Lippincott; 1990:269–272.

Rudolph AJ, Desmond MM. Clinical manifestations of the congenital rubella syndrome. *Int Ophthalmol Clin* 1972;12:3–19. *A good review of the congenital rubella syndrome with emphasis on the systemic manifestations.*

Wolff SM. The ocular manifestations of congenital rubella. *Trans Am Ophthalmol Soc* 1972;70:577–614. *A prospective study of the ocular findings seen in 328 patients with the congenital rubella syndrome.*

Chapter 63

SUBACUTE SCLEROSING PANENCEPHALITIS

Jean-Jacques De Laey

I. GENERAL

1. Degenerative disease of the central nervous system in children and adolescents
2. History of measles in 93% of patients with confirmed subacute sclerosing panencepalitis (SSPE)
3. Two to four times more common in boys than in girls
4. Incidence almost six times higher in rural (and especially farm) areas than in large cities
5. The incidence of SSPE has dropped dramatically in populations that have received mass antimeasles vaccination.
6. High titers of measles antibody in the blood and cerebrospinal fluid (CSF)
7. Viral particles have been isolated from brain tissue as well as from the retina.
8. Most patients die within 5 to 12 months.

II. SYSTEMIC MANIFESTATIONS

1. Central nervous system
   - Stage 1 (behavioral signs)
     - Poorer school performances
     - Mental regression
     - Increased irritability
   - Stage 2
     - Myoclinic jerks with typical electroencephalographic changes
   - Stage 3
     - Increased spasticity
     - Decerebrate rigidity
     - Coma
   - Stage 4
     - Loss of all central functions
2. Nonspecific
   - Fever (dysregulation of autonomic function)

III. OCULAR MANIFESTATIONS

1. Retina
   - Necrotizing retinitis (uni- or bilateral) may precede the neurologic signs by several months.
2. Neuroophthalmology
   - Hallucinations
   - Cortical blindness
   - Motility problems
     - Ocular muscle palsies
     - Supranuclear palsies
     - Ptosis
     - Nystagmus
   - Papilledema
   - Papillitis
   - Optic atrophy
3. Orbit
   - Exophthalmos (exceptional)

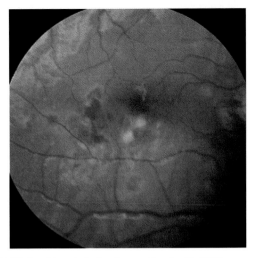

FIGURE 63.1. Macula lesion in a patient with SSPE: appearance in June 1980.

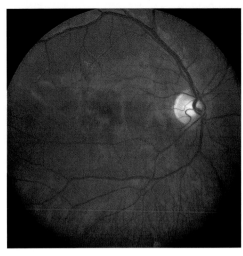

FIGURE 63.2. Appearance of the same fundus as Fig. 63.1 in September 1980.

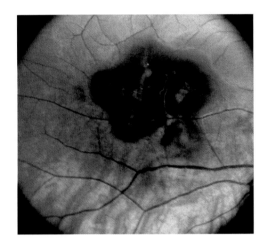

FIGURE 63.3. Red-free appearance of the same fundus as Fig. 63.1 and Fig. 63.2 in November 1981. Courtesy of Dr. A. Leys.

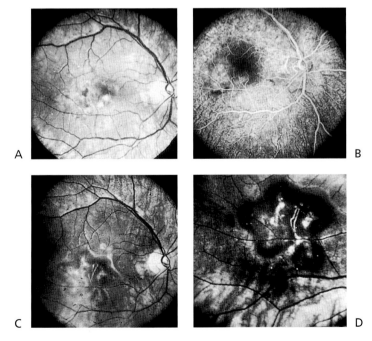

FIGURE 63.4. Composite slide of the same patient. (**A**) Appearance in June 1980; (**B**) fluorescein angiography in June 1980; (**C**) appearance in September 1980; (**D**) appearance in November 1981.

SUGGESTED READINGS

Cochereau-Massin F, Gaudric A, Reinert P, et al. Altérations du fond d'oeil au cours de la panencéphalite sclérosante subaigue. A propos de 23 cas. *J Fr Ophtalmol* 1992;15:255–261.

De Laey JJ, Hanssens M, Colette P, et al. Subacute sclerosing panencephalitis: Fundus changes and histopathologic correlations. *Doc Ophthalmol* 1983;56:11– 21.

Horta-Barbosa L, Fucillo DA, Sever JL. Subacute sclerosing panencephalitis: Indication of measles virus from a brain biopsy. *Nature* 1969;221:974.

Jabbour JT, Garcia JH, Lemmi H, et al. Subacute sclerosing panencephalitis. A multidisciplinary study of eight cases. *JAMA* 1969;207:2248–2254.

Modlin JF, Halsey MA, Eddins DL, et al. Epidemiology of subacute sclerosing panencephalitis. *J Pediatr* 1979;94:231–236.

Chapter 64

VARICELLA

John E. Sutphin

I. GENERAL

1. Highly communicable childhood disease with a generalized vesicular rash
2. Caused by the varicella-zoster virus of the Herpesviridae family
3. Contagious from prior to rash to 5 days after onset, incubation is 14 days, spread by droplets in air or on direct contact, hematogenous dissemination
4. Peak age is 2 to 8 years; 98% of population is seropositive by age 20 years.
5. Capable of inducing latency after the primary infection
6. Oral or systemic acyclovir may be useful in selected cases including immunocompromised children or adults; hyperimmune varicella-zoster gamma globulin may prevent disease in immunocompromised, seronegative patients if given after known exposure before onset of rash.
7. Avoid aspirin and other salicylates in children because of the danger of Reye's syndrome.
8. Live, attenuated, varicella vaccine has completed successful clinical trials, but its effect on zoster and duration of immunity are unknown.

II. SYSTEMIC MANIFESTATIONS

1. Skin
   - Rash begins as erythematous macules, progresses to papules, vesiculates, and then crusts over. Rash begins in scalp, face, and trunk and then spreads to limbs, and resolves in 10 to 14 days, sometimes leaving small pock scars.
   - Bacterial superinfection is most common complication.
   - Pruritus
2. Nonspecific
   - Fever
   - Muscle ache
   - Malaise
   - Headache
3. Pulmonary
   - Diffuse interstitial pneumonia
4. Neurologic
   - Encephalitis in adults
   - Reye's syndrome in children (not reported in adults)
   - Transverse myelitis
   - Guillain-Barré syndrome
5. Visceral
   - Hepatitis
   - Pancreatitis
6. Hemorrhagic
   - Thrombocytopenic purpura
   - Purpura fulminans
7. Congenital varicella syndrome
   - Varicella early in first trimester
   - Microcephaly
   - Limb deformities
   - Deafness
   - Cardiac abnormalities
   - Ocular, including microphthalmia, chorioretinitis, cataracts

III. OCULAR MANIFESTATIONS

1. Conjunctiva
   - Mild papillary conjunctivitis
   - Vesicles
2. Cornea
   - Punctate epithelial or dendritic keratitis
   - Disciform keratitis
   - Both are self-limited and do not recur
3. Rare
   - Uveitis
   - Glaucoma
   - Eyelid necrosis
   - Cranial nerve palsies
   - Focal chorioretinitis
   - Optic neuritis
   - Cataracts

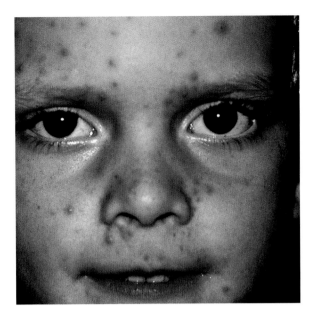

FIGURE 64.1. Facial macules and papules in 5-year-old boy.

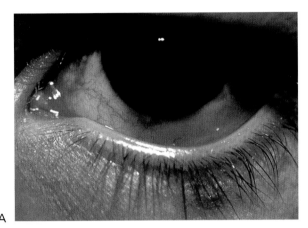

A

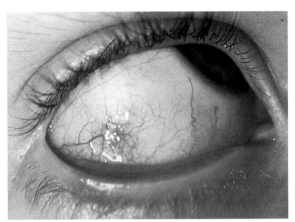

B

FIGURE 64.2. Lid (**A**) and conjunctival vesicles (**B**) in same boy.

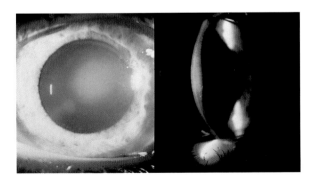

FIGURE 64.3. Disciform keratitis occuring 2 months after varicella in a 10-year-old boy.

SUGGESTED READINGS

Flugfelder SC. Varicella chicken pox. In: Gold DH, Weingeist TA, eds. *The Eye in Systemic Disease.* Philadelphia: JB Lippincott; 1990:275–276.

Liesgang TJ. Biology and molecular aspects of herpes simplex and varicella-zoster virus infections. *Ophthalmology* 1992;99:781–799. *Review of the mechanisms for latency.*

Brunell PA. Varicella. In: Wyngaarden JB, Smith LH, Bennett JC, eds. *Cecil Textbook of Medicine,* 19th ed. Philadelphia: WB Saunders; 1992:1840–1842.

PART 9. INFLAMMATORY DISEASES OF UNKNOWN ETIOLOGY

Chapter 65

BEHÇET'S SYNDROME

William J. Dinning
Elizabeth M. Graham

I. GENERAL

1. First described by Hippocrates but recognized as clinical entity by the Turkish dermatologist Hulusi Behçet in 1937
2. Rare in Western Europe and the United States but found with increasing frequency from Eastern Europe and the Mediterranean across Asia. Japan has the highest incidence (7–8/100,000).
3. Onset commonly in third decade
4. Sexes are equally affected although males generally have more severe disease.

II. SYSTEMIC MANIFESTATIONS

1. The diagnosis is clinical. It is traditionally based on the presence of two or more major criteria in combination with any of the minor criteria. However, validation of diagnostic criteria is under continuous dispute.
2. Major criteria
   - Oral ulceration—clinically and histologically indistinguishable from aphthous ulcers
   - Genital ulceration—similar to oral ulcers but leave more scars
   - Ocular disease
   - Nonulcerative skin lesions
     - Acneiform
     - Folliculitis
     - Erythema nodosum
     - Superficial thrombophlebitis
2. Minor criteria
   - Musculoskeletal
     - Arthritis
       - Mono- or oligoarticular, knees, ankles, wrists, elbows, nonerosive, nondeforming
   - Cardiovascular
     - Thrombophlebitis 25% patients, particularly calf

5. HLA B51
6. Pathophysiology
   - Etiology unknown; suspicion that disease is triggered by herpes virus in susceptible individual
   - Vasculitis of small blood vessels, which produces thromboses and infarcts
   - In acute phase there are raised circulating immune complexes, increased fibrinolysis with raised fibrinogen, raised factor VII and von Willebrand factors as well as activated T cells and polymorphs.

   vessels but rarely may involve axillary veins, iliac veins, or both venae cavae
   - Arterial lesions are less common than venous ones but any part of the arterial tree may be involved with occlusive disease or aneurysm formation.
   - Pulmonary infarcts produce hemoptysis.
   - Gastrointestinal
     - Ulcerative lesions in gut particularly in caecum and terminal ileum, rarely esophagus
   - Central nervous system
     - Dural sinus thrombosis leads to papilledema.
     - Brain stem, hemispheric, meningeal and spinal cord lesions, and neuropsychiatric problems
     - Peripheral neuropathy is unusual.
     - Magnetic resonance imaging is examination of choice and acute lesions produce high-intensity signal on T2-weighted images.
   - Genitourinary
     - Epididymitis
   - Family history

III. OCULAR MANIFESTATIONS

1. Anterior uveitis
   - Nongranulomatous
   - Fibrinous
   - Hypopyon
2. Vitritis
3. Retina
   - Ischemic
     - Minor branch vein occlusion (Fig. 65.1)
     - Hemorrhages
     - Neovascularization
     - Peripheral retinal capillary closure
     - Late-stage disease characterized by optic atrophy and obliterated retinal vasculature (Fig. 65.4)
   - Inflammatory
     - Infiltrates—self resolving (Fig. 65.2)

   - Fluorescein angiography
     - Diffuse capillary leakage (Fig. 65.3)
     - Disc leakage
     - Cystoid macular edema
     - Capillary closure
     - Macular ischemia
4. All other ocular manifestations are rare.
   - Conjunctivitis
   - Episcleritis
   - Scleritis
   - Neuroophthalmologic disease
     - Papilledema secondary to sinus thrombosis
     - Eye movement disorders

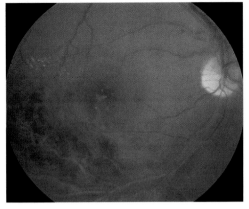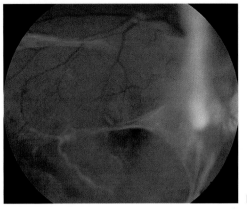

A   B

FIGURE 65.1. **(A)** Inferior retinal vein occlusion in 20-year-old white woman with severe orogenital ulceration, arthritis, and gastrointestinal disease. **(B)** Same eye 3 years later with epiretinal membrane formation and occluded retinal vessels.

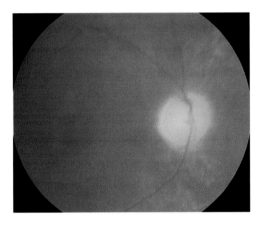

FIGURE 65.2. End-stage disease shows atrophic optic disc and obliterated retinal vessels.

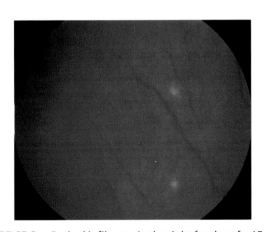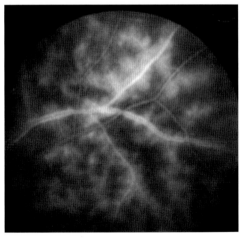

FIGURE 65.3. Retinal infiltrates in the right fundus of a 15-year-old boy. These resolved spontaneously within 7 days.

FIGURE 65.4. Fluorescein angiogram shows diffuse capillary leakage in fern leaf pattern in active phase of Behçet's disease.

SUGGESTED READINGS

Hashimoto T, Takeuchi A. Treatment of Beçhet's disease. *Curr Opin Rheumatol* 1992;4:31–34.
Michelson JB, Friedlaender MH. Behçet's disease. *Int Ophthalmol Clin* 1990;30:271–278.
O'Duffy JD. Behçet's disease. *Curr Opin Rheumatol* 1994;6:39–43.

Chapter 66

CHRONIC GRANULOMATOUS DISEASE

Andrew N. Blatt
Jay S. Pepose

I. GENERAL

1. Chronic granulomatous disease (CGD) clinically presents with recurrent, life-threatening infections with catalase-positive bacteria and fungal microorganisms in the first 2 years of life.
2. Blood neutrophils, monocytes, and eosinophils lack the respiratory burst required to generate microbicidal oxidants during phagocytosis.
3. The disease is transmitted as an X chromosome–linked recessive trait in 70% to 80%, and as an autosomal recessive trait in 20% to 30%.
4. The abnormal gene of the X-linked form was cloned in 1986. Antibodies targeted to a synthetic peptide derived from the abnormal gene's complementary DNA sequence identified the missing neutrophil proteins in CGD.
5. In the majority of X-linked CGD, the neutrophil membrane component b cytochrome is absent. In autosomal CGD, soluble cofactors in the cytosol of neutrophils are typically deficient.
6. Abnormal phagocyte oxidative metabolism can be diagnosed by abnormal chemiluminescence, deficient superoxide and hydrogen peroxide production by stimulated granulocytes, and failure of stimulated CGD cells to reduce nitroblue tetrazolium dye.
7. Treatment involves long-term antibiotic therapy; investigational therapies include recombinant interferon-γ, granulocyte-colony stimulating factor, allogeneic bone marrow transplantation, and gene therapy to rescue defective bone marrow cells.

II. SYSTEMIC MANIFESTATIONS

1. Lungs (70–80%)
   - Chronic/recurrent pneumonia
2. Lymph nodes (60–80%)
   - Cervical and generalized lymphadenopathy and lymphadenitis
3. Skin and soft tissues (60–70%)
   - Subcutaneous abscesses
   - Recurrent skin furunculosis
   - Eczematoid dermatitis
   - Impetigo around orifices
4. Liver (30–40%)
   - Hepatomegaly
   - Hepatic and perihepatic abscesses
5. Gastrointestinal (25–40%)
   - Stomatitis
   - Esophagitis
   - Esophageal outlet narrowing
   - Gastric antral narrowing
   - Chronic diarrhea
   - Perianal abscess
   - Perirectal fistula
6. Bone (20–30%)
   - Osteomyelitis
7. Genitourinary (15–25%)
   - Obstructive uropathy
   - Cystitis
   - Pyelonephritis
   - Renal/perinephric abscess
8. Central nervous system (<10%)
   - Brain abscess
   - Meningitis
9. Miscellaneous
   - Otitis media (20%)
   - Pericarditis (<5%)
   - Sinusitis (<10%)
   - Septicemia (10–20%)

III. OCULAR MANIFESTATIONS

1. Lids
   - Chronic blepharitis (staphylococcal)
2. Conjunctiva/sclera
   - Chronic conjunctivitis
   - Granulomatous scleral inflammation
3. Cornea
   - Marginal or punctate keratitis
   - Pannus formation
   - Perilimbal infiltration
4. Uvea
   - Granulomatous choroidal inflammation
   - Choroidal atrophy
5. Vitreous
   - Vitritis
   - Endophthalmitis
6. Retina
   - Chorioretinal scars (peripapillary, perivascular, not macular)

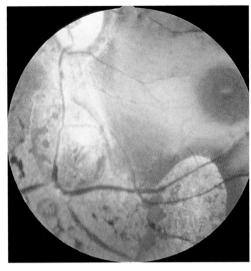

FIGURE 66.1. Perivascular, peripapillary, macular sparing chorioretinal scars in chronic granulomatous disease. Courtesy of M. Smith and S. Valluri.

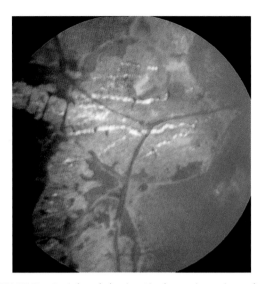

FIGURE 66.2. Peripheral chorioretinal scars in perivascular pattern in chronic granulomatous disease. Courtesy of M. Smith and S. Valluri.

SUGGESTED READINGS

Baehner RI. Chronic granulomatous disease of childhood: Clinical, pathological, biochemical, molecular, and genetic aspects of the disease. *Pediatr Pathol* 1990;10:143–153.

Berendes H, Bridges RA, Good RA. A fatal granulomatosis of childhood: The clinical study of a new syndrome. *Minn Med* 1957;40:309–312.

Curnutte JT. Disorders of granulocyte function and granulopoiesis. In: Nathan DG, Oski FA, eds. *Hematology of Infancy and Childhood.* Philadelphia: WB Saunders; 1993:922–932.

Pepose JS. Chronic granulomatous disease. In: Gold DH, Weingest TA, eds. *The Eye in Systemic Disease.* Philadelphia: JB Lippincott; 1990:282–284.

Royer-Polora B, Kunkel LM, Monacò AP, et al. Cloning the gene for an inherited human disorder—chronic granulomatous disease—on the basis of its chromosomal location. *Nature* 1986;322:32–38.

Chapter 67
REYE'S SYNDROME

Stephen P. Kraft

I. GENERAL

1. An acute biphasic potentially fatal illness of unknown cause.
2. Encephalopathy and fatty infiltration of multiple organs develop after a viral illness, such as influenza B and varicella.
3. May be caused by a viral-host interaction such that genetic makeup renders the patient more susceptible to modification by exogenous factors
4. Ingestion of salicylates is now felt to be a potent factor in the causation of this disease.
5. Seen most often in children ages 4 to 12, but reported in ages ranging from infancy to age 60

6. Manifestations are felt to be due to a self-limited derangement of mitochondria in liver, muscle, and brain.
7. Pathology consistently shows acute hepatocellular failure, with microvesicular panlobular accumulation of fat in hepatocytes and swelling and distortion of mitochondria.
8. Fatty infiltration can invade kidney tubules cells, myocardium, pancreas, brain endothelial cells, and lymph nodes. Brain develops diffuse cerebral edema.
9. Therapy is directed to two most life-threatening problems—hypoglycemia and elevated intracranial pressure.

II. SYSTEMIC MANIFESTATIONS

1. The disease manifests as a biphasic disorder consisting of a prodromal illness followed within days by a rapidly progressive encephalopathy.
2. Prodromal illness
   - Ear/nose/throat
     - Sore throat
     - Rhinorrhea
     - Otitis
   - Gastrointestinal
     - Diarrhea
     - Anorexia
   - Nonspecific
     - Fever
     - Irritability
     - Drowsiness
3. Acute encephalopathy
   - Central nervous system
     - Mental confusion
     - Delirium
     - Seizures
     - Coma
     - Elevated intracranial pressure

   - Pulmonary
     - Hyperventilation
     - Tachypnea
     - Wheezing
     - Apnea
   - Gastrointestinal
     - Hepatomegaly
     - Vomiting
     - Nausea
   - Metabolic
     - Hypoglycemia
     - Elevated serum ammonia
     - Elevated serum aspartate aminotransferase or alanine aminotransferase
     - Elevated prothrombin time
     - Hyperaminoacidemia
     - Elevated serum fatty acids
     - Hyperbilirubinemia
     - Metabolic acidosis
   - Nonspecific
     - Personality change
     - Lethargy

III. OCULAR MANIFESTATIONS

1. There are no pathognomonic ocular signs.
2. Neuroophthalmologic
   - Pupillary dilatation with reduced reactivity to light
   - Cortical blindness
   - Facial nerve palsy (one case)
3. Optic nerve
   - Papilledema
   - Optic atrophy

4. Retina
   - Bilateral central retinal vein occlusions (one case)
5. Ocular motility
   - Nystagmus
   - Exotropia (one case)
6. Cornea
   - Exposure keratitis (one case)

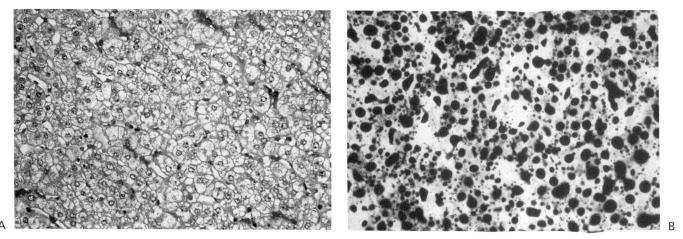

A

B

FIGURE 67.1. (**A**) Medium-power magnification of liver biopsy specimen from a patient with Reye's syndrome. Portion of a liver lobule is shown. Note that the liver parenchymal cells are swollen and vacuolated (hematoxylin-eosin; original magnification, × 20). (**B**) Medium-power magnification of a liver biopsy from the same patient. This specimen has been stained histochemically to show fat globules (orange color). Note abundant distribution of fat (oil-red-O stain; original magnification, ×20). Courtesy of V. Edwards, PhD.

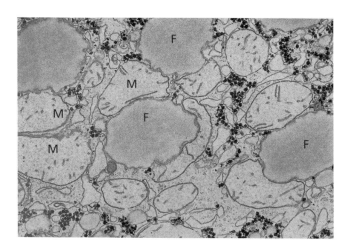

FIGURE 67.2. Electron micrograph of liver biopsy specimen from a patient with Reye's syndrome. Note presence of fat (F) and pleomorphic, swollen mitochondria (M), which show distorted cristae (uranyl acetate and lead citrate stain; original magnification, ×32,000). Courtesy of V. Edwards, PhD.

SUGGESTED READINGS

Glasgow JFT. Clinical features and prognosis of Reye's syndrome. *Arch Dis Child* 1984;59:230–235.

Hurwitz ES, Barrett MJ, Bregman D, et al. Public health service study on Reye's syndrome and medications. *New Engl J Med* 1985;313:849–857.

Kraft SP. Reye's syndrome. In: Gold DH, Weingeist TA, eds. *The Eye in Systemic Disease.* Philadelphia: JB Lippincott; 1990:287–289.

Massey JY, Roy FH, Bornhofen JH. Ocular manifestations of Reye syndrome. *Arch Ophthalmol* 1974;91:441–444.

Mowat AP. Reye's syndrome: 20 years on. *BMJ* 1983;286:1999–2001.

Smith P, Green WR, Miller NM, Terry JM. Central retinal vein occlusion in Reye's syndrome. *Arch Ophthalmol* 1980;98:1256–1260.

Chapter 68

SARCOIDOSIS

Gordon K. Klintworth
Charles J. Bock

I. GENERAL

1. Incidence peak ages 20 to 30 years; second, minor peak, ages 50 to 60 years
2. Women outnumber men 2:1 according to some authors, although others report equal incidence.
3. In the United States, the disease is more common in African-Americans (40–82/100,000 population) than in whites (5–8/100,000).
4. In Europe, sarcoidosis is predominantly a disease of whites.
5. All racial groups have been affected.
6. Up to 80% of patients are asymptomatic and go undiagnosed.
7. Disease is likely initiated by an as yet unidentified airborne agent.
8. Disease is first manifest by the accumulation of T lymphocytes at affected sites.
9. The hallmark noncaseating granulomas form, consisting of a center of epithelioid cells, macrophages, and giant cells surrounded by a thin layer of T and B lymphocytes, monocytes, and fibroblasts.
10. Secondary effects of immunomodulation include a peripheral T-cell lymphopenia due to pooling at active lesions.

II. SYSTEMIC MANIFESTATIONS

1. Pulmonary
   - Hilar adenopathy in 70%
   - Abnormal pulmonary function tests
     - Early: limited diffusion capacity
     - Late: decreased static lung volume; restrictive lung disease
   - Pulmonary infiltrates
   - Pulmonary fibrosis
   - Hemoptysis (rare)
2. Nonspecific
   - Lymphadenopathy
   - Hypergammaglobulinemia
   - Hypercalcemia
   - Fever
   - Malaise
   - Anorexia
   - Chest pain
   - Anergy
3. Cardiac
   - Pulmonary insufficiency (number one cause of death)
   - Arrhythmias, including sudden cardiac death
   - Papillary muscle dysfunction
   - Pericarditis
   - Congestive heart failure
4. Neurologic
   - Cranial neuropathies (in decreasing order of frequency)
     - Facial nerve palsy, lower motor neuron type
     - Optic nerve (see Ocular Manifestations)
     - Acoustic nerve
       Deafness
       Vertigo
     - Any other cranial nerve
   - Peripheral neuropathies
     - Paresthesias
     - Muscle weakness and wasting
     - Decreased deep tendon reflexes
     - Neuralgias
   - Seizures
   - Meningitis, acute or chronic
   - Hydrocephalus
   - Pseudotumor cerebri
   - Focal deficits due to granulomas
   - Hypothalamic and pituitary granulomas
   - Cerebellar ataxia
   - Psychiatric symptoms
5. Mucocutaneous
   - Erythema nodosum
   - Lupus pernio
   - Subcutaneous skin nodules
   - Maculopapular or vesicular eruptions
6. Gastrointestinal
   - Abnormal liver enzymes
   - Hepatomegaly
   - Splenomegaly
   - Granulomas
7. Musculoskeletal
   - Muscle granulomas
   - Bone cysts
   - Arthritis, acute or chronic
   - Acute myositis
   - Slowly progressive myopathies

1. Lids
   - Granulomas
2. Lacrimal gland
   - Painless granulomatous dacryoadenitis
3. Conjunctiva
   - Granulomas
4. Cornea/sclera
   - Mutton fat keratic precipitates
   - Keratoconjunctivitis sicca
   - Calcific band keratopathy
   - Scleritis
5. Lens
   - Cataract
6. Uvea
   - Anterior granulomatous uveitis, acute or chronic
   - Intermediate uveitis
   - Chorioretinitis
   - Koeppe (pupil margin) and Busacca (stromal) iris nodules
   - Choroidal granulomas
7. Retina/vitreous
   - Vitritis
   - Retinal neovascularization

- Retinal vasculitis
  - Focal perivascular exudates (candlewax drippings)
  - Branch retinal venous thrombosis
  - Focal venous sheathing
  - Macular edema
  - Epiretinal membranes
8. Optic nerve
   - Disc edema
   - Neovascularization
   - Optic neuritis
   - Optic atrophy
   - Granulomas
7. Neuroopthalmic
   - Pupil
     - Internal ophthalmoplegia
     - Argyll-Robertson pupil
     - Adie's pupil
   - Third, fourth, and sixth cranial nerve palsies
8. Orbit
   - Granulomas
   - Proptosis
9. Other
   - Glaucoma

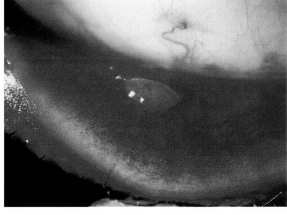

FIGURE 68.1. Conjunctival granuloma of the lower eyelid. Courtesy of Glenn J. Jaffe, MD.

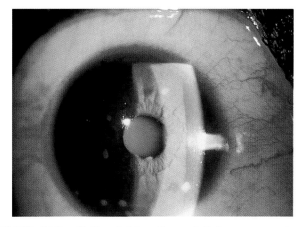

FIGURE 68.2. Mutton fat keratic precipitates on corneal endothelium and iris nodules in anterior uveitis due to sarcoidosis. Courtesy of Glenn J. Jaffe, MD.

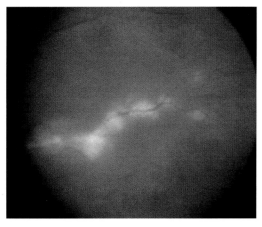

FIGURE 68.3. Focal perivascular exudates (candlewax drippings) in retinal vasculitis in sarcoidosis. Courtesy of Glenn J. Jaffe, MD.

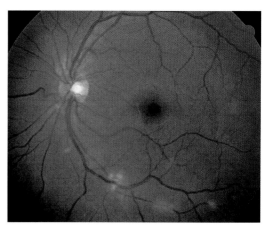

FIGURE 68.4. Focal venous sheathing secondary to retinal vasculitis. Courtesy of Glenn J. Jaffe, MD.

SUGGESTED READINGS

Crystal RG. Sarcoidosis. In: Isselbacher KJ, Braunwald E, Wilson JD, et al, eds. *Harrison's Principles of Internal Medicine,* 13th ed. New York: McGraw-Hill; 1994:1679–1684.

Hunter DG, Foster CS. Systemic manifestations of sarcoidosis. In: Albert DM, Jakobiec FA, eds. *Principles and Practice of Ophthalmology.* Philadelphia: WB Saunders; 1994:3132–3142.

Klintworth GK. Sarcoidosis. In: Gold DH, Weingeist TA, eds. *The Eye in Systemic Disease.* Philadelphia: JB Lippincott; 1990:289–293.

Weissler JC. Southwestern Internal Medicine Conference: Sarcoidosis: Immunology and clinical management. *Am J Med Sci* 1994;307:233–245.

Chapter 69

VOGT-KOYANAGI-HARADA SYNDROME

Manabu Mochziuki

I. GENERAL

1. An autoimmune disease against melanocytes
2. Affecting systemic tissues containing melanocytes, such as the eyes, meninges, hair, and skin
3. Nontraumatic bilateral uveitis with sudden onset
4. Age and sex: primarily adults between 20 and 50 years old, and no sex difference
5. Ethnic group: more frequent in Asian and pigmented races than in whites
6. Immunogenetics: association with HLA-DR4 and HLA-DRw53
7. Ocular complications following persistent uveitis: cataract, glaucoma, chorioretinal atrophy, chorioretinal neovascularization
8. Treatment: local and systemic corticosteroids

II. SYSTEMIC MANIFESTATIONS

1. Central nervous system
   - Headache
   - Nausea
   - Pleocytosis in cerebrospinal fluid
2. Ear
   - Tinnitus
   - Vertigo
   - Dysacousia (sensory neural hearing loss)
3. Hair
   - Tingling sensation of the head hair
   - Alopecia
   - Poliosis (head hair, eyebrow, eyelash)
4. Skin
   - Vitiligo (face, hand, chest, and back)
5. Nonspecific
   - Slight fever

III. OCULAR MANIFESTATIONS

1. Conjunctiva
   - Perilimbal depigmentation at the convalescent stage (Sugiura's sign)
2. Uvea/retina/optic nerve
   - Early ophthalmic acute stage
     - Bilateral uveitis with sudden onset
     - Iridocyclitis (cells and flare in the anterior chamber)
     - Choroiditis
     - Exudative retinal detachment
     - Multifocal dye leakage from retinal pigment epithelium (RPE) by fluorescein angiography
     - Hypermia and edema of the optic disc
   - Convalescent stage
     - Depigmentation of the iris
     - Mutton fat–like keratic precipitates
     - Koeppe's nodules at the pupillary pargin
     - Sunset glow fundus
     - Dalen-Fuchs nodules
3. Ocular complications
   - Posterior synechia
   - Complicated cataract
   - Secondary glaucoma
   - Chorioretinal degeneration
   - Subretinal neovascularization

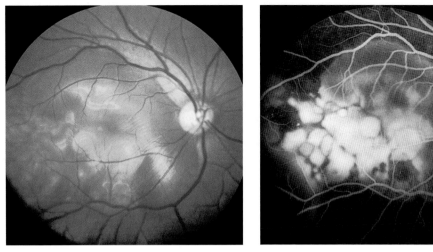

FIGURE 69.1. Exudative retinal detachment in the posterior pole of the fundus (**A**) and multifocal dye leakage from RPE by fluorescein angiography (**B**) in a 38-year-old woman with Vogt-Koyanagi-Harada syndrome. The pictures were taken 7 days after the onset of bilateral uveitis.

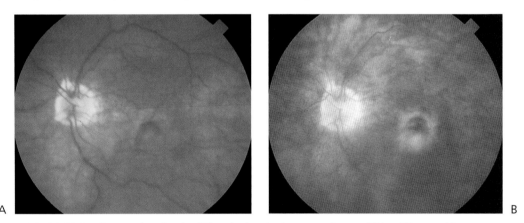

FIGURE 69.2. Sunset glow fundus (**A**) and subretinal neovascular net (**B**) in a 59-year-old woman with Vogt-Koyanagi-Harada syndrome. The patient developed the disease in March 1992 and the pictures were taken in February 1993.

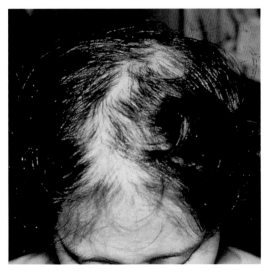

FIGURE 69.3. Hair loss seen in a 34-year-old woman at 3 months after the onset of Vogt-Koyanagi-Harada syndrome.

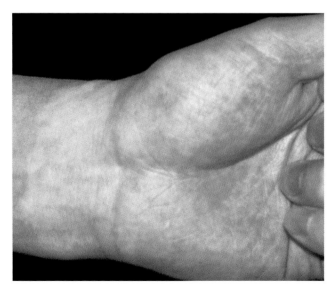

FIGURE 69.4. Vitiligo at the wrist skin of the left hand in a 42-year-old man who had developed Vogt-Koyanagi-Harada syndrome 8 months before.

SUGGESTED REFERENCES

Inomata H, Kato M. Vogt-Koyanagi-Harada disease. In: Vinken PJ, Bruyn GW, Klawans, eds. *Hand-book of Clinical Neurology,* Amsterdam: Elsevier Science Publishers; 1989;12:611–625. *A review of the clinical findings and ocular pathology of the disease.*

Mizuki N, Inoko H, Ohno S. Role of HLA and T lymphocytes in the immune response. *Ocular Immunol Inflammation* 1994;2:57–91. *A good review of the role of HLA and T lymphocytes in the immune response in relation to ocular diseases including Vogt-Koyanagi-Harada syndrome.*

Mochizuki M. Vogt-Koyanagi-Harada syndrome. In: Gold DH, Weingeist TA, eds. *The Eye in Systemic Disease.* Philadelphia: JB Lippincott; 1990:293–295. *A review of systemic and ophthalmic manifestations of the disease.*

Nussenblatt RB, Palestine AG, eds. Vogt-Koyanagi-Harada syndrome. In: *Uveitis: Fundamentals and Clinical Practice.* Chicago: Year Book Medical Publishers; 1989:274–289. *A good review of the clinical findings, laboratory tests, etiology, and treatment of the disease.*

Rao NA, Forster DJ, Augsburger JJ, eds. Vogt-Koyanagi-Harada syndrome. In: *The Uvea: Uveitis and In-traocular Neoplasms.* New York: Gower Medical Publisher; 1992. *A review of the ocular findings with clinical color pictures.*

PART 10. MALIGNANT DISORDERS

Chapter 70

METASTATIC MALIGNANT TUMORS (EYE)

Jerry A. Shields
Carol L. Shields

I. GENERAL

1. A malignant neoplasm that spreads to the ocular structures from a distant primary malignancy
2. Most are carcinomas. Melanoma is relatively rare and sarcomas are extremely rare.
3. May affect the eyelid, conjunctiva, intraocular structures, or orbit
4. Most affect the uveal tract. The posterior uvea (choroid) is the most common site of uveal metastasis. Iris and ciliary body metastasis are considerably less common.
5. Orbital, eyelid, and conjunctival metastasis are less common.
6. Occurs almost exclusively in adulthood; extremely rare in childhood
7. More common in women because breast cancer accounts for most ocular metastasis
8. No racial predisposition
9. Reaches the ocular area via hematogenous routes
10. About 25% of patients with uveal or orbital metastasis who present to the ophthalmologist have no prior history of a primary cancer. Hence, the ophthalmologist must be familiar with the systemic and ophthalmic manifestations of ocular metastasis.

II. SYSTEMIC MANIFESTATIONS

1. Depends on location of primary tumor. If there is no history of a primary cancer, systemic symptoms and signs may suggest the primary site.
2. Ocular metastasis from breast cancer: concurrent evidence of a breast mass
3. Ocular metastasis from lung cancer: cough, hemoptysis
4. Ocular metastasis from gastrointestinal cancer: abdominal discomfort and distention
5. Ocular metastasis from kidney cancer: abdominal or back pain, hematuria
6. Ocular metastasis from cutaneous melanoma: history of prior excision of a pigmented lesion or concurrent presence of a cutaneous pigmented lesion
7. Patients with ocular metastasis from other primary neoplasms may have symptoms related to the primary site.

III. OCULAR MANIFESTATIONS

1. The ocular manifestations of metastatic cancer vary with whether the metastasis occurs in the uveal tract, optic disc, orbit, eyelids, or conjunctiva.
2. Choroidal metastasis (Fig. 70.1) occurs as one or more yellow, sessile, or dome-shaped tumors deep to the retina. Secondary serous retinal detachment is common.
3. Iris metastasis (Fig. 70.2) presents as a yellow-white friable lesion that may seed diffusely through the anterior chamber and simulate uveitis or endophthalmitis.
4. Ciliary body metastasis may attain a large size because of its hidden location behind the iris. It can seed tumor cells into the surrounding structures and clinically simulate an iridocyclitis.
5. Optic disc metastasis (Fig. 70.3) presents as an infiltrative swelling of the optic nerve head with ipsilateral visual loss. In contrast to papilledema, it is almost always unilateral.
6. Orbital metastasis generally occurs as proptosis, often associated with pain and oculomotor palsies.
7. Eyelid metastasis (Fig. 70.4) usually occurs as a rapidly enlarging, firm, subepidermal mass that may initially suggest a chalazion.
8. Conjunctival metastasis occurs as a diffuse red-yellow mass usually in the bulbar conjunctiva.

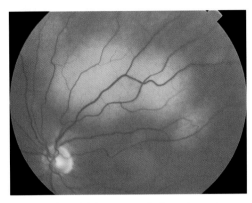

FIGURE 70.1. Choroidal metastasis from breast cancer. Note the creamy yellow sessile subretinal masses.

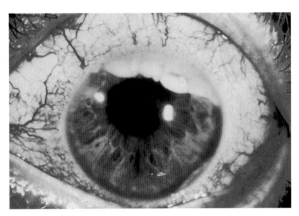

FIGURE 70.2. Iris metastasis from breast cancer. The superior tumor in the anterior chamber is loosely cohesive.

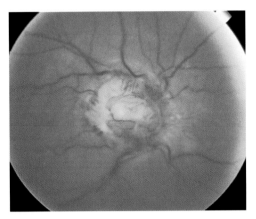

FIGURE 70.3. Metastatic lung cancer to the optic disc. A fine-needle aspiration biopsy established the diagnosis and the primary lung cancer was found on a repeat systemic evaluation.

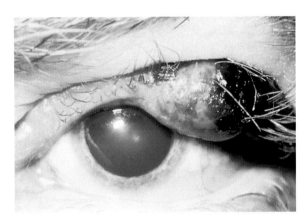

FIGURE 70.4. Metastatic renal cell carcinoma to the upper eyelid. The lesion was initially diagnosed as a chalazion, but biopsy revealed metastatic renal cell carcinoma. Subsequent systemic evaluation revealed a mass in the kidney.

SUGGESTED READINGS

Kiratli H, Shields CL, Shields JA, De Potter P. Metastatic tumors to the conjunctiva. Report of ten cases. *Brit J Opthalmol* 1996;80:5–8.

Shields CL, Shields JA, Gross N, Schwartz G, Lally S. Survey of 520 uveal metastases. *Opthalmology* 1997;104:1265–1276.

Shields JA, Shields CL. *Atlas of Eyelid and Conjuctival Tumors.* Philadelphia: Lippincott Williams and Wilkins, 1999.

Shields JA, Shields CL. *Atlas of Intraocular Tumors.* Philadelphia: Lippincott Williams and Wilkins, 1999.

Shields JA, Shields CL. *Atlas of Orbital Tumors.* Philadelphia: Lippincott Williams and Wilkins, 1999.

Shields JA, Shields CL, Kiratli H, De Potter P. Metastatic tumors to the iris in 40 patients. *Am J Opthalmol* 1995;119:422–430.

Shields JA, Shields CL, Singh AD. Metastatic neoplasms in the optic disc. The 1999 Bjerrum Lecture. Part 2. *Arch Opthalmol* 2000; 118:217–224.

Chapter 71

LYMPHOMA

James Augsburger
Ingrid E. Zimmer-Galler
Andrew P. Schachat

I. GENERAL

1. Systemic
   - Heterogeneous group of lymphoid malignancies characterized by uncontrolled proliferation of neoplastic lymphocytic cells; highly variable clinical presentation, response to therapy and prognosis
   - Distinguished clinically and pathologically from acute and chronic lymphoid leukemias and the immunoglobulin-synthesizing lymphoproliferative diseases (such as multiple myeloma and Waldenström's macroglobulinemia)
   - Frequent cause of death in affected individuals
   - Two major categories of disease: Hodgkin's disease and non-Hodgkin's lymphoma (NHL)
   - Many subcategories of NHL according to histopathologic and immunohistochemical features and clinical course. All exhibit monoclonal expansion of either malignant B (most common) or T lymphocytes.
   - Hodgkin's disease rarely has ophthalmic manifestations, whereas several forms of NHL frequently involve the eyes and/or orbits.
   - Cause of this malignancy is unknown, but genetic factors, environmental factors, and immunodeficiency have all been implicated.
   - Affects men and women in similar proportions, and occurs in all races
   - Annual number of new cases in the United States is approximately 18,000 for NHL and 7500 for Hodgkin's disease.
   - Peak of incidence for NHL occurs during fourth to fifth decades of life, but is substantially earlier in Hodgkin's disease.

2. Intraocular non-Hodgkin's lymphoma
   - Much less common than other forms of NHL.
   - Average age at diagnosis of ocular involvement is 60 years.
   - Intraocular involvement may be more common in women than men.
   - Intraocular disease can be isolated (22%), but more commonly occurs in association with central nervous system (56%) or visceral (16%) involvement or both (6%).
   - Is bilateral or becomes bilateral in approximately 80% of cases
   - Median survival time from the onset of ocular symptoms is less than 2 years.

II. SYSTEMIC MANIFESTATIONS

1. Lymphatic
   - Painless, persistent, peripheral lymphadenopathy
   - Retroperitoneal, pelvic, mesenteric, mediastinal node involvement
2. Pulmonary
   - Chronic cough
   - Pleural effusions
   - Parenchymal involvement
3. Gastrointestinal
   - Painless abdominal mass
   - Hepatosplenomegaly
4. Neurologic
   - Intracranial mass
   - Increased intracranial pressure
   - Higher cortical function deficits (confusion, memory loss)
   - Focal neurologic deficits (hemiparesis, dysphagia)
   - Seizures
   - Headache
   - Cranial nerve dysfunction
5. Hematologic
   - Bone marrow involvement
   - Peripheral blood involvement
   - Anemia (usually associated with bone marrow replacement by lymphoma cell)
6. Renal
   - Renal insufficiency (obstruction by retroperitoneal tumor)
7. Cutaneous
   - Multiple cutaneous or subcutaneous lesions
8. Nonspecific
   - Fever
   - Night sweats
   - Weight loss
   - Weakness
   - Fatigue

III. OCULAR MANIFESTATIONS*

1. Orbit
- Space-occupying mass causing proptosis, motility problems, diplopia
- Lacrimal gland mass

2. Lids
- Puffiness or swelling, ptosis
- Solid palpable mass

3. Conjunctiva
- Pink subepithelial conjunctival tumor

4. Cornea
- Keratic precipitates

5. Uvea
- Anterior segment inflammation
- Diffuse or localized lymphoid infiltrates of iris, ciliary body, and/or choroid
- Pseudohypopyon
- Iris mass
- Iris neovascularization

6. Retina
- Fuzzy white superficial retinal infiltrates ("retinitis")
- Intraretinal hemorrhages
- Perivascular infiltrates of lymphoid cells ("perivasculitis")
- Nonrhegmatogenous retinal detachment
- Multiple solid subretinal pigment epithelial masses
- Retinal anteriolar occlusions
- Macular edema
- Exudative retinal detachment

7. Vitreous
- Diffuse infiltration by finely dispersed white cells
- Large intravitreal cellular clumps in some patients
- Vitreous hemorrhage

8. Optic disc/Neuroophthalmologic
- Congestion due to infiltration by lymphoma cells
- Papilledema due to lymphoma in brain
- Cranial nerve palsy

9. Nonspecific
- Painless, blurred vision
- Floaters

---

* Two general clinical forms of NHL have been associated with ophthalmic manifestations: (1) primary lymphoma of the CNS and retina is a multicentric malignancy (usually diffuse large-cell lymphoma by histopathologic and immunologic analysis) that is frequently confined to the eyes and brain; it is principally characterized by vitreous cells and retinal and subretinal pigment epithelial infiltrates; rarely is it associated with lid, orbital, conjunctival, or uveal infiltrates; (2) primary visceral lymphoma with ophthalmic manifestations is the more common form of systemic NHL; this form is characterized by orbital, lid, and conjunctival tumors and occasionally by focal or diffuse uveal infiltrates; involvement of the retina and vitreous are uncommon, and brain involvement occurs almost exclusively as metastatic disease.

SUGGESTED READINGS

Char DH, Ljung BM, Miller T, Phillips T. Primary intraocular lymphoma (ocular reticulum cell sarcoma): Diagnosis and management. *Ophthalmology* 1988;95:625–630.

Fine HA, Mayer RJ. Primary central nervous system lymphoma. *Ann Intern Med* 1993;119:1093–1104. *A comprehensive review of diagnosis and treatment in central nervous system lymphoma.*

Freeman LN, Schachat AP, Knox DL, et al. Clinical features, laboratory investigations, and survival in ocular reticulum cell sarcoma. *Ophthalmology* 1987;94:1631–1639. *A large clinical series from the ophthalmic literature.*

Garner A. Orbital lymphoproliferative disorders. *Br J Ophthalmol* 1992;76:47–48. *A nice "mini review" of orbital lymphoid tumors with a current bibliography.*

Longo DL, DeVita VT, Jaffe ES, et al. Lymphocytic Lymphomas. In: DeVita VT, Hellman A, Rosenberg SA, eds. *Cancer: Principles and Practice of Oncology,* 4th ed. Philadelphia: JB Lippincott; 1993:1859–1927. *One of the classic oncology textbooks.*

Peterson K, Gordon KB, Heinemann MH, DeAngelis LM. The clinical spectrum of ocular lymphoma. *Cancer* 1993;72:843–849.

Non-Hodgkin's Lymphoma Pathologic Classification Project: National Cancer Institute sponsored study of classifications of non-Hodgkin's lymphomas. *Cancer* 1982;49:2112–2135. *Outlines the National Cancer Institute Working Formulation.*

Ridley ME, McDonald HR, Sternberg P, et al. Retinal manifestations of ocular lymphoma (reticulum cell sarcoma). *Ophthalmology* 1992;99:1153–1161. *Describes the "retinitic" type of intraocular non-Hodgkin's lymphoma.*

Whitcup SM, deSmet MD, Rubin BI, et al. Intraocular lymphoma. Clinical and histopathological diagnosis. *Ophthalmology* 1993;100:1399–1406.

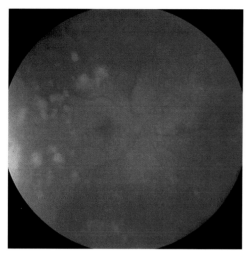

FIGURE 71.1. Diffuse intravitreal cells in large clumps in 62-year-old woman with primary intraocular lymphoma.

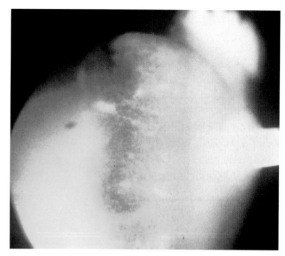

FIGURE 71.2. Vitreous infiltrate in non-Hodgkin's lymphoma.

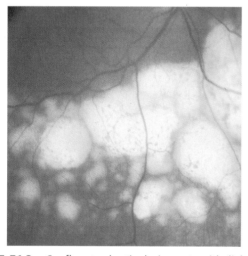

FIGURE 71.3. Confluent subretinal pigment epithelial masses outside the inferior arcade of the right eye in intraocular non-Hodgkin's lymphoma. Courtesy of Michael Novak, MD.

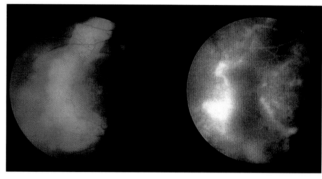

A   B

FIGURE 71.4. Classic geographic subretinal pigment epithelial lesion of primary intraocular lymphoma. **(A)** Amelanotic subretinal pigment epithelial infiltrate with surrounding smaller "satellite lesions." **(B)** Late phase frame of fluorescein angiogram showing hypofluorescence of lesion proper and leakage of dye from its margins.

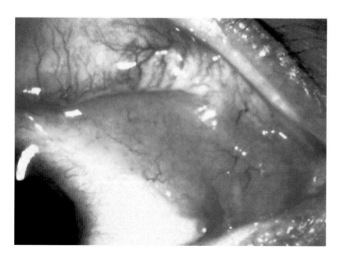

FIGURE 71.5. Subepithelial lymphoma of conjunctiva arising in superonasal fornix of 59-year-old man with primary visceral non-Hodgkin's lymphoma.

PART II.   METABOLIC DISORDERS

Section A.   Disorders of Amino Acid Metabolism

Chapter 72

ALBINISM

Scott W. Hyver
Everett Ai

I. GENERAL

1. Heterogeneous group of genetically determined disorders of the melanocyte pigmentary system affecting the skin and eye
2. Variable phenotypic expression depending on syndrome
3. Incidence: 1/5000 to 1/20,000 births
4. Absence or dysfunction of tyrosinase—enzyme involved in melanin synthesis (tyrosinase-negative oculocutaneous albinism, autosomal recessive)
5. Abnormal melanosome maturation with normal tyrosinase activity (tyrosinase-positive oculocutaneous albinism, autosomal recessive)
6. Decreased number of melanocytes with normal melanosomes and tyrosinase activity (ocular albinism, X-linked, and autosomal recessive)
7. Dermatologic without ocular abnormalities (albinoidism, autosomal dominant)
8. Hair bulb incubation test for tyrosinase activity

II. SYSTEMIC MANIFESTATIONS

1. Dermatologic
   - Skin and hair hypopigmentation
   - Easy sunburning
   - Cutaneous sqaumous cell carcinoma
2. Hematologic
   - Bleeding diathesis (Hermansky-Pudlak)
   - Reticuloendothelial incompetence (Chediak-Higashi)
   - Lymphohistiocytic malignancies (Chediak-Higashi)
   - Generalized lymphadenopathy (Chediak-Higashi)
3. Pulmonary
   - Pulmonary fibrosis (Hermansky-Pudlak)
4. Gastrointestinal
   - Granulomatous colitis (Hermansky-Pudlak)
   - Gingival fibromatosis (Cross)
5. Renal
   - Renal failure (Hermansky-Pudlak)
6. Neurologic
   - Mental retardation (Chediak-Higashi, Cross)
   - Peripheral neuropathy (Chediak-Higashi)
   - Athetosis (Cross)
7. Psychological
   - Social stress from unusual appearance

III. OCULAR MANIFESTATIONS

1. Iris
   - Pale color
   - Diaphanous
   - Transillumination
2. Fundus
   - Hypopigmentation
   - Foveal hypoplasia
3. Neuroophthalmologic
   - Congenital nystagmus
   - Strabismus
   - Abnormal chiasmal decussation
   - Other visual pathway abnormalities
   - Absence of binocularity
4. Nonspecific
   - Decreased vision
   - Protanomaly
   - Photophobia
   - Refractive errors
   - Anterior segment dysgenesis
   - Microphthalmia (Cross)

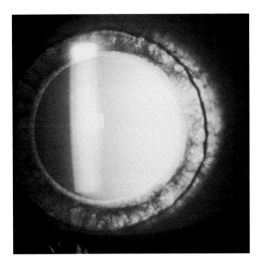

FIGURE 72.1. Iris transillumination.

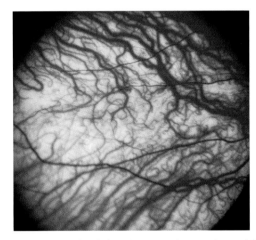

FIGURE 72.2. Fundus hypopigmentation and resulting increased visibility of choroidal vasculature.

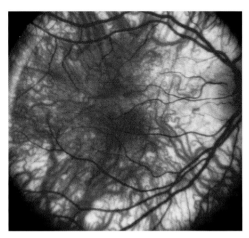

FIGURE 72.3. Foveal hypoplasia—absence of the foveal reflex as well as a defined foveal avascular zone.

SUGGESTED READINGS

Ai E, Coonan P. Albinism. In: Gold DH, Weingeist TA, eds. *The Eye in Systemic Disease.* Philadelphia: JB Lippincott; 1990:311–314.

McHam ML, Fulton A. Albinism. *Int Ophthalmol Clin* 1992;32:185–200.

Spencer WH. *Ophthalmic Pathology: An Atlas and Textbook.* Philadelphia: WB Saunders; 1985:607–613.

Witkop CJ Jr, Quevedo WC Jr, Fitzpatrick TB. Albinism and other disorders of pigment metabolism. In: Stanbury JB, Wyngaarden JB, Frederickson DS, et al, eds. *The Metabolic Basis of Inherited Disease,* 5th ed. New York: McGraw-Hill; 1983:301–346.

Chapter 73

CYSTINOSIS

Muriel I. Kaiser-Kupfer
William A. Gahl

I. GENERAL

1. Cystinosis is an autosomal recessive disorder occurring in most populations.
2. Cystine accumulates within cellular lysosomes due to impaired transport into the cytoplasm.
3. Cystine crystallizes because of its poor solubility, destroying parenchymal cells of various organs.
4. Laboratory diagnosis relies on measurement of intracellular cystine, specifically in polymorphonuclear leucocytes or cultured fibroblasts.
5. Symptomatic therapy includes replacement of renal losses due to tubular Fanconi syndrome, as well as kidney transplantation once renal failure develops.
6. The treatment of choice for the primary defect is oral cysteamine, which lowers the intracellular cystine content by over 90%, preserves renal function, allows growth, and may prevent progression of the nonrenal complications.
7. Cysteamine eye drops remove corneal crystals.

II. SYSTEMIC MANIFESTATIONS

1. Renal
   - Polyuria/dehydration/polydipsia
   - Proximal tubular acidosis
   - Hypokalemia
   - Phosphaturia/hypophosphatemia
   - Hypercalciuria
   - Hyponatremia
   - Hypomagnesemia
   - Uremia
2. Endocrine
   - Hypothyroidism
   - Hypogonadism (males)
   - Insulin-dependent diabetes mellitus
3. Musculoskeletal
   - Growth retardation
   - Hypophosphatemic, vitamin D–resistant rickets
   - Poor muscular development
   - Vacuolar myopathy
4. Gastrointestinal
   - Vomiting
   - Penchant for salty, spicy foods
   - Pancreatic exocrine insufficiency
5. Mucocutaneous
   - Decreased salivation
   - Decreased sweating
   - Hypopigmentation
6. Ear/nose/throat
   - Dysphagia
   - Hypophonia
7. Hematologic
   - Increased sedimentation rate
   - Anemia
8. Neurologic
   - Cerebral atrophy
   - Basal ganglia calcification
9. Nonspecific
   - Failure to thrive

III. OCULAR MANIFESTATIONS

1. Conjunctiva
   - Crystals
2. Cornea
   - Crystals
   - Corneal erosions
   - Band keratopathy (late complication)
3. Iris
   - Crystals
   - Posterior synechia (late complication)
4. Intraocular pressure
   - Glaucoma (late complication)
5. Retina
   - Pigment epithelial depigmentation
   - Elevated cone thresholds (late complication)
   - Reduced or extinguished electroretinogram (late complication)
   - Color vision defects (late complication)
6. Nonspecific
   - Extreme photophobia
   - Blepharospasm

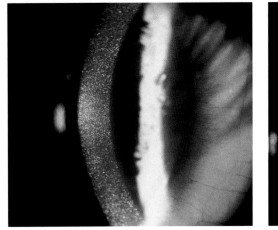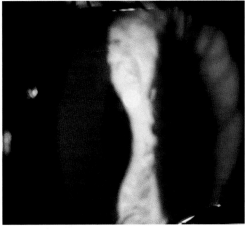

FIGURE 73.1. Slit lamp photographs of the cornea in a patient with nephropathic cystinosis who was part of a study conducted at the National Institutes of Health to determine the efficacy of cysteamine eye drops in the removal of corneal crystals. **(A)** Right cornea at age 2 years 4 months at the time of initiation of topical cysteamine 0.5% eye drops showing moderate deposition of corneal crystals. **(B)** Right cornea after 3 months of treatment with topical cysteamine 0.5% eye drops (10 drops/day) showing complete resolution of the corneal crystals.

SUGGESTED READINGS

Gahl WA, Schneider JA, Aula PP. Cystinosis and sialic acid storage disorders. In: Scriver CR, Beaudet AL, Sly WS, Valle D, eds. *The Metabolic Basis of Inherited Disease.* New York: McGraw-Hill; 1994: Chapter 126. *A comprehensive review of the medical scientific fund of knowledge concerning cystinosis.*

Kaiser-Kupfer MI, Caruso RC, Minckler DS, Gahl WA. Long-term ocular manifestations in nephropathic cystinosis: Post renal transplantation. *Arch Ophthalmol* 1986;104:706–711.

Kaiser-Kupfer MI, Gazzo MA, Datiles MB, et al. A randomized placebo-controlled trial of cysteamine eye drops in nephropathic cystinosis. *Arch Ophthalmol* 1990;108:689–693.

Chapter 74

HARTNUP DISORDER

Kathryn M. Brady-McCreery
David A. Hiles

I. GENERAL

1. This rare autosomal recessive familial metabolic disorder is characterized by impaired neutral amino acid transportation involving the renal tubules and columnar epithelial cells of the jejunum.
2. Parental consanguinity is a predisposing factor.
3. Diagnosis is based on biochemical rather than clinical abnormalities. A characteristic pattern of neutral hyperaminoaciduria is considered the *sine qua non* for diagnosis.
4. Although the intestinal transport of affected monoamino acids is reduced, separate unaffected transport systems exist for the absorption of these same amino acids as peptides. Therefore, only a relative amino acid deficiency exists, which becomes clinically important in times of inadequate dietary intake.
5. There is defective absorption of tryptophan; intestinal flora convert this to indole compounds that are excreted in excess in the urine.
6. The "pellagra-like" features of the disorder and the clinical response to the administration of nicotinamide suggest that there may be nicotinic acid deficiency. However, serum niacin and nicotinic acid derivative levels have been found to be normal. It appears to be due to a reduction in available tryptophan as opposed to a block in the catabolism of tryptophan to nicotinic acid.
7. Most carriers of the disorder as identified by routine newborn urine screening are asymptomatic. It is felt that clinical expression of the disease requires complicating factors such as diarrhea or poor diet.
8. Clinical exacerbations are thought to be due to a combination of the systemic accumulation of toxic indole compounds and a relative nicotinamide deficiency.

II. SYSTEMIC MANIFESTATIONS

1. The disease is characterized by exacerbations and remissions with its onset in late infancy.
2. A photosensitive rash on exposed areas of the body may be eczematous or on occasion bullous. This is followed by desquamation and depigmentation.
3. Severe cerebellar ataxia usually appears after the rash. Complete recovery generally occurs over several weeks.
4. Mental disturbances occur and range from emotional lability to psychosis and usually resolve completely. However cases of progressive neurologic deterioration have been reported.
5. Mental retardation was present in the first two reported cases; however, very few of the subsequently reported cases have evidence of this.
6. Edema, hypoproteinemia, diarrhea, atrophic glossitis, and fatty degeneration of the liver have been reported.
7. Small stature is a common feature.
8. Neurologic findings include headaches, increased muscle tone and deep tendon reflexes, seizures, choreiform movements associated with ataxia, vasovagal attacks, and dystonia.
9. The electroencephalogram may be abnormal in patients with neurologic involvement. These abnormalities are nonspecific and generalized.
10. Treatment consists of oral nicotinamide 50 to 300 mg/day in patients who have signs suggestive of deficiency. This often results in the disappearance of the rash and improves ataxia and psychotic behavior in many instances.
11. Protein supplementation is beneficial in patients with low plasma amino acids. Oral neomycin, by clearing the intestine of flora, may result in reduced indole compound accumulation and clinical improvement. Tryptophan ethyl ester may also be effective.

III. OCULAR MANIFESTATIONS

1. Nystagmus, which may be horizontal or vertical in association with exacerbations of ataxia
2. Ptosis
3. Photosensitive skin rash involving the lids
4. Conjunctival xerosis with skin rash
5. Diplopia and strabismus with acute exacerbations
6. Optic atrophy and diffuse cerebral atrophy most marked in the occipital lobes

SUGGESTED READINGS

Darras BT, Ampola MG, Dietz WH, Gilmore HE. Intermittent dystonia in Hartnup disease. *Pediatr Neurol* 1989;5:118–120.

Hiles DA, Hered RW. Hartnup disease. In: Gold DH, Weingeist TA, eds. *The Eye in Systemic Disease.* Philadelphia: JB Lippincott; 1990:316–318.

Jonas AJ, Butler IJ. Circumvention of defective neutral amino acid transport in Hartnup disease using tryptophan ethyl ester. *J Clin Invest* 1989;84:200–204.

Levy HL. Hartnup disorder. In: Scriver CR, Beaudet AL, Sly WS, Valle D, eds. *The Metabolic Basis of Inherited Disease.* New York: Mc Graw-Hill; 1989:2515–2527.

Schmidtke K, Endres W, Roscher A, et al. Hartnup syndrome, progressive encephalopathy and allo-albuminaemia. A clinico-pathological case study. *Eur J Pediatr* 1992;151:899–903.

Chapter 75

HOMOCYSTINURIA

Aki Kawasaki
Forrest D. Ellis

1. Homocystinuria refers to a group of inherited disorders of metabolism characterized by markedly elevated plasma and urine homocysteine levels.
2. "Classical" homocystinuria, the best known and most common type, is due to deficiency of cystathionine β-synthase (CBS), the enzyme that converts homocysteine to cystathionine. Other types are defect in vitamin B_{12} metabolism, deficiency of N(5,10)-methylenetetrahydrofolate reductase, and selective intestinal malabsorption of vitamin B_{12}.
3. The gene for CBS is on chromosome 21. CBS deficiency is inherited as an autosomal recessive trait and occurs 1/335,000 births.
4. Elevated plasma homocysteine leads to defective collagen cross-linking. Ocular zonular fibers are composed of glycoprotein with high concentrations of cysteine. Lens dislocation is common (50% to nearly 100%) and bony abnormalities such as long thin bones and scoliosis are characteristic.
5. Elevated homocysteine is toxic to endothelial cells, increases platelet adhesiveness, and promotes intravascular thrombus formation. Premature thromboembolic disease is the chief cause of morbidity and mortality among homocystinurics with an incidence of 60% by age 40 years.
6. In newborns, urinary cyanide-nitroprusside reaction is positive and quantitative blood analysis shows severe elevation of homocysteine and methionine. Skin biopsy confirms deficient CBS activity in cultured fibroblasts.
7. Treatment involves dietary restriction of methionine with supplementation of pyridoxine (vitamin B_6), folate, and betaine.

II. SYSTEMIC MANIFESTATIONS

1. Cardiac
   - Coronary artery disease
2. Vascular
   - Premature atherosclerosis
   - Arterial occlusion (thrombi, emboli)
   - Venous thrombosis
3. Pulmonary
   - Pulmonary embolus
   - Cor pulmonale
4. Renal
   - Renal infarction
   - Hypertension
5. Gastrointestinal
   - Pancreatitis
   - Fatty liver
6. Genitourinary
   - Inguinal hernia
7. Neurologic
   - Developmental delay
   - Mental retardation
   - Behavioral problems
   - Psychiatric disorders
   - Seizures
   - Extrapyramidal signs (dystonia)
   - Cerebrovascular disease (stroke)
8. Hematologic
   - Platelet dysfunction
   - Clotting factor abnormalities
9. Endocrine
   - Hypoglycemia
10. Musculoskeletal
    - Marfanoid features
      - Thinning and lengthening of long bones (dolichostenomelia)
      - Pes cavus
      - High arched palate
      - Pectus carinatum or excavatum
      - Genu valgus
      - Arachnodactyly
      - Scoliosis
      - Kyphosis
      - "Fish" vertebrae (biconcave)
    - Osteoporosis
    - Short fourth metacarpal
    - Widened metaphyses
    - Myopathy
11. Mucocutaneous
    - Malar flush
    - Livedo reticularis
    - Hypopigmentation, skin and hair (reversible in pyridoxine-responsive patients)
    - Thin, brittle hair
12. Ear/nose/throat
    - Dental anomalies

III. OCULAR MANIFESTATIONS

1. Conjunctiva/sclera
   - Thin or blue sclera
2. Cornea
   - Peripheral iridocorneal adhesions
3. Intraocular pressure
   - Acute pupillary block glaucoma
4. Lens

- Bilateral subluxation (ectopia lentis)
- Cataracts
- High myopia
5. Retina
   - Central retinal artery occlusion
   - Peripheral retinal degeneration
   - Retinal detachment

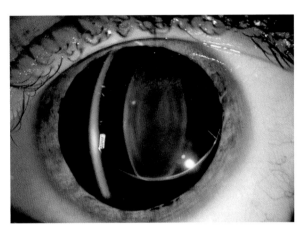

FIGURE 75.1. Superiorly dislocated lens.

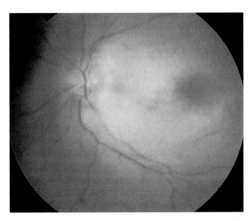

FIGURE 75.2. Retinal edema and cherry-red macula from central retinal artery occlusion.

SUGGESTED READINGS

Cross HE, Jensen AD. Ocular manifestations in the Marfan syndrome and homocystinuria. *Am J Ophthalmol* 1973; 75:405–420.

Mudd SH, Levy HL, Skovby F. Disorders of transsulfuration. In: Scriver CR, Beaudet AL, Sly WS, Valle D, eds. In: *The Metabolic and Molecular Basis of Inherited Disease*, 7th ed. New York: McGraw-Hill; 1995:1279–1327.

Chapter 76

HYPERORNITHINEMIA

Muriel I. Kaiser-Kupfer
David L. Valle

I. GENERAL

1. Autosomal recessive disorder occurring in all populations but most commonly in Finns
2. The primary defect is deficiency of ornithine-δ-aminotransferase (OAT), which catalyzes the interconversion of ornithine and Δ^1 pyrroline-5-carboxylate, an intermediate in proline and glutamate metabolism. OAT activity can be measured in cultured skin fibroblasts.
3. OAT deficiency results in accumulation of ornithine in all body fluids to levels that are 10- to 15-fold normal. For example, normal plasma ornithine is 75 ± 23 μM (mean $\pm$ SD), whereas in gyrate atrophy patients on a regular diet, plasma ornithine values are 848 ± 180 μM (range 400–1339 μM).

4. The *OAT* gene is located at 10q26 and more than 60 mutations have been described in gyrate atrophy patients.
5. Current treatment involves an initial trial of pyridoxine (vitamin B_6). A few patients (<5%) respond with a significant (>50%) reduction in fasting plasma ornithine. For pyridoxine nonresponders, an arginine-restricted diet can be used to reduce ornithine levels to near normal. Long-term studies suggest that chronic reduction of ornithine slows or prevents further chorioretinal degeneration; however, only about 20% of patients are able to maintain this highly restrictive diet.

II. SYSTEMIC MANIFESTATIONS

1. A few patients have mild proximal muscle weakness. Nonspecific histologic (type 2 fiber atrophy) and electron microscopic (tubular aggregates) abnormalities are present in the skeletal muscle of most patients.

2. About one-third of patients have mild to moderate diffuse slowing on electroencephalography. Seizures do not occur with increased frequency and intelligence is normal.

III. OCULAR MANIFESTATIONS

1. Lens
   - Posterior subcapsular cataracts (late-term)
   - Anterior polar, mixed cataracts
2. Vitreous
   - Syneresis, ropy
3. Retina
   - Peripheral chorioretinal atrophy, 360°
   - Circumferential garland appearance with
   - Hyperpigmentation at margins of atrophy
   - Peripapillary atrophy

4. Myopia
5. Psychophysical and electroretinography (ERG)
   - Constricted fields
   - Nyctalopia
   - Abnormal color vision
   - Markedly decreased ERG amplitude
6. Progressive loss of function

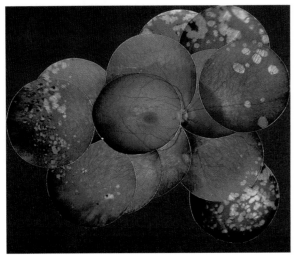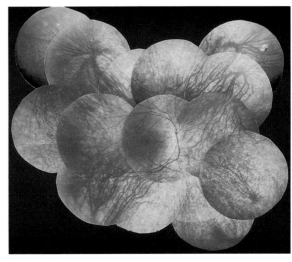

A

B

FIGURE 76.1. Photomontages of the retina. (**A**) right retina at age 6 years 4 months of the older sibling at the time of diagnosis of gyrate atrophy showing multiple peripheral atrophic lesions. (**B**), right retina at age 9 years and 10 months of the younger sibling showing only a peripheral solitary atrophic lesion (1 o'clock position). The younger sibling had been receiving the low arginine diet for 84 months, beginning at 2 years 10 months at the time this photomontage was taken. Three years have elapsed since these photos and no subsequent atrophic lesions have developed. This minimal involvement should be compared with the multiple lesions in her sibling at age 6 years and 4 months.

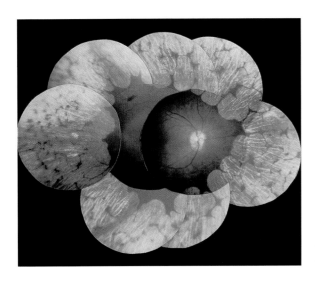

FIGURE 76.2. Photomontage of retina. Right retina in patient in late teens with 360° scalloped chorioretinal atrophy.

SUGGESTED READINGS

Kaiser-Kupfer MI, Caruso RC, Valle D. Gyrate atrophy of the choroid and retina: Long-term reduction of ornithine slows retinal degeneration. *Arch Ophthalmol* 1991;109:1539–1548.

Valle D, Simmell O. The hyperornithinemias. In: Scriver RC, Beaudet AL, Sly WS, Valle D, eds. *The Metabolic Basis of Inherited Disease.* New York: McGraw-Hill; 1989:599–627. *A comprehensive review of the medical scientific fund of knowledge concerning gyrate atrophy.*

Chapter 77
OCHRONOSIS
Mary Seabury Stone

I. GENERAL

1. Usually associated with the rare autosomal recessive disorder, alkaptonuria (incidence <1:250,000)
2. In alkaptonuria, the enzyme homogentisic acid oxidase, required for phenylalanine and tyrosine degradation, is absent. Homogentisic acid accumulates and is metabolized to ochronotic pigment.
3. Ochronosis without underlying alkaptonuria, called exogenous ochronosis, has been reported following prolonged application of carbolic acid to leg ulcers. Skin-limited exogenous ochronosis can result from topical hydroquinone bleaching creams and from antimalarial drug ingestion.

II. SYSTEMIC MANIFESTATIONS

1. Cutaneous
    - Blue-gray pigmentation is seen most prominently on ears, nose, extensor tendons of hands, and costochondral junctions.
    - It generally appears in the fourth decade.
    - Discolored sweat may stain skin and clothing.
2. Musculoskeletal
    - Arthropathy of spine and large joints
    - Tendon rupture
    - Black cartilage, tendons, and ligaments
3. Cardiac
    - Pigment in heart valves and atherosclerotic plaques
    - Aortic stenosis
4. Pulmonary
    - Pigment deposition may cause stiffening of rib cartilage.
5. Genitourinary
    - Urine turns dark with alkalinization or on standing.
    - Dark-stained diapers may be the first sign of disease.
    - Black prostatic, renal, and bladder stones
6. Ear/nose/throat
    - Black cerumen
    - Blue tympanic membranes
    - External ear is often first area of obvious pigmentation.
    - Hoarseness
7. Nonspecific
    - Despite disabling problems, life expectancy is normal.

III. OCULAR MANIFESTATIONS

1. Conjunctiva/sclera
    - Scleral pigmentation, most pronounced near rectus muscle insertions, begins in the third to fourth decade.
    - Pigmented pinguecula-like changes
2. Cornea
    - Pigmented globules in the peripheral stroma

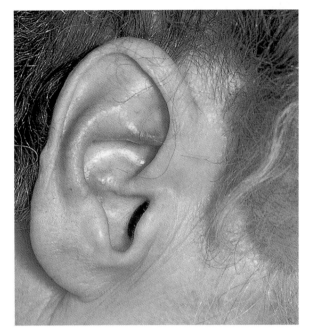

FIGURE 77.1. Bluish gray auricular cartilage in a patient with alkaptonuria. Courtesy of Richard M. Caplan, MD.

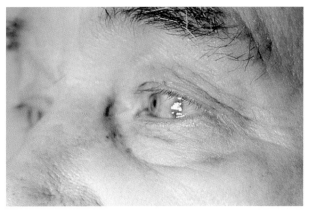

FIGURE 77.2. Ocular ochronosis with scleral pigmentation.

SUGGESTED READINGS

Albers SE, Brozena SJ, Glass LF, Fenske NA. Alkaptonuria and ochronosis: Case report and review. *J Am Acad Dermatol* 1992;27:609–614. *An excellent, concise, clinical review.*

LaDu BN. Alcaptonuria. In: Stanbury JB, Wyngaarden JB, Fredrickson DS, eds. *The Metabolic Basis of Inherited Disease,* 6th ed. New York: McGraw-Hill; 1989:775–790. *An in-depth review of clinical and biochemical aspects of alkaptonuria.*

Stone MS. Ochronosis. In: Gold DH, Weingeist TA, eds. *The Eye in Systemic Disease.* Philadelphia: JB Lippincott; 1990:325–326.

Section B. Disorders of Carbohydrate Metabolism

Chapter 78

GALACTOSEMIA

Harold Skalka

I. GENERAL

1. Autosomal recessive disease
2. May be caused by one of three enzyme deficiencies in galactose metabolic pathway:

$$\text{Galactose ATP} \xrightarrow[\text{(GK)}]{\text{Galactokinase}} \text{Galactose-1-phosphate} + \text{ADP}$$

Galactose-1-phosphate 1 UDP glucose

$$\xrightarrow[\text{(GPUT)}]{\text{Galactose-1-phosphate 1 uridyl transferase}}$$

Glucose-1-phosphate + UDP galactose

$$\text{UDP galactose} \xrightarrow{\text{UDP Galactose-4-epimerase UDP glucose}}$$

3. Manifestations depend on enzyme involved, homo- or hererozygosity (GK), allelic variants (GPUT), and possibly diet.
4. Diagnosis—reducing substances in urine (galactose); distinguish by enzyme assays
5. Cataract—osmotic secondary to dulcitol accumulation in lens
   If galactose cannot be metabolized:

$$\text{Galactose} + \text{NADPH} \xrightarrow[\text{reductase}]{\text{aldose}} \text{dulcitol} + \text{NADP}$$

(Dulcitol does not cross lens cell membranes.)
6. Treatment: lactose-free diet

II. SYSTEMIC MANIFESTATIONS

1. GK deficiency
   - Galactosemia
   - Galactosuria
2. GPUT deficiency
   - Renal
     - Proximal renal tubular acidosis
     - Renal tubular defects
     - Proteinuria
     - Glycosuria
     - Aminoaciduria
     - Phosphaturia
     - Ascites
   - Gastrointestinal
     - Vomiting
     - Diarrhea
     - Hepatosplenomegaly
     - Cirrhosis
     - Jaundice
   - Neurologic
     - Lethargy
     - Mental retardation
     - Extrapyramidal dysfunction
   - Hematologic
     - Galactosemia
     - Hypoglycemia
   - Nonspecific
     - Neonatal sepsis
     - Death if untreated
3. Epimerase deficiency
   - Some may show GPUT-like symptoms.

III. OCULAR MANIFESTATIONS

1. GK
   - Homozygote: cataracts in first few years of life
   - Heterozygote: increased susceptibility to presenile cataracts
2. GPUT
   - Cataracts, often in first few days of life
3. Epimerase
   - Possible increased cataract incidence

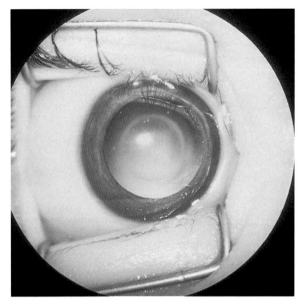

FIGURE 78.1. "Oil-droplet" galactosemic cataract in infancy. Courtesy of Thomas D. France, MD.

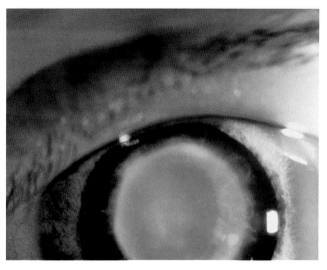

FIGURE 78.2. Nuclear cataract due to galactosemia. Courtesy of Thomas D. France, MD.

SUGGESTED READINGS

Gitzelmann R. Deficiency of eythrocyte galactokinase in a patient with galactose diabetes. *Lancet* 1965; 2:670–671. *The first report identifying GK deficiency in galactosemia.*

Gitzelmann R. Deficiency of uridine diphosphate galactose-4-epimerase in blood cells of an apparently healthy infant. *Helv Paediatr Acta* 1972; 27:125–130. *The first report of epimerase deficiency.*

Isselbacher RJ, Anderson EP, Kurahashi K, et al. Congenital galactosemia, a single enzymatic block in galactose metabolism. *Science* 1956; 123:635–636. *The first report identifying GPUT deficiency in galactosemia.*

Stambolian D. Galactose and cataract. *Surv Ophthalmol* 1988; 32:333–349. *Good review of galactose metabolism and relationship to cataract, with extensive reference list.*

Skalka HW, Prchal JT. Presenile cataract formation and decreased activity of galactosemic enzymes. *Arch Ophthalmol* 1980; 98:269–273. *Report strongly linking GK heterozygosity with "idiopathic" presenile cataract formation.*

Chapter 79

GLYCOGENOSES

Richard S. Smith

I. GENERAL

1. Inherited disorders of altered glycogen metabolism and storage
2. Liver and muscle are most often affected due to their normally abundant stores of glycogen.
3. Hepatomegaly and hypoglycemia are most common liver manifestations.
4. Muscle effects include exercise-induced pain, easy fatigueability, weakness, muscle atrophy, and myoglobinuria.
5. Types I through VII are well characterized genetically and enzymatically. Other varieties have also been described.
6. Only glycogenoses I and II have ocular manifestations.
7. Glycogenosis type I (von Gierke's disease) is characterized by glucose-6-phosphatase deficiency and is inherited as an autosomal recessive. Several subvarieties (types Ia–Id) have been described.
8. Glycogenosis type II (Pompe's disease) is caused by lysosomal acid α-glucosidase deficiency and is inherited as an autosomal recessive. Several subvarieties have been described, including defects caused by missense and nonsense substitutions and by partial chromosomal deletions. The gene for human acid α-glucosidase has been found on human chromosome 17, at 17q23.

II. SYSTEMIC MANIFESTATIONS

ORGAN/SYSTEM MANIFESTATIONS

	Type I	Type II
1. Cardiac	None	Cardiomegaly[a]
2. Vascular	Hypertension	
3. Pulmonary	Pulmonary hypertension	Respiratory failure
4. Renal	Enlarged kidneys	
5. Gastrointestinal	Intermittent diarrhea Mucosal ulceration Chronic inflammatory bowel disease Increased risk of pancreatitis Hepatomegaly Hepatic adenomas and carcinomas	Macroglossia[a] Hepatomegaly
6. Genitourinary	Proteinuria Nephrocalcinosis Proteinuria, albuminuria Glomerulosclerosis Amyloidosis Fanconi-like syndrome	
7. Hematologic	Prolonged bleeding time Impaired platelet aggregation Epistaxis Easy bruising Neutropenia	
8. Musculoskeletal	Osteoporosis Short stature	Scoliosis and lordosis Proximal muscle weakness Respiratory muscle impairment Progressive weakness[a] Hypotonia[a]
9. Mucocutaneous	Skin xanthomas Excess adipose tissue in cheeks	
10. Nonspecific	Hyperlipidemia Hypoglycemia and lactic acidosis Hyperuricemia and gout Elevated cholesterol, triglycerides Elevated phospholipids	

[a] Limited to infantile form

TYPES

	Type I	Type II
1. Cornea	Marginal corneal clouding	None
2. Retina	Yellow paramacular lesions	Glycogen deposits in ganglion cells Glycogen deposits in mural cells
3. Ocular motility	None	Glycogen deposits in extraocular muscles and ocular smooth muscle ?? Strabismus

SUGGESTED READINGS

Conti JA, Kemeny M. Type I-a glycogenosis associated with hepatocellular carcinoma. *Cancer* 1992;69:1320–1322.

Hermanns MM, DeGraff E, Kroos MA, et al. The effect of a single base pair deletion (delta T525) and a C1634T missense mutation (pro545leu) on the expression of lysosomal alpha-glucosidase in patients with glycogen storage disease type II. *Hum Mol Genet* 1994;3:2213–2218.

Scriver CR, Beaudet AL, Sly WS, Valle D, eds. *The Metabolic and Molecular Bases of Inherited Disease.* New York: McGraw-Hill; 1995: *Chapters 24 and 77.*

Shin YS. Diagnosis of glycogen storage disease. *J Inherit Metabol Dis* 1990;13:419–434.

Smith RS. Glycogenoses. In: Gold DH, Weingeist TH, eds. *The Eye in Systemic Disease.* Philadelphia: JB Lippincott; 1990:332–334.

Chapter 80

OXALOSIS

Travis A. Meredith
Richard Alan Lewis

I. GENERAL

1. Primary hyperoxaluria is a rare autosomal recessive inborn error of glyoxylate metabolism.
2. Two different forms have been described based on different enzyme defects.
   - Type 1 has a deficiency of peroxisomal alanine: glyoxylate aminotransferase.
   - Type 2 is characterized by deficient D-glyceric dehydrogenase.
3. Widespread deposition of calcium oxalate crystals in many tissues.
4. Clinical onset is usually in childhood but may be delayed into adulthood.
5. Renal failure due to nephrolithiasis may lead to early death.
6. Infantile onset is strongly correlated with presence of retinopathy.
7. Presence of retinopathy may be correlated with earlier death.
8. Secondary hyperoxaluria is rare. Reported causes include ingestion of ethylene glycol and methoxyflurane anesthesia.

II. SYSTEMIC MANIFESTATIONS

1. Renal
   - Calcium oxalate nephrolithiasis
     - Renal colic
     - Gross hematuria
   - Uremia
   - Terminal renal failure
   - Urolithiasis
2. Musculoskeletal
   - Acute arthritis, sometimes associated with hyperuricemia
   - Osteodystrophy
3. Vascular
   - Conduction abnormalities
   - Crystal deposition related to organ vascularity in thyroid, spleen, liver, thymus, pituitary, adrenal, pancreas, parathyroid, and central nervous system
4. General
   - Growth retardation secondary to uremia

III. OCULAR MANIFESTATIONS

1. Retina
   - Calcium oxalate crystal deposition in retina with predilection for retinal arteries and arterioles
   - Small pigmented retinal pigment epithelial lesions, which coalesce in some patients to form larger irregular black macular lesions
   - Subretinal fibrosis
   - Retinal ischemia with nerve fiber layer infarcts
   - Retinal and optic nerve neovascularization
   - Fluorescein may show small hyperfluorescent rings surrounding relatively hypofluorescent cores.
2. Optic nerve
   - Optic atrophy
3. Ciliary body
   - Calcium oxalate deposition
4. Extraocular muscles
   - Calcium oxalate deposition

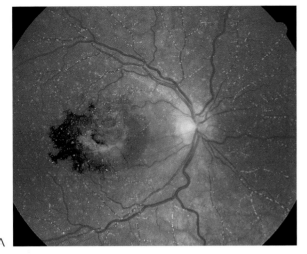 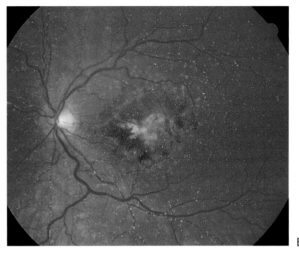

A   B

FIGURE 80.1. **(A)** In the right eye of a 14-year-old girl calcium oxalate crystals are prominent with a golden appearance. There is a predilection of periarterial distribution. The central macular area is dominated by a large irregular black lesion with white central areas that stain late on fluorescein angiography. **(B)** The left eye demonstrates a similar black macular lesion with a "Chinese figure" configuration. Some oxalate crystals appear to lie in the superficial retina partially obscuring larger vessels; fluorescein angiography demonstrates pigment epithelial changes suggesting deposition at that level.

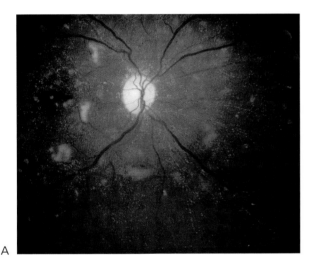 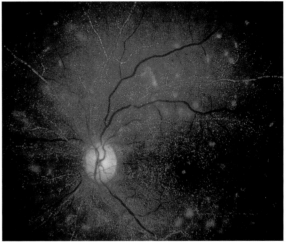

A   B

FIGURE 80.2. **(A)** The right eye demonstrates prominent crystalline deposits with an arterial predilection. The arteries are narrowed and cotton-wool spots are present. The pigment epithelium demonstrates multiple yellow lesions scattered sporadically throughout the posterior pole. **(B)** Findings are similar in the left eye. Both eyes later developed optic nerve neovascularization with subsequent vitreous hemorrhage and irretrievable loss of vision.

SUGGESTED READINGS

Hillman RE. Primary hyperoxaluria. In: Scriver CR, Beaudet AL, Sly WS, et al, eds. *The Metabolic Basis of Inherited Disease.* New York: McGraw-Hill; 1989:933–944. *An excellent summary of primary hyperoxaluria.*

Meredith TA, Wright JD, Gammon A, et al. Ocular involvement in primary hyperoxaluria. *Arch Ophthalmol* 1984;102:584–587.

Small KW, Letson R, Schneinman J. Ocular findings in primary hyperoxaluria. *Arch Ophthalmol* 1990;108:89–93. *A review of ocular findings of 24 patients with hyperoxaluria and correlation with the systemic manifestations of the diseases process.*

Section C. Disorders of Lipoprotein and Lipid Metabolism

Chapter 81

CEREBROTENDINOUS XANTHOMATOSES AND OTHER XANTHOMAS

Ahmad M. Mansour

I. GENERAL

1. Xanthomas are tumors composed of lipid-laden foam cells, which are histiocytes containing cytoplasmic lipid material. Lipids found in xanthomas are composed of free and esterified cholesterol, although other lipids may be found occasionally. Xanthomas result from decreased triglyceride catabolism due to abnormal lipoprotein lipase activity, abnormal remnant catabolism by the liver, or abnormal low-density lipoprotein catabolism.

2. Various types of xanthomas may be seen in patients having primary hyperlipoproteinemia and also in patients with systemic disorders and secondary hyperlipoproteinemia (such as diabetes mellitus, hypothyroidism, uremia, liver diseases, pancreatitis, obesity, nephrotic syndrome, multiple myeloma, lymphoma, as well as ingestion of estrogens, corticosteroids, and Accutane).

3. Cutaneous xanthomas are classified on the basis of location and appearance as tendinous, planar, tuberous, disseminated, and eruptive. There is an association between tendinous xanthoma and β-lipoprotein disease, tuberous xanthoma and broad β-lipoprotein disease, eruptive xanthoma and severe hypertriglyceridemia, as well as planar xanthoma and hypercholesterolemia.

4. Cerebrotendinous xanthomatosis is a rare autosomal recessive condition characterized by tissue deposition of cholestanol and cholesterol from a primary biochemical defect in bile acid synthesis. Intake of chenodeoxycholic acid results in the reduction of plasma cholestanol level and in the improvement in the neurologic signs.

II. SYSTEMIC MANIFESTATIONS

1. Cutaneous
   - Tendinous xanthoma: freely movable firm nodules over extensor tendons of hands, knees, elbows, and Achilles tendons
   - Cerebrotendinous xanthomatosis: tendon xanthomas especially over Achilles tendons
   - Planar xanthoma: xanthelasma palpebrae, creases of palms and fingers
   - Tuberous xanthoma: yellow papules can enlarge to the size of a nodule over extensor surfaces and areas subjected to trauma such as elbows, knuckles, buttocks, knees, and heels.
   - Eruptive xanthoma: yellow papules with erythematous halo over extensor surfaces (elbows, knees) and pressure sites (buttocks, back)
   - Disseminated xanthoma: dark mahogany-brown papules over flexural creases (axilla, neck, elbows, knees), and mucous membranes

2. Cardiovascular
   - Coronary atherosclerotic heart disease (premature death in cerebrotendinous xanthomatosis and tendinous xanthoma)

3. Central nervous system
   - Seen only with cerebrotendinous xanthomatosis
     - Dementia
     - Mental retardation
     - Cerebellar ataxia
     - Pyramidal paresis
     - Pseudobulbar paresis

III. OCULAR MANIFESTATIONS

1. Lids
   - Xanthelasma palpebrum (usually associated with tendinous xanthoma, planar xanthomas, and cerebrotendinous xanthomatosis)

2. Cornea
   - Arcus
   - Xanthoma (associated with disseminated xanthoma)

3. Sclera
   - Xanthoma (associated with disseminated xanthoma)

4. Lens
   - Juvenile cataract (associated with cerebrotendinous xanthomatosis)

5. Retina
   - Lipemia retinalis (associated with eruptive xanthoma)
   - Lipemic diabetic retinopathy (Coats-like picture of hard retinal exudates occurring in patients with diabetes mellitus and lipid disorders such as eruptive and tendinous xanthomas)

6. Optic nerve
   - Optic pallor (associated with cerebrotendinous xanthomatosis)

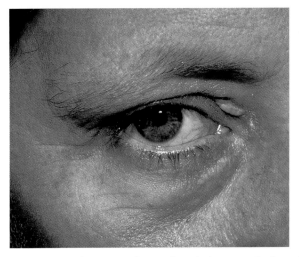

FIGURE 81.1. Planar xanthoma (xanthelasma palpebrum). Courtesy of Sharon Raimer, MD.

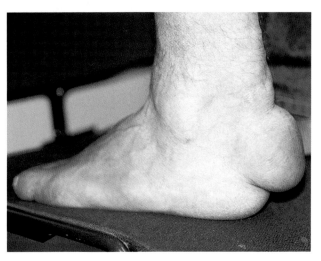

FIGURE 81.2. Tendinous xanthoma of Achilles tendon. Courtesy of Sharon Raimer, MD.

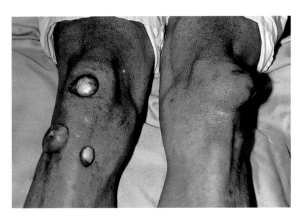

FIGURE 81.3. Tuberous xanthoma of knees. Courtesy of Sharon Raimer, MD.

SUGGESTED READINGS

Kearns WP, Wood WS. Cerebrotendinous xanthomatosis. *Arch Ophthalmol* 1976;94:148–150.

Parker F. Xanthomas and hyperlipidemias. *J Am Acad Dermatol* 1985;13:1–30.

Rosenman RH, Brand RJ, Shultz RI, et al. Relation of corneal arcus to cardiovascular risk factors and the incidence of coronary disease. *N Engl J Med* 1924;291:1322–1324.

Chapter 82

HISTIOCYTOSIS X (LANGERHANS CELL HISTIOCYTOSIS)

Diva R. Salomao
Robert Folberg

I. GENERAL

1. Group of rare disorders characterized by a clonal proliferation of Langerhans cells
2. Langerhans cells, special subset of histiocytes or dendritic antigen-presenting cells, are normally found in the epithelium (skin, cornea, and conjunctiva).
3. Langerhans cells secrete interleukin-1 (IL-1), prostaglandin-E_2 (PGE_2), and stimulate T4 lymphocytes to release IL-1, and γ-interferon (γIFN).
4. Excessive cytokine production may explain most of the clinical and pathologic features, but the initiating mechanism is still unknown.
5. More common in children, peak age 1 to 2 years, range from birth to older age
6. Males are affected twice as frequently as females.
7. Wide spectrum of clinical manifestations: acute, leukemialike disorder affecting infants (Letterer-Siwe disease); curable solitary lesion of bone (eosinophilic granuloma); intermediate forms characterized by osseous, cutaneous, or visceral lesions, with indolent course
8. Uniform pathologic presentation: accumulation of histiocytes with abundant vacuolated cytoplasm and elongated grooved nuclei, admixed with variable number of eosinophils, plasma cells, and lymphocytes.
9. Characteristic immunophenotype: S100 protein, CD1a, and CD68 positivity
10. Ultrastructural finding: Birbeck granules (tennis racket–shaped cytoplasmic inclusion bodies)

II. SYSTEMIC MANIFESTATIONS

1. Bone
   - Most common presentation: painful swelling
   - Skull, long bones, flat bones, and vertebrae are involved, in this order.
   - Extension to adjacent soft tissues
   - Ulceration of overlying skin and mucous membrane, rarely
2. Skin
   - Typical skin rash in inguinal region, necklace, and axillary folds mimicking seborrheic keratosis
   - Papules with depigmented scar in the trunk
3. Reticuloendothelial system
   - Lymphadenopathy
   - Cervical lymph nodes are most often affected, followed by mediastinal and abdominal lymph nodes.
   - Splenomegaly
4. Ears
   - Aural discharge is common, maybe due to otitis externa.
   - Aural polyps
   - Middle ear involvement
5. Peripheral blood and bone marrow
   - Mild anemia of the "chronic disorders," most common presentation
   - Pancytopenia in infants with hepatosplenomegaly and bone marrow infiltrate
6. Liver
   - Hepatomegaly
   - Reduced albumin production resulting in ascites
   - Reduced production of clotting factors (prolonged prothrombin time and activated partial thromboplastin time)
7. Lungs
   - Can be the only manifestation in adults, provoked by smoking
   - Tachypnea and rib recession in young children
   - Pleural effusion
   - Restrictive pattern in pulmonary function tests
8. Central nervous system
   - Involvement of pituitary gland and hypothalamus, causing diabetes insipidus
   - Involvement of cerebellar white: nystagmus, ataxia, and incoordination
   - Extension to dura matter from overlying bone lesion
   - Hydrocephalus
   - Solitary intracerebral lesion simulating tumor
9. Endocrine
   - Diabetes insipidus
   - Growth failure
   - Panhypopituitarism
   - Solitary lesion of the thyroid gland or pancreas
10. Gastrointestinal tract
    - Involvement of the oral mucosa, commonly adjacent to the upper molars
    - Diarrhea due to small bowel or colonic involvement
    - Malabsorption

1. Solitary eosinophilic granuloma involving the frontal bone is the most common presentation.
2. It is usually a painful lesion. Associated signs of inflammation can lead to the clinical diagnosis of dacryoadenitis or preseptal cellulitis.
3. Radiolucent lesion with serrated borders and sclerotic margins on x-rays.
4. Secondary involvement of the adjacent orbital soft tissue can result in proptosis.
5. Optic nerve compression with optic disc edema and optic nerve atrophy are observed in extraconal orbital involvement.
6. Optic chiasm may be involved by direct extension in pituitary-hypothalamic lesions.
7. Choroidal lesions are demonstrated in cases of disseminated disease.
8. Complications of ocular histiocytosis X are corneal ulceration, secondary open angle glaucoma, iritis, and posterior scleritis.

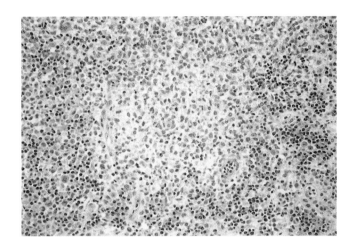

FIGURE 82.1. Eosinophilic granuloma. An aggregate of large cells with pale cytoplasm is surrounded by many eosinophils. The large cells stained appropriately with Langerhans cell markers (hematoxylineosin; original magnification, ×320).

SUGGESTED READINGS

Erly WK, Carmody RF, Dryden RM. Orbital histiocytosis. *Am J Neuroradiol* 1995;16:1258–1261.

Favara, BE. Histiocytosis syndromes: Classification, diagnostic features and current concepts. *Leuk Lymphoma* 1990;2:141–150.

Hage C, Willman CL, Favara BE, Isaacson PG. Langerhans cell histiocytosis (histiocytosis X): Immunophenotype and growth fraction. *Hum Pathol* 1993;24:840–845.

MacCumber MW, Hoffman PN, Wand GS, et al. Ophthalmic involvement in aggressive histiocytosis X. *Ophthalmology* 1990;97:22–27.

Moore AT, Pritchard J, Taylor DSI. Histiocytosis X: An ophthalmological review. *Br J Ophthalmol* 1985;69:7–14.

Williman CL, Busque L, Griffith BB, et al. Langerhans cell histiocytosis (histiocytosis X)—A clonal proliferative disease. *N Engl J Med* 1994;331:154–160.

Chapter 83
HYPERLIPOPROTEINEMIA
Robert J. Schechter

I. GENERAL

1. Plasma lipids are transported in soluble complexes called lipoproteins
   - Chylomicrons
   - Very low-density lipoproteins (VLDL)
   - Low-density lipoproteins (LDL)
   - High-density lipoproteins (HDL)
2. Causes of hyperlipoproteinemia
   - Primary
     - Genetic
   - Secondary
     - Diet
       - Excessive calories, cholesterol, or saturated fat
     - Alcohol
     - Nephrotic syndrome
     - Chronic renal failure
     - Glycogen storage disease
   - Acute intermittent porphyria
   - Hepatoma
   - Hypothyroidism
   - Biliary obstruction or primary biliary cirrhosis
   - Dysglobulinemia: autoimmune disease
   - Uncontrolled diabetes
   - Anorexia nervosa
   - Systemic lupus erythematosus
   - Cushing's syndrome
   - Drug induced
     - Corticosteroids
     - Estrogens
     - Thiazides
     - β-Blockers
     - 13-*cis*-Retinoic acid

II. SYSTEMIC MANIFESTATIONS

1. Cardiac
   - Premature coronary artery disease
   - Aortic stenosis (homozygous familial hypercholesterolemia)
   - Mitral valve xanthoma (familial hypercholserolemia)
2. Vascular
   - Atherosclerosis: coronary, femoral, carotid arteries
3. Gastrointestinal
   - Abdominal pains, pancreatitis, hepatosplenomegaly
4. Renal
   - Renovascular disease
   - Hyperuricemia
5. Neurologic
   - Peripheral neuropathy
   - Central nervous system dysfunction
6. Musculoskeletal
   - Painful joints
   - Tendon xanthomas, Achilles tendonitis
7. Mucocutaneous
   - Eruptive xanthomas
   - Palmar xanthoma
   - Xanthelasma
   - Tuberous xanthoma
8. Ear/nose/throat
   - Yellow plaques on buccal mucosa

III. OCULAR MANIFESTATIONS

1. Lids
   - Xanthelasma
2. Cornea
   - Arcus
   - Schnyder's crystalline stromal dystrophy (?)
3. Retina
   - Lipemia retinalis
   - Retinal vein occlusion
   - Hard exudates (related to cholesterol in insulin-dependent diabetics)
   - Age-related maculopathy (drusen, retinal pigment epithelium abnormalities)
     - Increases with HDL elevation
     - Decreases with serum cholesterol
4. Vitreous
   - Lipidosis vitrealis (if vitreous hemorrhage during lipemia retinalis)

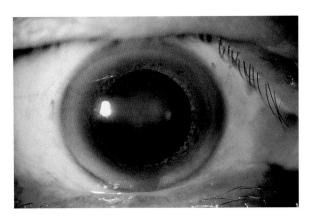

FIGURE 83.1. Corneal arcus. Note the clear periphery.

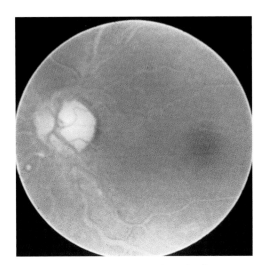

FIGURE 83.2. Lipemia retinalis.

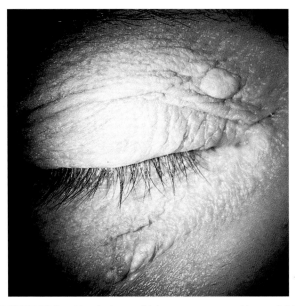

FIGURE 83.3. Xanthelasma (right eye, upper and lower lids).

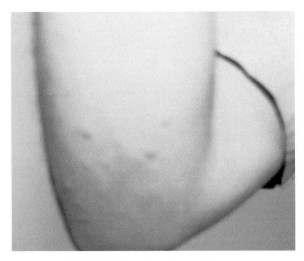

FIGURE 83.4. Eruptive xanthoma.

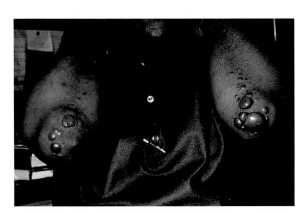

FIGURE 83.5. Tuberous xanthoma.

SUGGESTED READINGS

Klein BEK, Moss SE, Klein R, Surawicz TS. The Wisconsin Epidemiologic Study of Diabetic Retinopathy. Relationship of serum cholesterol to retinopathy and hard exudate. *Ophthalmology* 1991;98:1261–1265.

Klein R, Klein BEK, Franke T. The relationship of cardiovascular disease and its risk factors to age-related maculopathy. *Ophthalmology* 1993;100:406–414.

Rouhiainen P, Salonen R, Rouhiainen H, Salonen J. Association of corneal arcus with ultrasonographically assessed arterial wall thickness and serum lipids. *Cornea* 1993;12:142–145.

Chapter 84

HYPOLIPOPROTEINEMIA

Ann G. Neff
Guy W. Neff

I. GENERAL

1. Plasma lipids are transported by lipoproteins; the classes of lipoproteins include chylomicrons (CM), very low-density lipoproteins (VLDL), intermediate-density lipoproteins (IDL), low-density lipoproteins (LDL), and high-density lipoproteins (HDL).
2. The core of lipoproteins contain proteins termed apoproteins.
3. The hypolipoproteinemias are characterized by abnormally low levels of plasma lipoproteins.
   - Bassen-Kornzweig disease or abetalipoproteinemia
     - Autosomal recessive
     - Apo B not expressed
     - All plasma lipids decreased
     - Heterozygotes have normal levels of lipids.
     - Death in early adulthood without treatment
   - Familial hypobetalipoproteinemia
     - Similar clinically to homozygous abetalipoproteinemia
       - Homozygotes have decreased CM, VLDL, and LDL
       - Heterozygotes have half-normal levels
   - Tangier disease or familial HDL deficiency
     - Rare autosomal recessive
     - Deficient or absent HDL, with accumulation of cholesterol esters in tissues
     - Obligate heterozygotes clinically normal
   - Lecithin-cholesterol acyl transferase (LCAT) deficiency
     - Autosomal recessive
     - Unesterified cholesterol accumulates in plasma
     - Homozygotes have 30% normal levels of HDL
   - Fish-eye disease
     - Familial partial LCAT deficiency
     - Decreased HDL levels

II. SYSTEMIC MANIFESTATIONS

1. Bassen-Kornzweig disease
   - Gastrointestinal
     - Steatorrhea
     - Fat-soluble vitamin deficiency
   - Neurologic
     - Peripheral neuropathy
     - Ataxia
   - Hematologic
     - Acanthocytosis
     - Anemia
     - Coagulopathy
   - Cardiac
     - Cardiomyopathy
     - Arrhythmias
   - Musculoskeletal
     - Myopathy
2. Familial hypobetalipoproteinemia
   - Neurologic
     - Similar to Bassen-Kornzweig disease, but milder
3. Tangier disease
   - Gastrointestinal
     - Hepatosplenomegaly
   - Neurologic
     - Peripheral neuropathy
   - Ear/nose/throat
     - Hyperplastic yellow tonsils
   - Nonspecific
     - Lymphadenopathy
4. LCAT deficiency
   - Cardiac
     - Premature atherosclerosis and coronary artery disease
   - Renal
     - Renal insufficiency
     - Proteinuria
   - Hematologic
     - Hemolytic anemia
5. Fish-eye disease
   - Renal
     - Renal impairment

1. Bassen-Kornzweig disease
- Retina
  - Pigmentary retinopathy
  - Nyctalopia
  - Abnormal dark adaptation
- Neuroophthalmologic
  - Nystagmus
- Ocular motility
  - Strabismus

2. Tangier disease
- Cornea
  - Bilateral, punctate stromal opacities
- Lid
  - Orbicularis weakness
  - Ectropion

- Conjunctiva/sclera
  - Conjunctival deposits

3. LCAT deficiency
- Cornea
  - Bilateral, diffuse stromal haze, accentuated at periphery
- Conjunctiva/sclera
  - Cholesterol deposition

4. Fish-eye disease
- Cornea
  - Bilateral, severe corneal clouding due to diffuse dotlike opacities

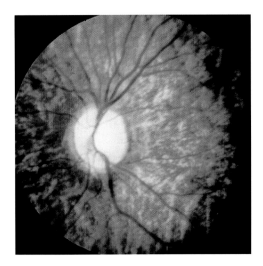

FIGURE 84.1. Fundus of 13-month-old child with abetalipoproteinemia. Note the generalized granular pigmentary retinopathy with patchy pigment loss.

SUGGESTED READINGS

Barchiesi BJ, Eckel RH, Ellis PP. The cornea and disorders of lipid metabolism. *Surv Ophthalmol* 1991;36:1–22.

Brewer HB, Santamarina-Fojo S, Hoeg JM. Disorders of lipoprotein metabolism. In: DeGroot LJ, ed. *Endocrinology.* Philadelphia: WB Saunders; 1995:2731–2753.

Pulido JS, Judisch GF, Vrabec MP. Hypolipoproteinemias. In: Gold DH, Weingeist TA, eds. *The Eye in Systemic Disease.* Philadelphia: JB Lipincott; 1990:344–348.

Section D. Disorders of Lysosomal Enzymes

Chapter 85

FARBER'S DISEASE

Marco A. Zarbin

I. GENERAL

1. Autosomal recessive inheritance
2. Associated with deficiency in lysosomal ceramidase (catalyzes breakdown of sphingosine and fatty acid) and the accumulation of ceramide in the retina and elsewhere
3. Systemic histopathology is characterized by foam cell-containing granulomata in subcutaneous tissues, periarticular and synovial tissues, lymph nodes, thymus, and other solid viscera.
4. The foam cells contain lysosomes replete with curvilinear tubular bodies ("Farber bodies"), which represent accumulated ceramide and lamellar inclusions that represent a combination of ganglioside and phospholipid.
5. Ocular histopathology is characterized by intracellular inclusions of variable morphology in retinal ganglion cells, in retinal interneurons, in glia, and in phagocytic cells with relative sparing of the retinal pigment epithelium.

II. SYSTEMIC MANIFESTATIONS

1. Cardiac
   - Systolic murmurs
2. Neurologic
   - Mental retardation
   - Elevated cerebrospinal fluid protein
   - Hypotonia
   - Diminished deep tendon reflexes
   - Distended neurons and glia in brain
   - Intracellular lamellar inclusions (zebra bodies)
3. Skin and musculoskeletal
   - Subcutaneous periarticular nodules
   - Joint swelling
   - Progressive arthropathy
4. Ear/nose/throat
   - Hoarseness
   - Vocal cord thickening
   - Disturbances in swallowing
5. Pulmonary consolidation
6. Gastrointestinal
   - Hepatomegaly
7. Hematologic
   - Splenomegaly
8. Other
   - Elevation of ceramide levels in subcutaneous nodules
   - Variable phenotype: severe type is associated with rapid progression, visceral involvement, and death by age 5.
   - Poor growth and development
   - Fever
   - Irritability
   - Vomiting
   - Failure to thrive

III. OCULAR MANIFESTATIONS

1. Retina
   - Grayish parafoveal opacity
   - Macular cherry-red spot
2. Conjunctiva
   - Xanthomatoid growths
3. Cornea
   - Subepithelial nodular opacities
4. Nonspecific
   - Decreased vision

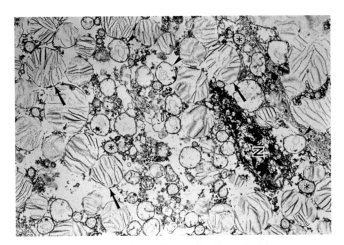

FIGURE 85.1. Retinal ganglion cells distended by numerous inclusions consisting of flattened stacks of osmophilic lamellae (*arrows*), round inclusions surrounded by bilaminar membrane (*arrowheads*), and circular inclusions (*asterisks*). The flattened stacks of osmophilic lamellae are most numerous. Nucleus (N) is displaced (original magnification, ×15,000).

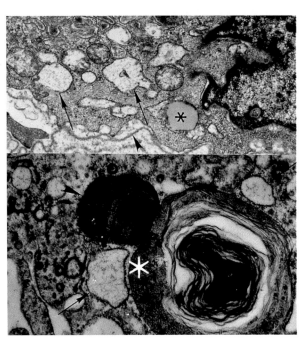

FIGURE 85.2. Conjunctiva. (**Top**) Lipidlike inclusion (*asterisk*) and circular inclusions (*arrows*) in endothelial cell (L, lumen of blood vessels; *arrowhead,* basement membrane) (×15,000). (**Bottom**) Probable macrophage containing single membrane-bound inclusion with granular material peripherally (*asterisk*) and 2.2-nm wide filaments organized in a concentric, roughly circular stacked array centrally. Adjacent inclusion (*arrowhead*) is composed of granular material, electron-dense lipofuscin, and lipidlike material. Circular inclusions (*arrows*) are also present (original magnification, ×32,000).

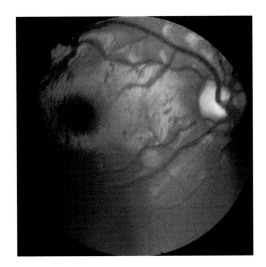

FIGURE 85.3. Macular cherry-red spot from a patient with Farber's disease who presented with dementia.

SUGGESTED READINGS

Farber S. A lipid metabolic disorder-disseminated lipogranulomatosis: A syndrome with similarity to, and important difference from, Niemann-Pick and Hand-Schuller-Christian disease. *Am J Dis Child* 1952;84:499–500.

Moser HW, Chen WW. Ceramidase deficiency: Farber's lipogranulomatosis. In: Stanbury JB, Wyngaarden JB, Frederickson DS, et al, eds. *The Metabolic Basis of Inherited Disease,* 5th ed. New York: McGraw-Hill; 1983:820–830.

Zarbin MA, Green WR, Moser HW, Morton SJ. Farber's disease—Light and electron microscopic study of the eye. *Arch Ophthalmol* 1985;103:73–80.

Zarbin MA, Green WA, Moser H, et al. Increased levels of ceramide in the retina of a patient with Farber's disease. *Arch Ophthalmol* 1988;106:1163.

Chapter 86

FABRY'S DISEASE (ANGIOKERATOMA CORPORIS DIFFUSUM)

Peter L. Sonkin

I. GENERAL

1. Caused by a deficiency of the enzyme α-galactosidase A, a lysosomal hydrolase, which results in an abnormal accumulation of the sphingolipid ceramide trihexosidase

2. Transmitted by X-linked inheritance; genetic defect localized to chromosome X q22-24

3. Incidence is approximately 1/40,000.

4. Prenatal diagnosis is possible by quantitative measurement of α-galactosidase A on chorionic villi biopsies.

5. Sphingolipid deposition occurs in all areas of the body, particularly within lysosomes of vascular endothelial and smooth muscle cells.

6. Female carriers can have corneal changes alone.

7. Characteristic Maltese cross pattern birefringent intracellular inclusions on histopathology of blood vessel–containing tissues; electron microscopy confirms the inclusion bodies.

8. Increased levels of sphingolipid and associated metabolites are measurable in tears, blood, and urine.

9. Foam cells or mulberry cells (free particles of glycolipid) can be found in the urinary sediment.

10. Affected males have near total enzyme deficiency; female carriers have an approximately 50% deficiency.

11. Individuals with Fabry's disease typically live into adulthood, with life expectancy into the third to fifth decades.

II. SYSTEMIC MANIFESTATIONS

1. Childhood (in symptomatic males)
   - Recurrent episodes of burning extremity pain (acroparasthesias) with associated fever and elevation of sedimentation rate.
   - Angiokeratoma corporis diffusum, which are characteristic dotlike telangiectatic skin lesions in the bathing-trunk area, develop around puberty and become more prominent with time.

2. Adult life
   - Renal
     - Failure
     - Proteinuria
     - Uremia
     - Hypertension
   - Cardiovascular complications
     - Arrhythmias
     - Valvular dysfunction (the mitral and tricuspid valves have been reported to be thickened due to deposition of glycosphingolipids, which may provide a source for small emboli)
     - Myocardial infarction
   - Gastrointestinal
     - Poor appetite
     - Vomiting
   - Central nervous system
     - Stroke
     - Cerebral hemorrhage
   - Dermatologic
     - Angiokeratomas
   - Paresthesias
   - Acral pain
   - Reduced sweating

3. Treatment
   - Symptomatic therapy
   - Dialysis
   - Renal transplant
   - Genetic counseling

1. Cornea

- Typical, fine powdery epithelial and subepithelial opacities, often in a whorl-like pattern (verticillata); can be diffuse epithelial haze early in disease
- Best seen with slit-lamp retroillumination
- Typically cream-colored and faint (can be white to golden brown)
- Usually do not affect visual acuity
- More commonly affect the inferior cornea
- Observed early in hemizygotes (before age 5, as early as 6 months) and around age 10 in heterozygotes
- Heterozygous females typically have mild systemic manifestations, but commonly have prominent subepithelial corneal changes (approximately 90% of carrier females with corneal changes).
- Possible causes
  - Intraepithelial lipid accumulation or epithelial basement membrane reduplication
  - Cytoplasmic aggregates of laminated dense material in lysosomal vacuoles of epithelial cells. These have been observed in conjunctival biopsies and are stainable with sudan black B in paraffin sections.
- Differential diagnosis: indomethacin, chloroquine, amiodarone, phenothiazines, striate melanokeratosis

2. Conjunctiva

- "Sausagelike" tortuous vascular changes
- Telangiectatic vascular changes
- Occurs in approximately 70% of affected males and 25% of carrier females

3. Lens

- Granular anterior subcapsular wedge-shaped or propellar-shaped opacity, reported to occur in 35% of affected males; not seen in carrier females
- Linear whitish, almost translucent spokelike deposit of granular material at or near the posterior capsule, reported to occur in 37% of affected males and 14% of carrier females

4. Retina

- "Sausagelike" tortuous vascular changes, much more common in affected males.
- Venules more commonly involved
- Retinal edema has been reported
- Rare cases of retinal vascular occlusion (central retinal vein, central retinal artery) have been reported.

5. Miscellaneous associations

- Lid edema
- Optic disc edema
- Optic disc atrophy
- Refractive error

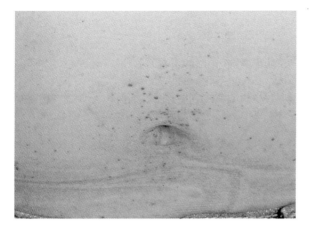

FIGURE 86.1. Clinical photograph illustrating angiokeratoma corporis diffusum associated with Fabry's disease.

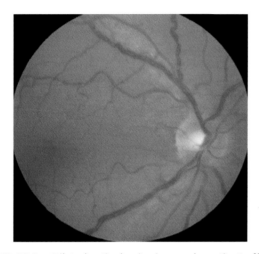

FIGURE 86.2. Dilated retinal veins in a male patient affected with Fabry's disease.

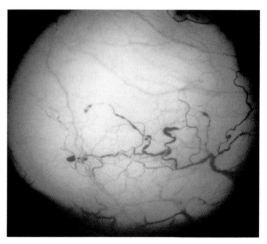

FIGURE 86.3. Tortuous vascular changes in the conjunctiva of a male patient affected with Fabry's disease.

SUGGESTED READINGS

Anderson MVN, Dahl H, Fledelius H, et al. Central retinal artery occlusion in a patient with Fabry's disease documented by scanning laser ophthalmoscopy. *Acta Ophthalmol* 1994;72:635–638.

Fabry disease. In: Isselbacher KI, Braunwald E, Wilson JD, et al., eds. *Harrison's Principles of Internal Medicine,* 13th ed. New York: McGraw-Hill; 1994:20.

Fabry's disease. In: Albert DM, Jakobiec FA, eds. *Principles and Practice of Ophthalmology.* Philadelphia: WB Saunders; 1994: vol. 1:305–6; vol. 4:2212–2213, 2782–2783.

Hasholt L, Wandall A, Sorensen SA. Fabry's disease. *Clin Genet* 1989;36:335–336.

Li-ling B, Ling-ling G, Shuang-nong L, et al. A family with Fabry's disease. *Chinese Medical Journal* 1990;103:134–141.

McCulloch C, Ghosh M. Fabry's disease. In: Gold DH, Weingeist JA, eds. *The Eye in Systemic Disease.* Philadelphia: JB Lippincott; 1990:355–358.

Sher NA, Letson RD, Desnick RJ. The ocular manifestations in Fabry's disease. *Arch Ophthalmol* 1979;97:671–676.

Weingeist TA, Blodi FC. Fabry's disease: Ocular findings in a female carrier. *Arch Ophthalmol* 1971;85:169–176.

Chapter 87

FUCOSIDOSIS

Jacques Libert

I. GENERAL

1. Autosomal recessive disease
2. Phenotypic heterogeneity
3. Deficiency of α-L-fucosidase
4. Intralysosomal storage of fucose-rich molecules
5. Diagnosis by enzyme analysis on blood, cultured cells, and tears and ultrastructural studies on skin and conjunctival biopsy
6. Prenatal diagnosis by amniocentesis

II. SYSTEMIC MANIFESTATIONS

1. Central nervous system
   - Muscle weakness, hypotonia
   - Later on hypertonia and spasticity
   - Psychomotor retardation
   - Death
     - Before the age of 6 in severe phenotype
     - Up to the third decade in mild phenotype
2. Hematologic
   - Hepatosplenomegaly
   - Vacuolated blood lymphocytes
   - Foam cells in bone marrow
3. Musculoskeletal
   - Coarse facies, macrocephaly
   - Thickness of the skull
   - Abnormalities of vertebral bodies
4. Mucocutaneous
   - Palmar telangiectasia
   - Papular rash

III. OCULAR MANIFESTATIONS

1. Conjunctiva
   - Tortuosities of capillaries
   - Saccular and fusiform aneurysms
2. Retina
   - Dilatation and tortuosities of veins
   - Contrasting with normal arteries

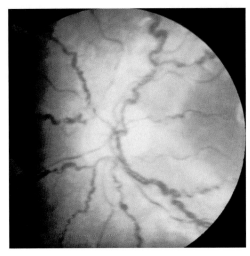

FIGURE 87.1. Dilated and tortuous retinal veins at age 4½ in a girl affected with the severe phenotype.

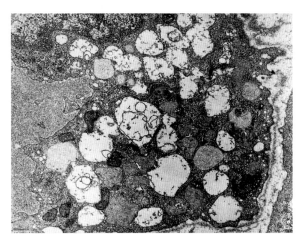

FIGURE 87.2. Severe disorganization of the cytoarchitecture of capillary endothelial cells with lysosomal massive overloading with oligosaccharides (original magnification, ×5000).

SUGGESTED READINGS

Durand P, Borrone C, Della Cella G, et al. Fucosidosis. *Lancet* 1968;1:1198.

Koussef BG, Beratis NG, Strauss L, et al. Fucosidosis type 2. *Pediatrics* 1976;57:205.

Libert J. La fucosidose. Ultrastructure oculaire. *J Fr Ophthalmol* 1984;7:519.

Libert J, Van Hoof F, Tondeur M. Fucosidosis: Ultrastructural study of conjunctiva and skin, and enzyme analysis of tears. *Invest Ophthalmol* 1976;15:626.

Section E. Disorders of Mineral Metabolism

Chapter 88

HEMOCHROMATOSIS

Robert A. Wiznia

I. GENERAL

1. Primary hemochromatosis is due to an autosomal recessive gene on chromasome 6 that is closely linked to the A locus of the HLA complex.
2. The hemochromatosis gene leads to an abnormally high rate of intestinal iron absorption.
3. In primary hemochromatosis iron is deposited mostly in parenchymal cells as hemosiderin.
4. Secondary or acquired hemochromatosis develops in cases of ineffective erythropoiesis due to a variety of anemias or thalassemias because of increased intestinal iron absorption or transfusions or both.
5. In secondary hemochromatosis, iron is first stored in the reticuloendothelial cells (systemic hemosiderosis), but eventually parenchymal cells also become involved leading to pathology similar to that noted in primary hemochromatosis.
6. Primary hemochromatosis is rarely diagnosed before age 40 because it takes many years for the body's normal iron content of 3 to 4 g to rise to the level of 20 g or more required for clinical manifestations to develop.
7. There is a 10:1 male predominance due to women's greater iron losses from menstruation, pregnancy, and lactation.

II. SYSTEMIC MANIFESTATIONS

1. Liver
   - Hepatomegaly is found in more than 90% of cases.
   - Cirrhosis is frequent in untreated cases.
   - Hepatocellular carcinoma develops in one-third of patients with cirrhosis; this is the most common cause of death.
2. Skin
   - Increased pigmentation due to iron and melanin deposition
3. Endocrine
   - Two-thirds of patients develop diabetes mellitus due to iron deposition in parenchymal cells of the pancreas.
   - Hypopituitarism with secondary testicular atrophy, adrenal insufficiency, hypothyroidism, and hypoparathyroidism
4. Musculoskeletal
   - Progressive polyarthritis develops in one-third to one-half of patients.
5. Cardiac
   - Cardiomegaly
   - Congestive heart failure
   - Cardiac arrythmias

III. OCULAR MANIFESTATIONS

1. Increased iron and secondary melanin deposits in
   - Conjunctiva
   - Sclera
   - Parapapillary retinal pigment epithelium (slate blue pigmentation around the optic disc)
   - Lid margins, especially surrounding the follicles
   - Nonpigmented epithelium of the ciliary body

SUGGESTED READINGS

Hudson JR. Ocular findings in haemochromatosis. *Br J Ophthalmol* 1953;37:242–246. *Good clinical description of ocular manifestation of hemochromatosis.*

Maddox K. The retina in haemochromatosis. *Br J Ophthalmol* 1933;17:393–394. *Classic report that includes description of slate blue pigment surrounding the optic disc.*

Motulsky AG. Hemochromatosis. In: Wyngaarden JB, Smith LH Jr, Bennett JC, eds. *Cecil Textbook of Medicine.* Philadelphia: WB Saunders; 1992:1133–1136. *A general review of primary hemochromatosis.*

Roth AM, Foos RY. Ocular pathologic changes in primary hemochromatosis. *Arch Ophthalmol* 1972;87:507–514.

Wiznia RA. Hemochromatosis. In: Gold DH, Weingeist TA, ed. *The Eye in Systemic Disease.* Philadelphia: JB Lippincott; 1990:385–387. *A general review of the ocular manifestations of primary and secondary hemochromatosis as well as of ocular hemosiderosis.*

Chapter 89

WILSON'S DISEASE

Thomas R. Hedges III
Thomas R. Hedges, Jr.

I. GENERAL

1. Autosomal recessive
2. Usually presents at 8 to 16 years of age with a range of 6 to 50 years.
3. Abnormalities caused by defective excretion of copper with copper deposition in various organ systems
4. Detected in laboratory by decreased serum ceruloplasmin (< 200 mg/L)
5. Morbidity primarily due to copper deposition in central nervous system (especially basil ganglia as well as frontal and cerebellar white matter) and in hepatocytes

II. SYSTEMIC MANIFESTATIONS

1. Neurologic
   - Incoordination
   - Dysarthria
   - Tremor
   - Athetosis
   - Chorea
   - Personality changes
2. Hepatic
   - Generalized liver dysfunction
   - Cirrhosis
3. Renal
   - Generalized renal failure

III. OCULAR MANIFESTATIONS

1. Cornea
   - Kayser-Fleischer ring of copper in Decemet's membrane
2. Lens
   - "Sunflower" deposition of copper in anterior and posterior subcapsular regions
3. Neuroophthalmologic
   - Saccadic slowing and dysmetria
   - Loss of normal pursuit
   - Convergence insufficiency
   - Myasthenialike syndrome secondary to penicillamine

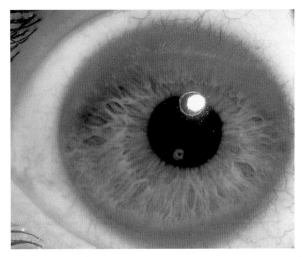

FIGURE 89.1. Kayser-Fleischer ring obscures peripheral iris details in a patient with Wilson's disease.

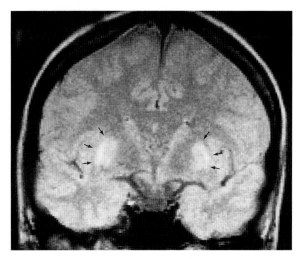

FIGURE 89.2. Magnetic resonance image shows increased intensity corresponding to areas of copper deposition in basal ganglia (*arrows*).

SUGGESTED READINGS

Curran RE, Hedges TR III, Boger WP III. Loss of accommodation and the near response in Wilson's disease. *J Pediatr Ophthalmol Strabismus* 1982;19:157–160.

Goldberg MF, Von Norden GK. Ophthalmologic findings in Wilson's hepatolenticular degeneration. *Arch Ophthalmol* 1966;75:162–170.

Kirkham TH, Kamin DF. Slow saccadic eye movements in Wilson's disease. *J Neurol Neurosurg Psychiatry* 1974;37:191–194.

Starosta-Rubinstein S, Young AB, Kluin K, et al. Clinical assessment of 31 patients with Wilson's disease. Correlations with structural changes on magnetic resonance imaging. *Arch Neurol* 1987;44:365–369.

Wiebers DO, Hollenhorst RW, Goldstein NP. The ophthalmologic manifestations of Wilson's disease. *Mayo Clin Proc* 1977;52:409–416.

Section F.   Miscellaneous Metabolic Disorders

Chapter 90

AMYLOIDOSIS

Joel Sugar

I. GENERAL

1. Amyloid is not a specific protein but rather an insoluble extracellular material made up of β-pleated sheets of fibrous protein.
2. Amyloid stains pink with Congo red and a birefringent apple green in polarized light.
3. Amyloidosis may be divided into
   - Primary (AL) made up of immunoglobulin light chains; also seen in multiple myeloma
   - Secondary (AA) from serum protein SAA
   - Heredofamilial (AF) from prealbumin
   - Localized
   - Age related
   - Hemodialysis associated

II. SYSTEMIC MANIFESTATIONS

1. Primary systemic amyloidosis (AL)—acquired, multiple organs involved
   - Multiple myeloma commonly associated
   - Hepatomegaly
   - Congestive heart failure
   - Nephrotic syndrome
   - Pulmonary involvement
   - Macroglossia
   - Cutaneous hemorrhages, papules, plaques
   - Peripheral neuropathy
   - Arthropathy
2. Secondary (AA)—seen with chronic infectious or inflammatory diseases (tuberculosis, leprosy, rheumatoid arthritis)
   - Renal disease
   - Multiple organ involvement histopathologically
3. Heredofamilial—autosomal dominant in all except familial Mediterranean fever, which is autosomal recessive. At least 14 types related to mutations in transthyretin (prealbumin) gene.
   - Peripheral neuropathy (some forms)
   - Cardiomyopathy (some forms)
   - Nephropathy (some forms)
   - Gastrointestinal dysfunction (some forms)
   - Fever, joint pain (familial Mediterranean fever)
4. Localized—isolated lesions, may appear anywhere
5. Age related—deposition in heart, kidneys, central nervous system
6. Hemodialysis related—joint involvement, carpal tunnel syndrome

III. OCULAR MANIFESTATIONS

1. Lids
   - Nodules
   - Ecchymosis (primary amyloidosis, myeloma associated amyloidosis)
   - Ptosis
   - Brow ptosis in heredofamilial forms
2. Conjunctiva
   - Subconjunctival masses (usually in localized amyloidosis)
3. Cornea
   - Lattice lines in corneal stroma in familial amyloid polyneuropathy—Finnish-type (Meretoja syndrome)—lattice dystrophy type II
   - Lattice lines in localized form—lattice dystrophies type I and III
   - Gelatinous droplike dystrophy—anterior corneal nodules (localized form)
   - Polymorphic amyloid stromal degeneration (age-related form)
   - Secondary—seen histopathologically in inflammatory corneal disease
4. Pupil
   - Irregular
   - Scalloped pupil has been described in the Portuguese form of hereditary familial amyloidosis.
5. Vitreous
   - Opacities
   - Veils
   - Sheets
   - "Strings of pearls" in vitreous (seen in some familial forms, especially Portuguese, Indiana-Swiss forms)

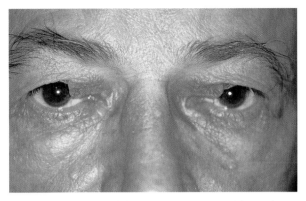

FIGURE 90.1. Upper eyelid lesions in a patient with myeloma associated systemic amyloidosis. Courtesy of H. Tessler, MD.

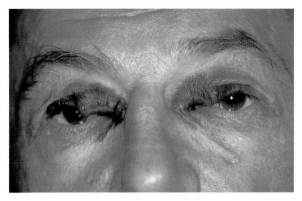

FIGURE 90.2. Same patient following bilateral spontaneous hemorrhage into the eyelid lesions. Courtesy of H. Tessler, MD.

SUGGESTED READINGS

Cohen AS. Amyloidosis. In: Isselbacher KJ, Braunwald E, Wilson JD, eds. *Harrison's Principles of Internal Medicine.* New York, McGraw-Hill; 1994:1625–1630. *A nice review of the subject.*

Cohen AS, Jones LA. Advances in amyloidosis. *Current Opin Rheumatol* 1993;5:62–76. *A more detailed review loaded with current references.*

Chapter 91
GOUT
Andrew P. Ferry

I. GENERAL

1. Gout is found exclusively in humans and in its full development is manifest by an increase in the serum urate concentration; recurrent attacks of acute arthritis; aggregated deposits of sodium urate monohydrate (tophi) occurring chiefly in and around the joints of the limbs; and renal disease, including uric acid urolithiasis.

2. A serum urate level above 7.5 to 8.0 mg/dL is abnormal.
3. In adults, serum urate levels correlate strongly with serum creatinine, body weight, height, age, blood urea nitrogen, blood pressure, and alcohol intake.

II. SYSTEMIC MANIFESTATIONS

1. Musculoskeletal
   - First attack of gouty arthritis usually occurs after at least 20 to 30 years of sustained hyperuricemia
   - Peak age at onset is between fourth and sixth decades
   - Marked propensity for men
   - Acute attacks of exquisitely painful arthritis, usually monoarticular at first
   - In at least one-half of initial acute attacks, the first metatarsophalangeal joint is the affected site.
   - Complete freedom from all symptoms between attacks is a prominent feature.
   - Chronic tophaceous gout is much less prevalent since advent of uricosuric agents. Sites of predilection for tophus formation include the helix and antihelix of ear, fingers, hands, knees, feet, olecranon bursae, and Achilles tendon.

2. Renal
   - After gouty arthritis, renal disease is the most frequent complication of hyperuricemia.
   - The two chief types of renal disease occurring in gout are urate nephropathy (attributed to the deposition of monosodium urate crystals in the renal interstitial tissue) and uric acid nephropathy (related to formation of uric acid crystals in the collecting tubules, pelvis, or ureter, with subsequent impairment of urine flow).
   - Renal calculi occur in 10% to 25% of patients who have primary gout, a prevalence more than 1000 times greater than that in the general population.
3. Nonspecific
   - Initial attacks are usually associated with few constitutional symptoms, but later episodes are often polyarticular and febrile.

III. OCULAR MANIFESTATIONS

1. Conjunctiva
   - Bilateral conjunctival redness is the most common form of ocular involvement in gout and occurs in about 60% of patients. It is caused by hyperemia of the conjunctival and episcleral vessels.
   - Pingueculas
2. Vitreous body
   - Asteroid hyalosis
3. Anterior chamber angle
   - Open-angle glaucoma
   - Ocular hypertension

4. Uvea
   - Uveitis is not more common in gouty patients than in the general population, many statements to the contrary in the older literature notwithstanding.
5. Sclera and episclera
   - Tophi have been reported, but are extremely rare.
6. Cornea
   - Crystals are a great rarity, and the nature of those in the several reported cases remains open to question.
   - Band keratopathy has been reported but is extremely rare.

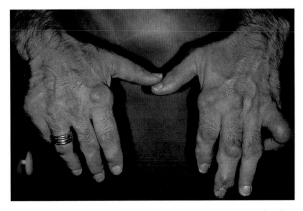

FIGURE 91.1. Chronic tophaceous gout involving the hands and wrists.

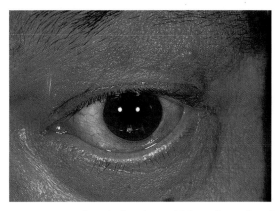

FIGURE 91.2. Conjunctival redness. (This patient's hands are depicted in Fig. 91.1.)

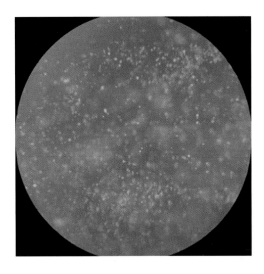

FIGURE 91.3. Asteroid hyalosis.

SUGGESTED READINGS

Ferry AP. Gout. In: Gold DH, Weingeist TA, eds. *The Eye in Systemic Disease.* Philadelphia: JB Lippincott; 1990:396–398.

Ferry AP. The eye and rheumatic diseases. In: Kelley WN, Harris ED, Ruddy S, Sledge CB, eds. *Textbook of Rheumatology,* 4th ed. Philadelphia: WB Saunders; 1993:507–518. *Covers ocular involvement in gout and various other rheumatic diseases.*

Ferry AP, Safir A, Melikian HE. Ocular abnormalities in patients with gout. *Ann Ophthalmol* 1985;17:632–635. *A detailed study of 69 patients who had particularly severe gout.*

Kelley WN, Schumacher HR. Gout. In: Kelley WN, Harris ED, Ruddy S, Sledge CB, eds. *Textbook of Rheumatology,* 4th ed. Philadelphia: WB Saunders; 1993:1291–1336. *An authoritative and detailed consideration of gout, with 667 references.*

Safir A, Dunn SN, Martin RG, Tate GW, Mincey GJ. Is asteroid hyalosis ocular gout? *Ann Ophthalmol* 1990;22:70–77. *Explores in detail the relationship between gout and asteroid hyalosis.*

Section G. Peroxisomal Disorders

Chapter 92

ADRENOLEUKODYSTROPHY

W. Bruce Wilson

I. GENERAL

There are several related disorders: all are associated because of peroxisomal enzymatic defects. Only childhood adrenoleukodystrophy (CALD), neonatal ALD (NALD), and adrenomyeloneuropathy (AMN) will be dealt with here.

1. Age of onset in years: CALD, 4 to 8; NALD, birth; AMN, 20 to 30. Inheritance is X-linked recessive (CALD, AMN) and autosomal recessive (NALD).
2. Lack of oxidative enzymes to degrade (oxidize) saturated unbranched very long-chain fatty acids (VLCFA)
3. Enzyme normally carried in cytoplasmic organelle, the peroxisome.
4. Enzymatic decrease can be measured in various tissues, such as liver, kidney
5. The VLCFA accumulate in tissue—brain, including optic nerve; retina (photoreceptors, ganglion cells, retinal pigment epithelium, etc.) at an early stage; also adrenal (atrophy)
6. Brain and optic nerve become atrophic secondary to demyelination and neuronal loss.

II. SYSTEMIC MANIFESTATIONS

1. Mucocutaneous
   - Bronzing of skin (CALD)
   - Atrophy of skin (NALD, AMN)
2. Liver
   - Congenital hepatomegaly and dysmorphia (NALD)
3. Endocrine
   - Atrophy of adrenal (all) with hypofunction
4. Central nervous system—see Ocular Manifestations

III. OCULAR MANIFESTATIONS

1. Skin of lids
   - Bronzing with atrophy (CALD, NALD)
2. Lens
   - Cataract (CALD)
3. Choroid/retina
   - Retinal pigmentlike fundus (NALD)
4. Neuroophthalmologic
   - Demyelination and atrophy of optic nerve (CALD, AMN)
   - Paresis cranial nerves 3, 4, 6 (CALD)
   - Loss of voluntary cerebral control of eye movement (Balint's syndrome) (CALD)
5. Other central nervous system
   - Seizure (NALD)
   - Dementia (CALD, NALD)
   - Behavioral change (CALD)
   - Motor signs
     - Gait
     - Paresis (CALD, AMN)
     - Hypotonia (NALD)
   - Peripheral neuropathy (CALD, AMN)
   - Sensorineural hearing loss (CALD, NALD)

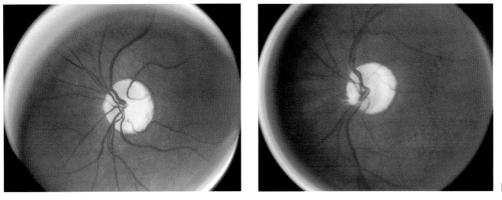

FIGURE 92.1. Right (**A**) and left (**B**) fundi of patient with CALD and far advanced optic atrophy.

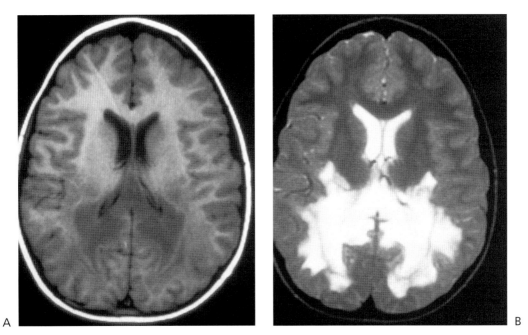

FIGURE 92.2. Magnetic resonance imaging scan of a patient with CALD. T1 (**A**) and T2 (**B**) images demonstrate marked white matter change posteriorly in the cerebrum (particularly white area on T2). Courtesy of Erin Prenger, DO, Swedish Medical Center, Denver, Colorado.

SUGGESTED READINGS

Aicardi J. The inherited leukodystrophies: A clinical overview. *J Inherit Metal dis* 1993:16:733–743. *A good review from a genetic/metabolic viewpoint.*

Brown FR III, Voigt R, Singh AK, Singh I. Peroxisomal disorders. Neurodevelopmental and biochemical aspects. *Am J Dis Child* 1993;147:617–626. *A good review from a neurologic viewpoint.*

Kamei A, Houdou S, Takashima S, et al. Peroxisomal disorders in children: Immunohistochemistry and neuropathology. *J Pediatr* 1993;122:573–579. *A good review from a pediatric viewpoint.*

Moser HW, Bergin A, Cornblath D. Peroxisomal disorders. *Biochem Cell Biol* 1991;69:463–474. *A good review from a biochemical viewpoint.*

Schaumburg HH, Powers JH, Raine CS, et al. Adrenoleukodystrophy. A clinical and pathological study of 17 cases. *Arch Neurol* 1975;32:577–591. *A pathologic review.*

Chapter 93

ADULT REFSUM'S DISEASE

Richard G. Weleber

1. The metabolic defect exists from early embryogenesis. Although congenital anomalies are not as common as is the case in infantile Refsum's disease, syndactyly when present is, of course, evident at birth. The acquired features of the disease begin in childhood. Symptoms of retinitis pigmentosa usually precede other features, such as neuropathy or cardiac defects, but rarely children can develop life-threatening cardiac conduction defects. Onset of clinically significant manifestations varies from early childhood to the fifth decade of life.

2. The disorder is autosomal recessive and affects males and females equally. Carriers are clinically normal.

3. There is no evidence of racial or ethnic predilection.

4. Pathologic mechanisms
   - Phytanic acid is a 20-carbon, branched-chain fatty acid (3,7,11,15-tetramethylhexadecanoic acid), which accumulates in blood and tissues and in affected individuals may account for 5% to 30% of total fatty acids in blood and up to 50% of fatty acids in tissues, such as liver.
   - Phytanic acid is not synthesized in the body and is ingested exclusively from the diet, being present in dairy products and ruminant fats. Free phytol is readily absorbed and converted to phytanic acid.
   - Phytol is present in chlorophyll and leafy vegetables and to some extent this bound phytol can be broken down into phytanic acid. However, plant phytol is a relatively unimportant source of phytanic acid in the diet.
   - Phytanic acid oxidation occurs in both mitochondria and to a 20-fold greater extent in peroxisomes. Phytanic acid cannot be broken down by β-oxidation because of the presence of a methyl group at the third carbon position. Instead phytanic acid undergoes a two-step process of α-oxidation: first, the formation of α-hydroxyphytanic acid followed by decarboxylation to form the n-1 carbon homologue, pristanic

   acid. Pristanic acid can be further catabolized by peroxisomal β-oxidation, which is normal in Refsum's disease.
   - Phytanic acid α-oxidation appears deficient in all tissues studied in Refsum's patients. Mitochondrial oxidation of phytanic acid is normal in Refsum's disease but insufficient to prevent disease. Refsum's disease is now considered a disorder involving a single, specific peroxisomal function, that of peroxisomal hydroxylation of phytanic acid to form α-hydroxyphytanic acid.
   - Refsum's disease, also called adult Refsum's disease, is distinct from the disorder of peroxisomal biogenesis called infantile Refsum's disease, which has multiple peroxisomal dysfunctions.
   - Phytanic acid can also accumulate in other peroxisomal disorders, such as Zellweger syndrome, neonatal adrenoleukodystrophy, and rhizomelic chondrodysplasia punctata. This accumulation is much less than in Refsum's disease and is related to loss of phytanic acid oxidation from defective peroxisomal biogenesis or defective import of multiple peroxisomal enzyme proteins.
   - Virtually all patients with Refsum's disease have or develop retinal degeneration, peripheral neuropathy, cerebellar ataxia, and high cerebrospinal fluid (CSF) protein concentrations.

5. Treatment
   - Dietary restriction of phytanic acid (and less importantly phytol) can reduce blood and tissue elevations.
   - If normal levels of plasma phytanic acid can be achieved, disease progression can be arrested.
   - Starvation, intercurrent illness, or marked weight loss may mobilize fatty stores of phytanic acid producing life-threatening cardiac abnormalities.
   - Plasmapheresis may be needed in severe cases or in conjunction with dietary control.

II. SYSTEMIC MANIFESTATIONS

1. Musculoskeletal
   - Epiphyseal dysplasia
   - Short fourth metatarsal
   - Syndactyly
   - Hammer toe
   - Pes cavus
   - Osteochondritis dissecans
2. Dermatologic
   - Ichthyosiform skin changes: from mild hyperkeratosis of palms and soles to frank truncal ichthyosis.
   - Accentuated palmar creases
   - Dermal nevus cell nevi, presenting as yellowish papules
3. Neurologic
   - Peripheral neuropathy with symmetric motor and sensory loss
   - Absent or decreased deep tendon reflexes
   - Cerebellar ataxia: dysmetria, unsteady gait, positive Romberg sign, intention tremor

4. Ear/nose/throat
   - Nerve deafness
   - Anosmia
5. Cardiologic
   - Nonspecific electrocardiographic changes
   - Impaired atrioventricular conduction and bundle branch block
   - Cardiac arrhythmia
6. Biochemical abnormalities in serum, plasma, and CSF
   - Markedly elevated serum or plasma levels of phytanic acid
   - Elevated CSF protein without pleocytosis
7. Histology
   - Lipid accumulation, presumably phytanic acid, within retinal pigment epithelium and other cells of the neural retina

III. OCULAR MANIFESTATIONS

1. Pupils
   - Pupillary abnormalities
2. Retina
   - Defective night vision
   - Constricted visual fields
   - Progressive retinal degeneration
   - Early macular degeneration
   - Attenuated vessels

   - Pigment dispersion and clumping of pigment
   - Severely subnormal electroretinogram
3. Optic nerve
   - Optic atrophy secondary to retinal degeneration
4. Lens
   - Posterior subcapsular cataract
5. Ocular motility
   - Nystagmus

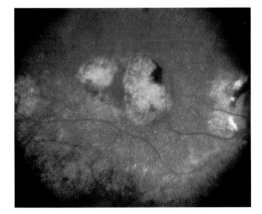

FIGURE 93.1. Retina of adult patient with Refsum's disease showing macular degenerative changes. Courtesy of Elias Traboulsi, MD and Irene H. Maumenee, MD.

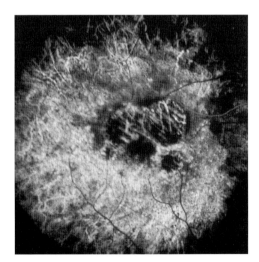

FIGURE 93.2. Fluorescein angiogram from same patient showing atrophy of pigment epithelium and choriocapillaris. Courtesy of Elias Traboulsi, MD and Irene H. Maumenee, MD.

SUGGESTED READINGS

Steinberg D. Refsum disease. In: Scriver CR, Beaudet AL, Sly WS, Valle D, eds. *The Metabolic and Molecular Bases of Inherited Disease,* 7th ed, vol 2. New York: McGraw-Hill; 1995:2351–2369.

Toussaint D, Danis P. An ocular pathologic study of Refsum's syndrome. *Am J Ophthalmol* 1971;72: 342–347.

Traupe H. Refsum's syndrome (heredopathia atactica polyneuritiformis). In: Traupe H, ed. *The Ichthyoses: A Guide to Clinical Diagnosis, Genetic Counseling, and Therapy.* Berlin: Springer-Verlag; 1989:81–87.

Weleber RG, Kennaway NG. Refsum's disease. In: Gold DH, Weingeist TA, eds. *The Eye in Systemic Disease.* Philadelphia: JB Lippincott; 1990:407–408.

Chapter 94

INFANTILE REFSUM'S DISEASE

Richard G. Weleber

I. GENERAL

1. Because dysmorphic features are evident at birth, the disease undoubtedly begins during intrauterine life.
2. The disorder is considered to be autosomal recessive and affects males and females equally. Carriers are normal.
3. There is no evidence of racial or ethnic predilection.
4. Pathologic mechanisms
   - Peroxisomes are deficient in number and size in most, if not all, tissues.
   - Peroxisomal functions include peroxisomal β-oxidation of very long-chain fatty acids (VLCFA), synthesis of plasmalogens and ether-phospholipids; synthesis of bile salts; catabolism of pipecolic acid, phytanic acid, dicarboxylic acids, and prostaglandins; and oxidation of polyamines, purines, and ethanol.
   - Virtually all peroxisomal functions that have been studied have been found to be deficient in infantile Refsum's disease (IRD).
   - IRD is related to Zellweger's syndrome and neonatal adrenoleukodystrophy, which are also disorders of generalized peroxisomal biogenesis. At least 13 different genes are required for formation of normal peroxisomes.
   - The exact biochemical deficiencies that cause the specific features seen in IRD are currently unknown.

II. SYSTEMIC MANIFESTATIONS

1. Musculoskeletal
   - Hypotony
   - Simian palmar creases
   - Muscle weakness and atrophy (late)
   - Osteopenia
   - Wheelchair bound by middle to end of second decade
2. Gastrointestinal
   - Neonatal jaundice
   - Hepatomegaly
   - Hepatic dysfunction
3. Neurologic
   - Severe to profound psychomotor retardation
   - Autistic behavior
   - Death in third decade
4. Ear/nose/throat
   - Sensorineural deafness
   - Craniofacial dysmorphism: low-set ears
   - Flat bridge of nose
   - Anosmia
5. Hematologic
   - Neonatal bleeding, often intracranial, secondary to hypovitaminosis K
   - Hemolytic anemia
6. Biochemical abnormalities in serum or plasma
   - Elevated VLCFAs
   - Elevated phytanic, pristanic, and pipecolic acids
   - Elevated bile precursors
   - Decreased plasmalogens and ether-phospholipids
   - Low cholesterol, high-density and low-density lipoprotein
   - Elevated liver function tests if hepatic dysfunction
7. Histology
   - Deficiencies in size and number of peroxisomes in virtually all cells
   - Lamellar neutral-lipid inclusions in hepatocytes
   - Micronodular and portal cirrhosis
   - Small, hypoplastic adrenals
   - Neutral lipid deposits between myofibrillar bundles
   - Single report of ocular and cochlear histology—severe degenerative changes with ganglion cell loss, gliosis of the nerve fiber layer and optic nerve, optic atrophy, and changes similar to those reported in retinitis pigmentosa

III. OCULAR MANIFESTATIONS

1. Lids
   - Epicanthal folds
2. Retina
   - Progressive retinal degeneration
   - Macular degeneration
   - Attenuated vessels
   - Pigment dispersion and clumping of pigment
   - Severely subnormal electroretinogram
3. Optic nerve
   - Optic atrophy
4. Lens
   - Posterior subcapsular cataract
5. Orbit
   - Microphthalmia
6. Ocular motility
   - Strabismus, amblyopia
   - Nystagmus

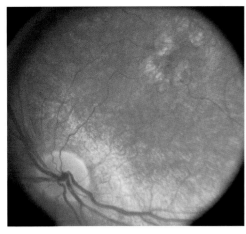

FIGURE 94.1 Retina of 3½-year-old child with IRD, demonstrating attenuated vessels and macular pigment epithelial defects. Reproduced with permission from Weleber RG, Tongue AT, Kennaway NG, Budden SS, Buist NRM. Ophthalmic manifestations of infantile phytanic acid storage disease. *Arch Ophthalmol* 1984;102:1317–1321. Copyright 1984, American Medical Association.

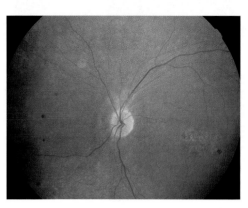

FIGURE 94.2 Retina of same child at 9⅓ years of age shows sparse pigment clumping in macula and nasal retina.

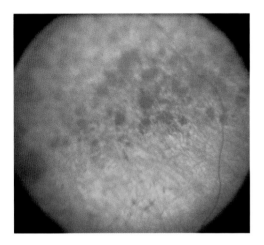

FIGURE 94.3 Retina of child with IRD at 10⅔ years of age shows dense pigment clumping in mid periphery.

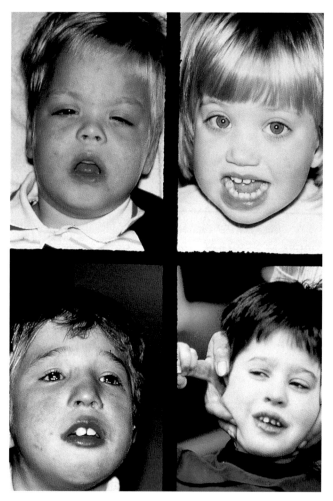

FIGURE 94.4 Facial appearance of four patients with IRD demonstrating similar features. Reproduced with permission from Budden SS, Kennaway NG, Buist NRM, Poulos A, Weleber RG. Dysmorphic syndrome with phytanic acid oxidase deficiency, abnormal very long chain fatty acids, and pipecolic acidemia: studies in four children. *J Pediatr* 1986;108:33–39.

SUGGESTED READINGS

Budden SS, Kennaway NG, Buist NRM, et al. Dysmorphic syndrome with phytanic acid oxidase deficiency, abnormal very long chain fatty acids, and pipecolic acidemia: Studies in four children. *J Pediatr* 1986;108:33–39.

Lazarow PB, Moser HW. Disorders of peroxisome biogenesis. In: Scriver CR, Beaudet AL, Sly WS, Valle D, eds. *The Metabolic and Molecular Bases of Inherited Disease,* 7th ed, vol 2. New York: McGraw-Hill; 1995:2287–2324.

Torvik A, Torp S, Kase BF, et al. Infantile Refsum's disease: A generalized peroxisomal disorder. Case report with postmortem examination. *J Neurol Sci* 1988;85:39–53.

Weleber RG, Kennaway NG. Infantile Refsum's disease. In: Gold DH, Weingeist TA, eds. *The Eye in Systemic Disease.* Philadelphia: JB Lippincott; 1990;409–411.

Weleber RG, Tongue AT, Kennaway NG, et al. Ophthalmic manifestations of infantile phytanic acid storage disease. *Arch Ophthalmol* 1984;102:1317–1321.

PART 12. MUSCULAR DISORDERS

Chapter 95

CONGENITAL MYOPATHIES (STRUCTURAL MYOPATHIES)

Jonathan D. Wirtschafter
Carlos Vazquez-Fermin

I. GENERAL

1. Group of congenital, usually nonprogressive myopathies, each of which displays a predominant histologic feature
2. Mitochondrial cytopathies are not included here and are discussed in Chapter 96.
3. Affected infants will manifest hypotonia during early childhood.
4. May present in adult life due to phenotypic heterogenicity within families
5. Some cases have a severe course.
6. Creatine kinase is usually normal or slightly elevated.
7. The electromyogram can be normal or myopathic, but it will not suggest an active neuropathy.
8. Only those congenital myopathies with reported ophthalmic manifestations are discussed: multicore with external ophthalmoplegia, congenital sex-linked myotubular, centronuclear (myotubular), congenital fiber-type disproportion, nemaline rod, reducing body (muscular dystrophy, late-onset distal), and central core.

II. SYSTEMIC MANIFESTATIONS

1. Muscular
   - Mostly proximal muscle weakness
   - Muscle hypotonia during early childhood
   - Deep tendon reflex depressed or absent
   - Weak crying, sucking, and swallowing
   - Nasal speech
2. Cardiac
   - Dilated cardiomyopathy
   - Atrioventricular septal defect
   - Heart block
3. Skeletal
   - Long, thin face
   - High arched palate
   - Thoracic wall abnormalities
   - Congenital dislocation of hips
   - Flat feet, pes cavus, club foot
4. Not all of these manifestations are present in each condition or patient.

III. OPHTHALMIC MANIFESTATIONS

Myopathy	Inheritance	Gene location	Ptosis/ ophthalmoplegia	Face weakness	Other
Multicore with external ophthalmoplegia	AR	—	+	+	
Congenital sex-linked myotubular	X-linked	Xq28	+	+	Cataract
Centronuclear (myotubular)	AD/AR, X-linked	—	+	+	Usually late onset; eye findings milder than in x-linked centronuclear myotubular
Congenital fiber-type disproportion	AR/AD	—	+	+	Type I muscle fibers are too small
Nemaline rod	AD/AR	1q-21-q23	Very rare	+	
Reducing body (muscular dystrophy, late-onset distal)	AR	2p13.3-p13.1	Very rare	Very rare	
Central core	AD	19q-13.1	Rare	+	Malignant hyperthermia cramps with exercise

AD, autosomal dominant; AR, autosomal recessive

SUGGESTED READINGS

McKusick V. *Online Medelian Inheritance in Man,* 2000.
Tome F, Fardeau M. *Congenital Myopathies.* In: Engel AG, Franzin-Armstrong C, eds. *Myology,* 2nd ed, vol. 2. New York: McGraw-Hill; 1994:1487–1532.
Miller NR, Newman NJ. *Walsh and Hoyt's Clinical Neuro-Ophthalmology,* 5th ed., vol. 1. Baltimore: Williams & Wilkins; 1998: 1354–1360.

Chapter 96

MITOCHONDRIAL CYTOPATHIES

Nancy J. Newman

I. GENERAL

1. Heterogeneous group of disorders
2. Primary defects in mitochondrial metabolism
3. Frequently have abnormal oxidative phosphorylation
4. May reflect nuclear or mitochondrial DNA defects
5. Inheritance will be mendelian if the primary defect is in nuclear DNA, maternal if the primary defect is in mitochondrial DNA.
6. Frequently have neurologic and ophthalmologic manifestations

II. SYSTEMIC MANIFESTATIONS

Disease	Systemic Manifestations
CPEO/KSS	Myopathy/ragged red fibers* Peripheral neuropathy Deafness Dementia Ataxia Vestibular dysfunction Basal gangliar lesions Cardiac conduction abnormalities* Short stature Gastrointestinal dysmotility Diabetes mellitus Delayed sexual maturation Hypogonadism Hypomagnesemia Hypoparathyroidism Hypothyroidism
LHON	Cardiac conduction abnormalities Multiple sclerosislike illness Minor neurologic/skeletal abnormalities Dystonia/basal gangliar lesions Encephalopathy
MELAS	Headache* Strokelike episodes* Seizures* Lactic acidosis* Psychiatric abnormalities Deafness Short stature Myopathy Basal gangliar lesions
\NARP/Leigh's syndrome	Neurogenic muscle weakness* Ataxia* Developmental delay* Sensory neuropathy Dementia Seizures Spongiform degeneration of basal ganglia and brainstem
MERRF	Myoclonus* Seizures Myopathy* Ataxia* Dementia* Developmental delay

* Commonly found.
CPEO, chronic progressive external ophthalmoplegia; KSS, Kearns-Sayre syndrome; LHON, Leber's hereditary optic neuropathy; MELAS, mitochondrial myopathy, encephalopathy, lactic acidosis, and strokelike episodes; NARP, neurogenic muscle weakness, ataxia, and retinitis pigmentosa; MERRF, myoclonic epilepsy and ragged red fibers

Disease	Ophthalmic Manifestations	Genetic Defect
CPEO/KSS	Ophthalmoplegia* Ptosis* Pigmentary retinopathy*	MtDNA deletions
LHON	Early: Disc microangiopathy* 　　　Pseudoedema* 　　　Vascular tortuosity* Late: Optic atrophy*	MtDNA point mutations
MELAS	Homonymous hemianopia* Cortical blindness* Pigmentary retinopathy Ophthalmoplegia Optic atrophy	MtDNA point mutations
NARP/Leigh's Syndrome	Pigmentary retinopathy* Optic atrophy Nystagmus	MtDNA point mutations
MERRF	Optic atrophy	MtDNA point mutations

* Commonly found.
CPEO, chronic progressive external ophthalmoplegia; KSS, Kearns-Sayre syndrome; LHON, Leber's hereditary optic neuropathy; MELAS, mitochondrial myopathy, encephalopathy, lactic acidosis, and strokelike episodes; NARP, neurogenic muscle weakness, ataxia, and retinitis pigmentosa; MERRF, myoclonic epilepsy and ragged red fibers; mtDNA, mitochondrial DNA.

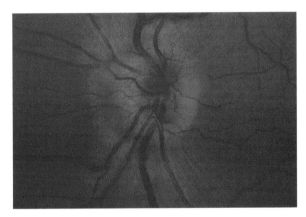

FIGURE 96.1. Optic disc appearance of a 20-year-old man with acute visual loss secondary to Leber's hereditary optic neuropathy. Note the hyperemia of the disc, the fine telangiectatic vessels on the disc surface, and the mild disc elevation (pseudoedema). The patient was positive for the mitochondrial DNA point mutation at position 11778.

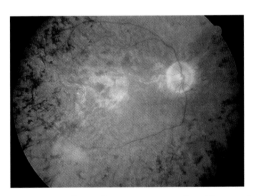

FIGURE 96.2. Funduscopic appearance of a 40-year-old man with profound visual loss, deafness, and mental retardation. He and his maternal relatives were found to harbor the mitochondrial DNA point mutation at position 8993 (so-called NARP mutation).

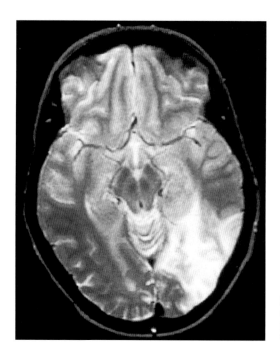

FIGURE 96.3. T2-weighted magnetic resonance image of the brain of a 12-year-old boy with MELAS and the mitochondrial DNA point mutation at position 3243. Note the abnormality in the posterior left brain, which does not respect major vascular territories, and which corresponds to his right homonymous hemianopia.

SUGGESTED READINGS

Newman NJ. Mitochondrial disease and the eye. *Ophthalmol Clin North Am* 1992;5:405–424. *Review of the most common neuroophthalmologic manifestations of mitochondrial disease.*

Newman NJ. Leber's hereditary optic neuropathy: New genetic considerations. *Arch Neurol* 1993;50:540–548. *Review of Leber's hereditary optic neuropathy and the mitochondrial DNA point mutations associated with the disease.*

Ortiz RG, Newman NJ, Shoffner JM, et al. Variable retinal and neurologic manifestations in patients harboring the mitochondrial DNA 8993 mutation. *Arch Ophthalmol* 1993;111:1525–1530. *Report of the ophthalmologic and neurologic manifestations of patients from two maternal pedigrees harboring the mitochondrial DNA point mutation 8993 associated with NARP and Leigh's syndrome.*

Shoffner JM IV, Wallace DC. Oxidative phosphorylation diseases. Disorders of two genomes. *Adv Hum Genet* 1990;19:267–330. *Review of mitochondrial biochemistry and genetics and its relation to human disease.*

Shoffner JM, Wallace DC. Oxidative phosphorylation diseases and mitochondrial DNA mutations: Diagnosis and treatment. *Annu Rev Nutr* 1994;14:535–568. *Review of the diseases currently associated with mitochondrial dysfunction and mitochondrial DNA abnormalities.*

Chapter 97

KEARNS-SAYRE SYNDROME

Edsel B. Ing
James A. Garrity
Thomas P. Kearns

I. GENERAL

1. The classic triad is external ophthalmoplegia, pigmentary retinopathy, and heart block.
2. Patients can be male or female and are usually less than 20 years of age at presentation.
3. Ptosis, usually bilateral, often precedes the ophthalmoplegia, and is the most frequent presenting ocular sign.
4. Progressive external ophthalmoplegia without diurnal variation is characteristic. Patients may not complain of diplopia. There is no response to oculocephalic maneuvers.
5. The pigmentary retinopathy of Kearns-Sayre syndrome differs from retinitis pigmentosa (see Ocular Manifestations).
6. Although cardiac problems can occur at any time, ptosis and ophthalmoplegia usually precede heart block. Patients should be regularly monitored by a cardiologist. Pacemaker implantation may be required.
7. Decreased brainstem ventilatory drive in response to hypoxia and hypercarbia can lead to respiratory failure. Fatal hyperglycemic metabolic acidosis with respiratory failure has been reported following systemic steroid administration.
8. Large-scale mitochondrial DNA deletions with decreased activities of mitochondrial respiratory chain enzymes are usually found. Because mitochondrial DNA is transmitted to progeny by the oocyte, Kearns-Sayre syndrome is thought to be maternally transmitted.
9. Muscle biopsy shows ragged red fibers.

II. SYSTEMIC MANIFESTATIONS

These systemic manifestations are not consistent findings in all cases
1. Cardiac
   - Cardiac conduction defects
   - Dilated cardiomyopathy
   - Asymmetrical septal hypertrophy
   - Mitral valve prolapse
   - Mitral regurgitation
2. Neurologic
   - Deficient brainstem respiratory control mechanisms
   - Spongiform encephalopathy
   - Elevated cerebrospinal fluid protein
   - Hearing loss
   - Subnormal intelligence
   - Cerebellar ataxia
   - Corticospinal tract signs
   - Somatic muscle weakness and elevated serum lactate
   - Continuous muscle fiber activity (Isaacs-Mertens syndrome)
3. Endocrine
   - Short stature
   - Gonadal dysfunction
   - Diabetes mellitus
   - Hypoparathyroidism (may have basal ganglia calcification)
   - Thyroid disease
   - Hyperaldonsteronism
   - Hypomagnesemia
   - Pearson syndrome (pancreas dysfunction, growth retardation, and pancytopenia)
   - Metabolic-endocrine failure with steroid treatment
4. Other
   - Renal tubular acidosis
   - Sideroblastic anemia
   - Skeletal abnormalities including metaphyseal dysplasia
   - Dental anomalies

III. OCULAR MANIFESTATIONS

1. Ptosis
   - May have compensatory chin-up posture
2. Progressive external ophthalmoplegia
   - No response to oculocephalic maneuvers
   - Poor Bell's phenomenon (to lid closure)
3. Pigmentary retinopathy
   - Changes tend to be centered in the posterior pole. In retinitis pigmentosa pigmentary changes are more peripheral, and bone spicules may be seen. Arteriolar narrowing, vitreous debris, posterior subcapsular cataracts, and "optic atrophy" are uncommon in Kearns-Sayre syndrome, but typical of retinitis pigmentosa.
   - Usually normal or minimally decreased on electroretinography and dark adaptation
4. Uncommon findings
   - Corneal edema
   - Primary open-angle glaucoma
   - Optic atrophy
   - Optic neuritis
   - Pendular nystagmus

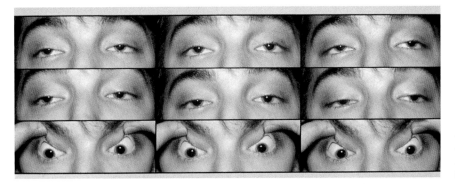

FIGURE 97.1. This 17-year-old boy had long-standing ptosis and markedly reduced vision in all fields of gaze. An enlarged left ventricle was seen on echocardiography. At age 20 the patient developed a subtle, non-specific intraventricular conduction delay.

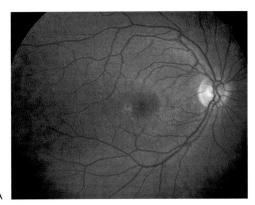
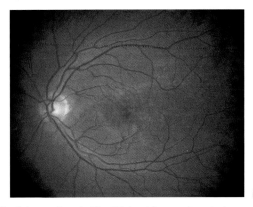

A   B

FIGURE 97.2. OD (**A**) and OS (**B**) show the fundi of the patient in Fig. 97.1, with prominent pigmentary retinopathy of the posterior pole.

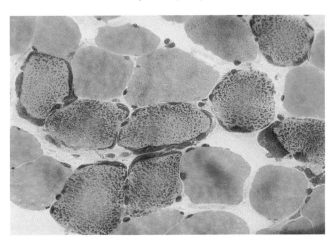

FIGURE 97.3. Skeletal muscle biopsy from another patient shows ragged red muscle fibers admixed with a population of relatively normal muscle fibers (Gomori trichrome stain). The ragged red fibers represent abnormal accumulations of mitochondria beneath the plasma membrane and between the myofibrils.

SUGGESTED READINGS

Bachynski BN, Flynn JT, Rodrigues MM, et al. Hyperglycemic acidotic coma and death in Kearns-Sayre syndrome. *Ophthalmology* 1986;93:391–396.

Barohn RJ, Clanton T, Sahenk Z, Mendell JR. Recurrent respiratory insufficiency and depressed ventilatory drive complicating mitochondrial myopathies. *Neurology* 1990;40:103–106.

Garrity JA, Kearns TP. Kearns-Sayre syndrome. In: Gold DH, Weingeist TA, eds. *The Eye in Systemic Disease*. Philadelphia: JB Lippincott; 1990:423–425. *A general review of Kearns-Sayre syndrome.*

Kearns TP, Sayre GP. Retinitis pigmentosa, external ophthalmoplegia, and complete heart block: Unusual syndrome with histologic study in one of two cases. *Arch Ophthalmol* 1958;60:280–289. *In this original article, "retinitis pigmentosa" was used to indicate the pigmentary retinopathy.*

Moraes CT, DiMauro S, Zeviani M, et al. Mitochondrial DNA deletions in progressive external ophthalmoplegia and Kearns-Sayre syndrome. *N Engl J Med* 1989;320:1293–1299.

Chapter 98

CONGENITAL MUSCULAR DYSTROPHIES WITH EYE FINDINGS

Jonathan D. Wirtschafter
Carlos Vazquez-Fermin

I. GENERAL

1. Genetically transmitted lissencephaly type II with other developmental brain abnormalities and progressive myopathy
2. Lack of specific histochemical and electron microscopic myopathic properties that characterize the congenital myopathies and/or Duchenne and myotonic dystrophies
3. Stationary or very slowly progressive muscular weakness with or without hypotonia
4. There are three recognized disorders with autosomal recessive inheritance:
   - Muscular dystrophy, congenital progressive with mental retardation (Fukuyama disease)
   - Hydrocephalus, agyria, and retinal dysplasia with or without encephalocele (HARD ± E syndrome) (Walker-Warburg congenital muscular dystrophy)
   - Muscle-eye-brain disease (Santauvori congenital muscular dystrophy)

II. SYSTEMIC MANIFESTATIONS

Disease	Systemic Manifestations
Fukuyama	Myopathy more proximal than distal Facial weakness with poor sucking Weak crying Developmental abnormalities of cerebral and cerebellar cortex Polymicrogyria Thick cortex and shallow sulci Ectopic glia and neurons Subarachnoid thickening Retarded intellectual development Seizures in 50% Funnel chest deformity Most cases are of Japanese ancestry Average life span: 9 years Gene map locus 9q31-q33
Walker-Warburg	Present at birth Generalized muscular weakness Weak crying and poor sucking Small cranial nerves Hydrocephalus Disorganized brain development with lack of cortical lamination, small brainstem and cerebellum Glial heterotopias with thick leptomeninges Life span: <4 months Gene map locus 9q31-q33
Santavouri	Clinical presentation about 5 years of age followed by progressive mental and muscular deterioration Proximal myopathy Spasticity Contractures of multiple joints Microcephaly without hydrocephalus Neuroimaging even at birth reveals developmental abnormalities Life span: 6–16 years Controversy if this is a distinct but milder form of Walker-Warburg syndrome

Disease	Ocular Manifestations
Fukuyama	Extraocular and orbicularis oculi muscle weakness Hypoplastic and abnormal development of optic nerve and retina Optic atrophy High myopia Cataract
Walker-Warburg	Features combine those of primary hyperplastic primary vitreous (PHPV) and Peter anomaly Extraocular muscle weakness Microphthalmos Central corneal opacities Shallow anterior chambers Iridolenticular synechiae Abnormal retinal differentiation (100%) Hypoplasia of optic nerve
Santavouri	Congenital myopia Retinal dysplasia and hyperplasia Optic atrophy Abnormal eye movements

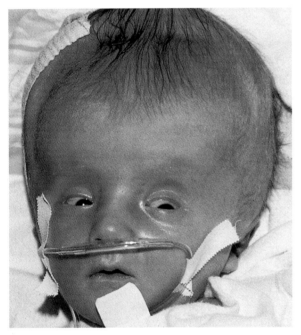

FIGURE 98.1.   Photograph of patient LP88-013 at age about 2 days showing recently shunted congenital hydrocephalus and sunset sign.

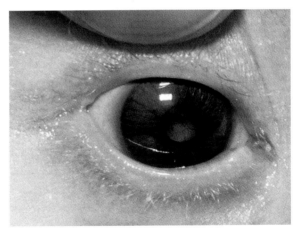

FIGURE 98.2.   Close-up of the right eye of patient LP88-013 showing leukocoria caused by a cataract or PHPV or both.

SUGGESTED READINGS

Banker BQ. The congenital muscular dystrophies. In: Engel AG, Franzin-Armstrong C, eds. *Myology,* 2nd ed, vol 2. New York: McGraw-Hill; 1994:1275–1286.

Chijiiwa T, Nishimura M. Ocular manifestations of congenital muscular dystrophy (Fukuyama type). *Ann Ophthalmol* 1983;15:921–928.

Dobyns WB, Pagon RA, Armstrong D, et al. Diagnostic criteria for Walker-Warburg syndrome. *Am J Hum Genet* 1989;32:195–210.

Fukuyama Y, Osawa M, Suzuki H. Congenital progressive muscular dystrophy of the Fukuyama type—Clinical, genetic and pathological considerations. *Brain Dev* 1981;3:1–29.

McKusick V. *Online Medelian Inheritance in Man,* 2000.

Miller NR, Newman NJ. *Walsh and Hoyt's Clinical Neuro-Ophthalmology,* 5th ed, vol. 1. Baltimore: Williams & Wilkins; 1998:1360–1363.

Chapter 99

OCULOPHARYNGEAL MUSCULAR DYSTROPHY

Carlos Vazquez-Fermin
Jonathan D. Wirtschafter

I. GENERAL

1. Autosomal dominantly inherited disorder (most frequently) with complete penetrance
2. Gene locus at 14q11.2-q13 with GCC repeat expansions in the poly (A) binding-protein 2 (PABP2) gene
3. Cases reported in French-Canadian families and in Spanish-Americans from Colorado, New Mexico, and Arizona
4. Symptoms and signs appear after age 40 years.
5. Morbidity due to impaired movement of pharyngeal muscle producing accumulation of secretions in the nasopharynx with increased risk for tracheobronchial and pulmonary disease
6. Death occurs as a result of starvation or aspiration pneumonia, but progress in palliative treatment (feeding gastrostomy) may prolong the life span and change the prognosis.
7. Muscle fibers contain rimmed vacuoles and small angulated intranuclear tubular filaments.
8. Mitochondrial abnormalities are found but may be nonspecific findings related to aging.

II. SYSTEMIC MANIFESTATIONS

1. Musculoskeletal
   - Dysphagia, due to pharyngeal and laryngeal weakness, usually precedes ptosis by years
   - Facial weakness, particularly involving orbicularis oculi muscles
   - Wasting and weakness of neck and distal limb muscles
   - Limb-girdle muscular weakness
   - Anal and vesicular sphincter weakness
2. Cardiac
   - Cardiac abnormalities are not a feature of this disease in contrast to Kearns-Sayre syndrome.

III. OCULAR MANIFESTATIONS

1. Ocular motility
   - Ptosis, usually bilateral and symmetrical
   - External ophthalmoplegia
   - Potential corneal complications can result from ptosis surgery due to absent Bell's phenomenon and orbicularis oculi weakness.
2. Retina
   - Pigmentary retinal degeneration may be infrequent because many earlier reports probably included cases of Kearns-Sayre syndrome.

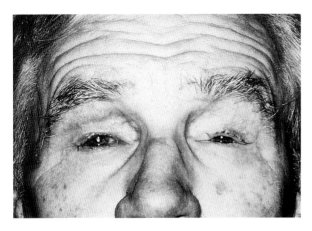

FIGURE 99.1. Bilateral ptosis in a 65-year-old man with oculopharyngeal muscular dystrophy.

SUGGESTED READINGS

Miller NR, Newman NS. *Walsh and Hoyt's Clinical Neuro-Ophthalmology,* 5th ed., vol. 1. Baltimore: Williams & Wilkins; 1998:1372–1376.

McKusick V. *Online Medelian Inheritance in Man,* 2000.

Tome F. *Oculopharyngeal muscular dystrophy.* In: Engel AG, Franzin-Armstrong C, eds. *Myology,* 2nd ed, vol 2. New York: McGraw-Hill; 1994:1241–1243.

Chapter 100

MALIGNANT HYPERTHERMIA (HYPERTHERMIA OF ANESTHESIA)

Jonathan D. Wirtschafter
Carlos Vazquez-Fermin

I. GENERAL

1. Autosomal dominant inheritance
2. Gene locus 19q13.1: *Ryanodine receptor-1* gene, which controls calcium-mediated release of calcium from the sarcoplasmic reticulum calcium release channel, is responsible for about 50% of cases. Some cases are due to a mutation in a calcium channel gene (*CACNAIS*).
3. Pharmacogenic disorder leading to hypertonicity of skeletal muscles leading to hyperpyrexia and rhabdomyolisis
4. Incidence is 1/15,000 anesthetic administrations in children and 1/50,000 in adults.
5. Anesthesia-related precipitating factors are succinylcholine, halothane, and increased potassium.
6. Some nonanesthetic precipitating factors are neuroleptic drugs, alcohol, infection, caffeine, and severe exercise in hot conditions.
7. Oral and intravenous dantrolene sodium inhibit the release of calcium ion from the sarcoplasmic reticulum and can be used for prophylaxis or treatment.
8. Other disorders affecting muscle manifest malignant hyperthermia as a result of anesthesia, particularly central core myopathy; King-Denborough syndrome; and possibly Noonan's syndrome.
9. King-Denborough syndrome and Native American myopathy are similar, except that the latter always has cleft palate; both have congenital muscular weakness and dysmorphic features.

II. SYSTEMIC MANIFESTATIONS

1. General
   - Muscular rigidity
   - Rhabdomyolysis
   - Elevated serum creatine phosphokinase, phosphate, and potassium
   - Lactic acidosis
   - Hyperthermia
   - Heat stroke
2. King-Denborough syndrome and Native American myopathy
   - Congenital muscle weakness
   - Myopathic facies
   - Low-set ears
   - Malar hypoplasia
   - Kyphosis/scoliosis
   - Abnormal sternum

III. OCULAR MANIFESTATIONS

1. General
   - Risk of anesthetic complications during "routine" ocular surgery
2. King-Denborough and Native American myopathy
   - Ptosis
   - Strabismus
   - Orbicularis oculi weakness

SUGGESTED READINGS

King JO, Denborough MA, Zapf PW. Inheritance of malignant hyperthermia. *Lancet* 1972;I:365–370.
McKusick V. *Online Medelian Inheritance in Man*, 2000.
Tome F, Fardeau M. *Congenital myopathies*. In: Engel AG, Franzin-Armstrong C, eds. *Myology*, 2nd ed, vol 2. New York: McGraw-Hill; 1994;1487–1532.

Chapter 101

PERIODIC PARALYSES

Jonathan D. Wirtschafter
Carlos Vazquez-Fermin

I. GENERAL

1. Group of diseases of different etiology characterized by episodes of flaccid muscular weakness or myotonia that recur at irregular time intervals
2. Patients can present with localized or generalized weakness that can last from less than 1 hour to several days.
3. Continued mild exercise may abort the weakness, but rest after exercise can induce the weakness.
4. Can present with malignant hyperthermia
5. Gene loci
   - Paramyotonia congenita—17q23.1-q25.3—probably allelic to hyperkalemic periodic paralysis; sodium channel gene mutation
   - Hyperkalemic periodic paralysis—17q23.1-q25.3—sodium channel gene mutations and allelic varients
   - Hypokalemic periodic paralysis—1q32—calcium channel gene mutation
   - Episodic muscle weakness—Xp22.3
6. *Note:* Only those periodic paralyses disorders with reported ophthalmic manifestations are discussed.

II. SYSTEMIC MANIFESTATIONS

1. Episodic skeletal muscle weakness, hypokalemic and hyperkalemic periodic paralyses
2. Episodic myotonia—hyperkalemic periodic paralysis and paramyotonia congenita
3. Precipitating factors
   - Paramyotonia congenita: cold
   - Hyperkalemic periodic paralysis: potassium
   - Hypokalemic periodic paralysis: administration of insulin or glucose; rest after exercise
   - Episodic muscle weakness: ferrile illness
4. Alleviating factors
   - Paramyotonia congenita: chlorothiazide, warmth
   - Hyperkalemic periodic paralysis: calcium
   - Hypokalemic periodic paralysis: potassium or exercise

III. OCULAR MANIFESTATIONS

1. Ocular muscle myotonia and lid lag during attacks
2. Inability to open eyelids during attacks
3. Facial weakness during attacks
4. Can be precipitated by cooling the eyelids with ice, cold water, or cold wind

SUGGESTED READINGS

Lettmon F, Engel AG. The periodic paralysis and paramyotonia congenita. In: Engel AG, Franzin-Armstrong C, eds. *Myology,* 2nd ed, vol 2. New York: McGraw-Hill; 1994:1303–1315.
McKusick V. *Online Medelian Inheritance in Man,* 2000.
Miller NR, Newman NJ. *Walsh and Hoyt's Clinical Neuro-Ophthalmology,* 5th ed, vol 1. Baltimore: Williams & Wilkins: 1998:1376–1377.
Ryan MM, Taylor P, Donald JA, et al. A novel syndrome of episodic muscle weakness maps to Xp22.3. *Am J Hum Genet* 1999;65:1104–1113.

Chapter 102

MYOPATHY AND ENCEPHALOPATHY OF VITAMIN E DEFICIENCY DISORDERS

Jonathan D. Wirtschafter
Carlos Vazquez-Fermin

I. GENERAL

1. Vitamin E (α-tocopherol) is essential for maintenance of neurologic and muscle structure
2. Causes of vitamin E deficiency
   - Malnutrition
   - Impaired intestinal absorption of lipids
   - Hepatic obstructive disorders
- Cystic fibrosis (gene locus 7q31.2)
- Abetalipoproteinuria (Bassen-Kornzweig syndrome)
   - Deficiency of microsomal-type triglyceride transfer protein
   - Gene locus 4q22-q24

II. SYSTEMIC MANIFESTATIONS

1. Neuropathologic features
   - Loss of oculomotor nuclei
   - Axonal dystrophy of long tracts
   - Premature lipofuscin accumulation in Schwann cells
2. Neurologic features
   - Progressive weakness
   - Loss of position and vibratory sense
   - Areflexia
   - Ataxia
   - Myopathy
3. Decreased ratio of vitamin E to total serum lipid
4. Acanthocytosis in abetalipoproteinemia

III. OCULAR MANIFESTATIONS

1. Ocular motility
   - External ophthalmoplegia
   - Internuclear ophthalmoplegia
   - Ptosis and "alternating" ptosis
   - Slow or absent fast components of optokinetic and vestibular nystagmus
   - Abnormal saccades
2. Retina
   - Night blindness
   - Pigmentary retinopathy that is less severe morphologically and functionally than classical retinitis pigmentosa

SUGGESTED READINGS

Miller NR, Newman NJ. *Walsh and Hoyt's Clinical Neuro-Ophthalmology,* 5th ed., vol 1. Baltimore: Williams & Wilkins: 1998;1331, 1391.

Neville HE, Ringel SP. Ultrastructural and histochemical abnormalities of skeletal muscle in patients with chronic vitamin E deficiency. *Neurology* 1983;33:483–488.

Satya-Murti S, Howard L. The spectrum of neurologic disorder from vitamin E deficiency. *Neurology* 1986;36:917–921.

Tomsai LG. Reversibility of human myopathy caused by vitamin E deficiency. *Neurology* 1979;29:1182–1186.

Victor M. Myopathies due to drugs, toxins and nutritional deficiency. In: Engel AG, Franzin-Armstrong, C, eds. *Myology,* 2nd ed, vol 2. New York: McGraw-Hill; 1994:1719–1720.

Werlin SL, Tlarb JM. Neuromuscular dysfunction and ultrastructural pathology in children with chronic cholestasis and vitamin E deficiency. *Ann Neurol* 1983;13:291–296.

Chapter 103

MYASTHENIA GRAVIS

Mark A. Ross
Richard K. Neahring

I. GENERAL

1. Pathogenesis
- Acquired myasthenia gravis (MG) is an autoimmune disorder.
- Antibodies damage the skeletal muscle acetylcholine receptor.
- Neuromuscular transmission failure causes muscle weakness and fatigability.
- Ocular MG: only the extraocular or levator palpebrae superioris muscles are affected.
- Generalized MG: limb, bulbar, or respiratory muscles are affected.
- Disorders of the thymus gland (thymic hyperplasia, thymoma) are associated.

2. Epidemiology
- Uncommon disorder affecting children and adults of all ages
- Annual incidence: 2 cases per million
- Prevalence: 50 to 125 cases per million
- Most often affects young adult women and older adult men
- Thyroid disease and other autoimmune disorders may be associated.

3. Management
- Individualized according to severity of clinical problems
- Cholinesterase inhibitors may suffice for mild cases.
- Immune-modulating therapies needed for more severe cases.
  - Thymectomy: reduce immunosuppressive therapy, increase chance of remission
  - Prednisone, azathioprine, cyclosporin, intravenous immunoglobulin (IVIG)
  - Plasmaphoresis used to improve symptoms rapidly

4. Prognosis
- Prognosis varies with the type and severity of MG.
- Ocular versus generalized MG usually determined in the first 3 years of the illness
- With treatment, most MG patients lead productive lives with few restrictions.
- Patients with severe MG may have persistent symptoms despite intensive treatment.
- Chronic use of immune-modulating therapies may lead to complications.
- Generalized MG can be fatal due to respiratory failure.

II. SYSTEMIC MANIFESTATIONS

Therapy causing the manifestation is in parentheses.

1. Cardiovascular
- Bradycardia (pyridostigmine)
- Deep venous thrombosis (IVIG)
- Hypertension (cyclosporin, prednisone)
- Hypotension (pyridostigmine, plasmaphoresis)
- Edema, congestive heart failure (prednisone, IVIG)

2. Central nervous system
- Aseptic meningitis (IVIG)
- Depression, psychosis (cyclosporin, prednisone)
- Epidural lipomatosis, spinal cord compression (prednisone)
- Encephalopathy (cyclosporin)
- Seizures (cyclosporin)
- Tremor (cyclosporin, prednisone)

3. Dermatologic
- Acne, hirsutism (cyclosporin, prednisone)
- Diaphoresis (pyridostigmine)
- Ecchymoses (prednisone)
- Lipomatosis (prednisone)
- Stria (prednisone)
- Rash (azathioprine, IVIG)

4. Endocrine
- Diabetes mellitus (prednisone)

5. Gastrointestinal
- Abdominal cramping, diarrhea (pyridostigmine)
- Acute pancreatitis (azathioprine)
- Hepatic toxicity (azathioprine, cyclosporin)
- Increased salivation (pyridostigmine)
- Peptic ulcer (prednisone)

6. Hematologic
- Bone marrow suppression (azathioprine)
- Possible risk of hematologic malignancy (azathioprine)

7. Musculoskeletal
- Aseptic necrosis of femur (prednisone)
- Compression fractures, osteoporosis (prednisone)
- Exacerbation of MG (initiation of prednisone therapy)
- Proximal muscle weakness (prednisone)

8. Pulmonary
- Myasthenic crisis, respiratory failure (excessive pyridostigmine)
- Bronchoconstriction (pyridostigmine)
- Increased bronchial secretions (pyridostigmine)
- Pneumothorax (central line for plasmaphoresis)

9. Renal
- Renal insufficiency or failure (IVIG, cyclosporin)

10. Nonspecific
    - Chills, fever (azathioprine, IVIG)
    - Headaches (cyclosporin, IVIG)
    - Insomnia (prednisone)
    - Irritability (prednisone)
    - Susceptibility to infection (prednisone, azathioprine, cyclosporin)
    - Systemic flulike illness (azathioprine)
    - Weight gain (prednisone)

III. OCULAR MANIFESTATIONS

1. Lids
    - Fluctuating blepharoptosis
    - Orbicularis oculi weakness/fatigability (peek sign)
    - Lid retraction
        - Retraction contralateral to blepharoptosis
        - Cogan's lid twitch
        - Transient spontaneous lid retraction
        - Lid retraction in patients with concomitant thyroid-related immune orbitopathy enhanced (seesaw) ptosis with manual elevation of one eyelid
2. Cornea
    - Exposure keratopathy
3. Intraocular pressure
    - Elevated intraocular pressure secondary to prednisone therapy in steroid responders
    - Use of β-blockers may worsen myasthenic symptoms in some patients
4. Lens
    - Cataracts as a side effect of prednisone therapy
5. Retina
    - Hypertensive sequelae related to prednisone or cyclosporin therapy
    - Immunosuppressive sequelae from prednisone or azathioprine therapy
    - Diabetes-related sequelae related to prednisone therapy

6. Optic nerve
    - Optic disc swelling as a side effect of cyclosporin therapy
7. Orbit
    - Thyroid-related immune orbitopathy is often seen in association with myasthenia gravis
8. Neuroophthalmologic
    - No clear pupillary involvement (except miosis from pyridostigmine therapy)
    - Fatigue of accommodation
    - Pseudomyopia secondary to spasm of convergence and accommodation (in an effort to overcome medial rectus weakness)
9. Ocular motility
    - Muscle paresis affecting one or all extraocular muscles
    - Diplopia, which varies with fatigue or which fluctuates with the course of the illness
    - Pseudo internuclear ophthalmoplegia
    - Pseudo gaze palsies
    - Pseudo pupil sparing oculomotor nerve paresis
    - Pseudo progressive external ophthalmoplegia
    - Slowing of the quick phase on optokinetic nystagmus testing
    - Hypometric large saccades
    - Hypermetric small saccades

SUGGESTED READINGS

Argov Z, Mastaglia FL. Disorders of neuromuscular transmission caused by drugs. *N Engl J Med* 1979;301:409–413. *A review of drugs that exacerbate myasthenia gravis.*

Kuncl RW, Hoffman PN. Myopathies and disorders of neuromuscular transmission. In: Miller NR, Newman NJ, *Walsh & Hoyt's Clinical Neuro-Ophthalmology,* 5th ed. Baltimore: Williams & Wilkins; 1998:1406–1444. *A current, in-depth review chapter of neuromuscular diseases affecting the eye, with many references.*

Lisak RP. *Handbook of Myasthenia Gravis and Myasthenic Syndromes.* New York: Marcel Dekker; 1994. *A thorough review of all aspects of myasthenia gravis.*

Massey JM. Acquired myasthenia gravis. *Neurol Clin* 1997;15:577–595. *A clinical review of myasthenia gravis including pathogenesis, clinical features, diagnosis, and management.*

Sergott RC. Myasthenia gravis. In: Gold DH, Weingeist TA, eds. *The Eye in Systemic Disease.* Philadelphia: JB Lippincott; 1990:431–432. *A general review of ocular myasthenia.*

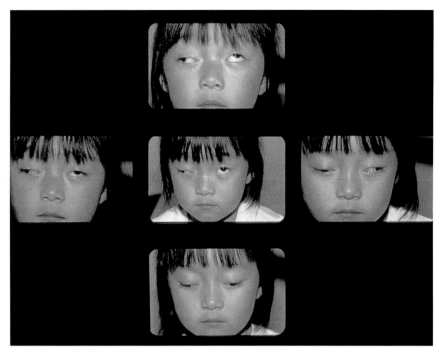

FIGURE 103.1. Blepharoptosis and extraocular muscle weakness in a 5-year-old girl with myasthenia gravis.

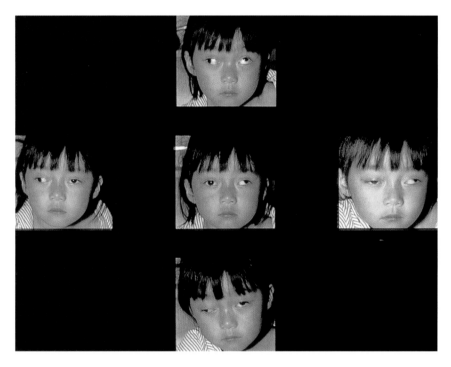

FIGURE 103.2. The patient shown in Figure 103.1 following a prostigmine test. Note the improvement in both the blepharoptosis and the extraocular muscle weakness.

PART 13. PHAKOMATOSES

Chapter 104

STURGE-WEBER SYNDROME

H. Culver Boldt

I. GENERAL

1. A neurooculocutaneous syndrome distinguished by facial port-wine nevus, ipsilateral leptomeningeal angiomatosis, and vascular malformations of the conjunctiva, episclera, choroid, and retina.
2. Also known as encephalotrigenminal (facial) angiomatosis and meningiofacial angiomatosis, this rare congenital vascular phakomatous condition has no sexual or racial predilection or genetic pattern.
3. A defective interaction during embryogenesis between neural crest-derived elements and the vascular endothelium leads to abnormalities of the facial dermal connective tissue, the choroid of the eye, and the perictes and smooth muscle cells of the vasculature.
4. Congenital glaucoma is often associated with involvement of the upper lid.
5. Seizures occur in 80% of patients (in 50% before 1 year of age).

II. SYSTEMIC MANIFESTATIONS

1. Mucocutaneous
   - Nevus flameus of the face (port-wine stain), usually unilateral and in the territory of the trigeminal nerve
2. Neurologic
   - Angioma of the pia and arachnoid mater
   - Cerebral gyriform calcifications—"tram lines"
   - Focal or generalized convulsions (80% of patients)
   - Mental retardation (54% of patients)
   - Hemiplegia contralateral to angiomas (31% of patients)
   - Transient ischemic attacks

III. OCULAR MANIFESTATIONS

1. Lids
   - Port-wine stain
2. Conjunctiva/sclera
   - Conjunctival and episcleral hemangiomas
   - Large, anomalous conjunctival and episcleral vessels
3. Intraocular pressure
   - Blood in Schlemm's canal
   - Malformation of the chamber angle
   - Glaucoma (30% of patients)
   - Bupthalmos
4. Uvea
   - Choroidal hemangioma—diffuse ("tomato catsup fundus") or focal
   - Heterchromia iridis
   - Melanocytic hamartomas of the iris
   - Prominent iris processes adherent to trabecular meshwork
5. Lens
   - Lens subluxation
6. Retina
   - Cystoid degeneration over choroidal hemangioma
   - Exudative retinal detachment
   - Tortuosity of retinal vessels
   - Retinitis pigmentosa
7. Nonspecific
   - Homolateral hyperopia

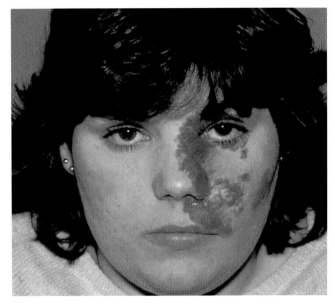

FIGURE 104.1. Nevus flammeus (port-wine stain) in Sturge-Weber syndrome.

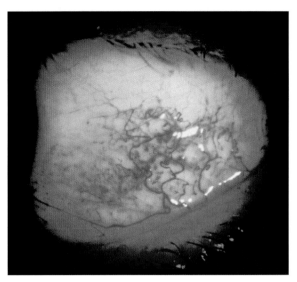

FIGURE 104.2. Dilated, telangiectatic conjunctival and episcleral vessels in a patient with Sturge-Weber syndrome.

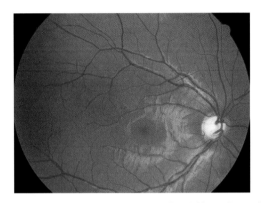

FIGURE 104.3. Fundus photograph of a diffuse choroidal hemangioma and glaucoma in Sturge-Weber syndrome. Note "tomato catsup" appearance to fundus and increased cupping of the optic nerve head when compared to fellow eye.

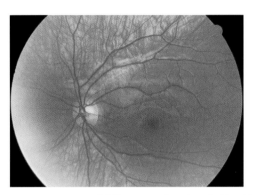

FIGURE 104.4. Normal fellow eye of patient in Fig. 104.2.

SUGGESTED READINGS

Pascual-Castroviejo I, Diaz-Gonzales C, Garcia-Melian RM, et al. Sturge-Weber syndrome: Study of 40 patients. *Pediatr Neurol* 1993;9:283–288.

Roach ES. Neurocutaneous syndromes. *Pediatr Clin North Am* 1992;39:591–620.

Sullivan TJ, Clarke MP, Morin JD. The ocular manifestations of the Sturge-Weber syndrome. *J Pediatr Ophthalmol Strabismus* 1992;29:349–356.

Tripathi BJ, Tripathi RC, Cibis GW. Sturge-Weber syndrome. In: Gold DH, Weingeist TA, eds. *The Eye in Systemic Disease.* Philadelphia: JB Lippincott; 1990:443–447. *A summary of the proposed pathogenesis and clinical findings of Sturge-Weber syndrome.*

Chapter 105

NEUROFIBROMATOSIS

Seymour Brownstein

I. GENERAL

1. Hereditary disseminated hamartomatous condition (phakomatosis)
2. Inherited as an autosomal dominant trait with high penetrance but with variable expressivity
3. Symptoms and signs develop progressively with onset usually in late childhood or early adulthood but may be earlier and even congenital.
4. Two major types
   - Type 1 (peripheral or von Recklinghausen's) neurofibromatosis
     - Prevalence rate of 1/3,000
     - Localized to the long arm of chromosome 17
     - Substantial mutation rate with a positive family history in about 50% of patients
     - Prenatal diagnosis with DNA markers
   - Type 2 (central) neurofibromatosis (or familial acoustic neuroma syndrome)
     - Prevalence rate of 1/50,000
     - Localized to the long arm of chromosome 22
   - Some overlap between the two types

II. SYSTEMIC MANIFESTATIONS

1. Cutaneous lesions (mainly in type 1)
   - Café-au-lait patches (six or more measuring over 15 mm in diameter is significant) (Fig. 105.1)
   - Superficial neurofibromas
     - Fibroma molluscum—proliferation of distal end of nerve (especially after puberty)
     - Plexiform neurofibroma—diffuse proliferation within nerve sheath ("bag of worms")
     - Elephantiasis neuromatosa—diffuse proliferation outside the nerve sheath
   - Multiple freckles in the axillary or inguinal regions
   - Malignant melanoma (rare)
2. Other neurologic tumors (mainly in type 2)
   - Multiple tumors involving brain, spinal cord, meninges, cranial nerves, peripheral nerves, and autonomic nervous system
   - Derived from Schwann cells, glial cells, nerve sheaths, and meninges
   - Neurofibrosarcoma, fibrosarcoma, or malignant schwannoma in 3% of patients
3. Learning disorders in substantial number of cases but rarely severe retardation
4. Skeletal manifestations (mainly in type 1)
   - Defects of the bones of the skull (eg, sphenoid dysplasia)
   - Vertebral anomalies including kyphoscoliosis
   - Congenital thinning of long bones with or without pseudoarthrosis
   - Macrocephaly
   - Short stature
5. Visceral abnormalities
   - Pheochromocytoma (10 times increased incidence)
   - Neurofibromas of intrathoracic and intraabdominal organs
   - Other neuroendocrine and malignant tumors

1. Café-au-lait spots of eyelids
2. Neurofibromas and neurilemmomas of lids, conjunctiva, cornea, and orbit
   - If plexiform neurofibroma of eyelid, S sign and 50% with ipsilateral congenital glaucoma (Fig. 105.2)
3. Thickened corneal, conjunctival, and ciliary nerves
4. Melanocytic hamartomas (nevi and rarely malignant melanomas) of the lids, trabecular meshwork, and uvea
   - Lisch nodules of iris in 90% of patients by age 6 years and older (mainly in type 1) (Figs. 105.3 and 105.4)
   - Choroidal hamartomas in 50%, which may be massive and contain both neuronal and melanocytic elements
5. Optic nerve gliomas (juvenile pilocytic astrocytoma)
   - 10% to 70% of these patients have neurofibromatosis.
   - If neurofibromatosis, 15% have optic nerve gliomas with two-thirds asymptomatic.
   - Circumferential perineural architectural pattern correlated with neurofibromatosis in contrast to expansile intraneuronal pattern, which did not.
   - Associated with proptosis, visual loss, optic atrophy, disc edema, and enlarged optic foramen
6. Glaucoma mechanisms include
   - Infiltration of anterior chamber angle by neurofibroma
   - Thickened ciliary body with neurofibroma
   - Fibrovascular and synechial angle closure
   - Congenital malformation of chamber angle
     - If congenital glaucoma, almost all have plexiform neurofibroma of ipsilatral (usually upper) eyelid.
     - Glaucoma usually is congenital and may be secondary.
7. Posterior subcapsular and cortical cataracts (in 40% of type 2)
8. Retinal findings
   - Astrocytic hamartomas
   - Sectoral pigmentation
   - Myelinated nerve fibers
   - Combined hamartoma of the retinal pigment epithelium and retina (mainly in type 2)
   - Epiretinal membranes (generally asymptomatic and usually in type 2)
9. Absence of greater wing of sphenoid bone with or without pulsating exophthalmos or enophthalmos without bruit (mainly in type 1); may have associated orbital encephalocele
10. Secondary to intracranial tumors
    - Visual field defects, ocular motor, autonomic, and sensory nerve deficits, papilledema, and optic atrophy
11. Increased incidence of orbital meningiomas

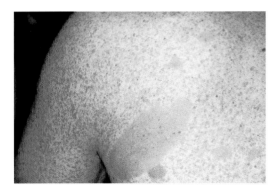

FIGURE 105.1. Multiple pigmented macules (café-au-lait spots) of various sizes on back of 25-year-old patient with neurofibromatosis.

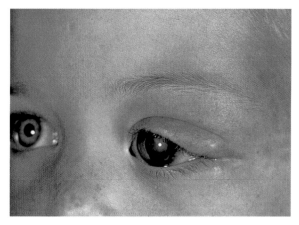

FIGURE 105.2. Plexiform neurofibroma mainly laterally in left eyelids with characteristic S-shaped contour of left upper lid, café-au-lait spots in left temple, and buphthalmic left globe displaying an enlarged cornea, dilated pupil, ectropion iridis, and cataract. From Brownstein S, Little JM. Ocular neurofibromatosis; used courtesy of *Ophthalmology* 1983;90:1595–1599.

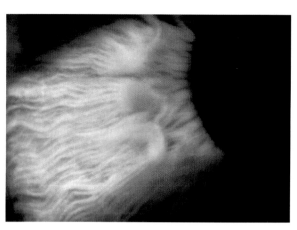

FIGURE 105.3. Lisch nodule of iris characterized by its elevation, smooth contour, and soft translucency. Courtesy of Trevor Krikham, MD, and from Brownstein S, Little JM. Ocular neurofibromatosis; used courtesy of *Ophthalmology* 1983;90:1595–1599.

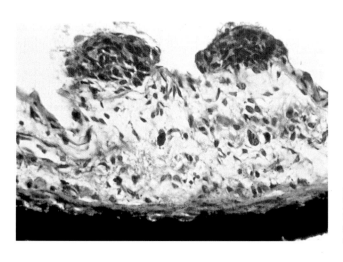

FIGURE 105.4. Melanocytic nodules covered by endothelium projecting into anterior chamber from anterior border layer of iris (hematoxylin-eosin; original magnification, × 400). From Brownstein S, Little JM. Ocular neurofibrosis; used courtesy of *Ophthalmology* 1983;90:1595–1599.

SUGGESTED READINGS

Brownstein S, Little JM. Ocular neurofibromatosis. *Ophthalmology* 1983;90:1595–1599.

Brownstein S. Neurofibromatosis. In: Gold DH, Weingeist TA, eds. *The Eye in Systemic Disease.* Philadelphia: JB Lippincott; 1990:447–450.

Ebert EM, Boger WP III, Albert DM. Phakomatoses. In: Albert DM, Jakobiec FA, eds. *Principles and Practice of Ophthalmology.* Philadelphia: WB Saunders; 1994:3298–3328.

Kaye LD, Rothner AD, Beauchamp GR, et al. Ocular findings associated with neurofibromatosis type II. *Ophthalmology* 1992;99:1424–1429.

Chapter 106

TUBEROUS SCLEROSIS

Mary A. Curtis

I. GENERAL

1. Except hypopigmented macules, findings may be age dependent. Brain "tubers" become evident on imaging under 2 years of age. Angiofibroma become evident at around 3 to 4 years old.
2. Prognosis is good except for symptomatic newborns. Large cardiac tumors (newborn) may obstruct blood flow. Myoclonic seizures/hypsarrythmia under 6 months suggest a high risk for retardation.
3. Prevalence is 1/12,000.
4. Treatment modalities include anticonvulsants, antihypertensives, dermabrasion, laser treatment, and renal or cardiac (newborn) surgery.
5. Dominantly inherited with variable expression, once present in the family.
6. More than one gene: 9q34 (40%), 16p13.3 (60%), though clinically indistinguishable.
7. Ungual fibromas, renal cysts/tumors, and giant cell astroacytomas, when present, become apparent later in childhood. Hypertension, hematuria, renal function impairment, and/or cerebrospinal fluid (CSF) obstruction may result.

II. SYSTEMIC MANIFESTATIONS

1. Cutaneous
   - Hypopigmented "ash leaf" macules (86%)
   - Facial angiofibroma (47%)
   - Fibrous plaques or Shagreen's patches (50%)
   - Ungual fibroma
2. Cardiac
   - Rhabdomyoma (40–50%)
3. Central nervous system
   - Cortical hamartomas (tubers) (40%)
   - Subependymal nodules (80%)
   - Giant cell astrocytomas (2%)
   - Seizures (82–90%)
   - Intellectual deficit (41–45%)
4. Renal
   - "Polycystic kidneys"
   - Angiomyolipoma (50–80%)
   - Hypertension
   - Hematuria
5. Skeletal/dental
   - Pitted enamel hypoplasia
   - Bone cysts

III. OCULAR MANIFESTATIONS

1. Retina
   - Achromatic patches (50%)
   - Astrocytic hamartoma (50–80%)
     - Flat, smooth, and translucent
     - Calcified, multinodular, elevated
   - Coloboma (rare)
2. Lids/lashes
   - Hypopigmented (white) patches
   - Angiofibromas
3. Intraocular pressure
   - Glaucoma (rare)
4. Vitreous
   - Hemorrhage (rare)
5. Optic nerve
   - Optic atrophy (rare)
   - Papilledema (rare) with CSF obstruction
6. Ocular motility
   - Paresis (rare) with CSF obstruction

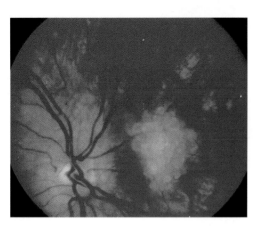

FIGURE 106.1. Multinodular astrocytic hemartoma in atypical location, obscuring underlying retinal vessel.

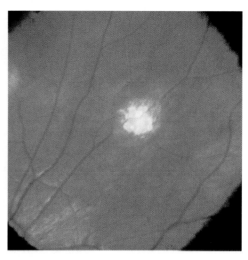

FIGURE 106.2. Smaller, multinodular, calcified astrocytic harmartoma of the retina.

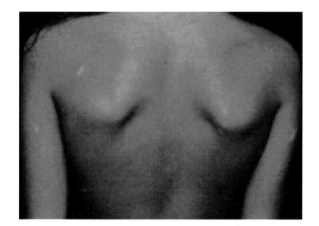

FIGURE 106.3. "Ash leaf" hypopigmented cutaneous signs of tuberous sclerosis.

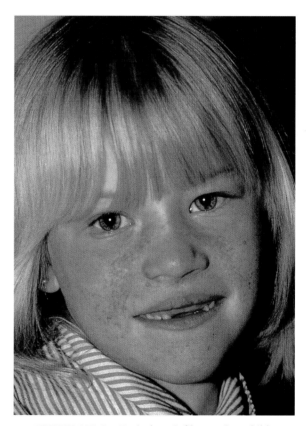

FIGURE 106.4. Typical angiofibroma in a child.

Tuberous Sclerosis   **419**

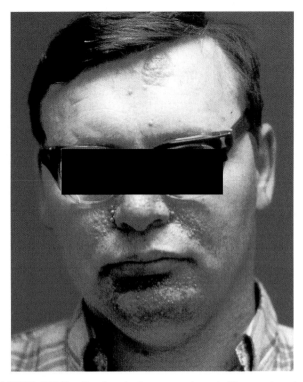

FIGURE 106.5. Forehead plaques and angiofibroma in adult (whose tuberous sclerosis went undiagnosed, until seen for renal complications in his early thirties).

SUGGESTED READINGS

Ahlsen G, Gillberg C, Lindblom R, Gillberg C. Tuberous sclerosis in western Sweden: A population study of cases with early childhood onset. *Arch Neurol* 1994;51:76–81. *The prevalence of tuberous sclerosis and its manifestations are investigated.*

Dotan SA, Trobe JD, Gebarski SS. Visual loss in tuberous sclerosis. *Neurology* 1991;41:1915–1917. *Periodic ophthalmologic examination and brain imaging are stressed to prevent visual loss secondary to obstructive hydrocephalus.*

Gomez MR, ed. *Neurocutaneous Diseases.* London: Butterworths; 1987. *Chapter 3 written by Dr. Gomez is the best summary available on tuberous sclerosis.*

Goodman M, Lamm SH, Engel A, et al. Cortical tuber count: A biomarker indicating neurological severity of tuberous sclerosis. *Child Neurology* 1997;12:85–9.

Maheshwar MM, Cheadle JP, Jones AC, et al. The GAP-related domain of tuberin, the product of the TSCZ gene is a target for missense mutations in tuberous sclerosis. *Hum Mol Genet* 1997;6:1991–1996.

Waziri M. Tuberous sclerosis. In: Gold DH, Weingeist TA, ed. *The Eye in Systemic Disease.* Philadelphia: JB Lippincott; 1990:450–452. *A summary for this text that focuses on systemic disorders that have effects on the eye.*

Chapter 107
VON HIPPEL-LINDAU DISEASE
Paul W. Hardwig

I. GENERAL

1. Genetics
   - Autosomal dominant
     - Incompletely penetrant
     - Variably expressed
     - Pleiotropic
   - Occasionally sporadic
   - Gene mapping available
2. Pathogenesis
   - Developmental dysgenesis of neuroectoderm and mesoderm
   - Basic defect unknown
3. Clinical manifestations
   - Protean

- Manifestations with significant morbidity
  - Angiomatosis retinae
  - Cerebellar, medullary, spinal hemangioblastomas
  - Clear cell carcinoma
  - Pheochromocytoma
4. Presymptomatic screening may identify patients at risk for significant morbidity.
   - Ophthalmoscopy
   - Urinary metanephrines
   - Cranial and spinal enhanced magnetic resonance imaging (MRI)
   - Abdominal enhanced computed tomography (CT) scanning

II. SYSTEMIC MANIFESTATIONS

1. Central nervous system
   - Almost always below the tentorium: cerebellum (hemangioblastoma), medulla oblongata (hemangioblastoma, syringobulbia), spinal cord (hemangioblastoma, syringomyelia)
   - Cerebellar dysfunction (gait ataxia, dysmetria, dysdiadochokinesia, vertigo, nystagmus)
   - Respiratory depression
   - Pyramidal tract, spinal cord compression
   - Increased intracranial pressure (headache, papilledema)
   - Cranial nerve palsies
2. Important visceral structures
   - Lesions common to all include simple cyst and/or adenoma
   - Renal
     - Clear cell carcinoma; hemangioblastoma
     - Hematuria
     - Obstructive nephropathy
     - Abdominal mass
     - Death from metastasis or uremia
   - Adrenal medulla and sympathetic chain
     - Pheochromocytoma, paraganglioma
     - Pheochyromocytoma clusters in predisposed families

- Pancreas
  - Hemangioblastoma
  - Islet cell tumor
3. Other
   - Polycythemia
     - Occasionally associated with cerebellar hemangioblastoma
     - Less often with clear cell carcinoma, pheochromocytoma
4. Miscellaneous sites
   - Cerebrum
   - Meninges
   - Lung
   - Liver
   - Spleen
   - Omentum, mesocolon
   - Ovary
   - Bladder
   - Bones
   - Skin
   - Epididymus

1. Angiomatosis retinae
- Incipient lesion like a diabetic microaneurysm
- Classic angioma a pinkish retinal tumor, with dilated, tortuous retinal artery/vein pair
- Usually midperipheral; occasionally, juxtapapillary or intraorbital portion of optic nerve
- Lipid exudation late

2. Reactive macular changes
- Circinate exudation
- Cystoid macular edema
- Epiretinal membrane
- Hole secondary to vitreous traction

3. Advanced reactive changes in eye
- Retinal detachment
- Retinal/iris neovascularization
- Vitreous hemorrhage secondary to neovascularization
- Rubeotic glaucoma
- Phthisis

4. Neuroophthalmologic
- Secondary to central nervous system involvement
- Papilledema
- Nystagmus
- Oculomotor nerve palsies
- Chiasmal compression from dilated third ventricle

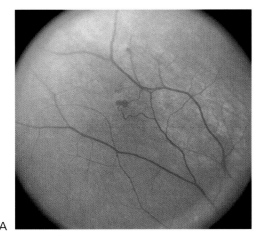
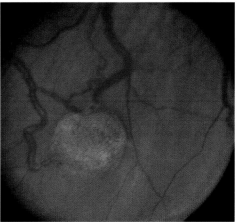

FIGURE 107.1. A preclassical capillary angioma (**A**) and a typical von Hippel angioma (**B**) found in the midperipheral retina.

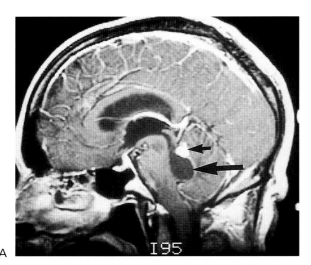
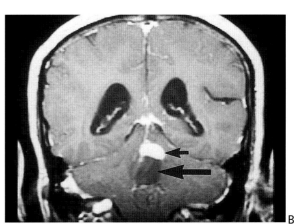

FIGURE 107.2. T1-weighted sagittal (**A**)and coronal (**B**) enhanced head MRIs demonstrate a superior vermian hemangioblastoma (*large arrow*). Within the 3-cm cystic cerebellar mass, there is a 1-cm densely enhancing mural nodule (*small arrow*). The cerebral aqueduct and fourth ventricle are compressed, and there is early obstructive hydrocephalus.

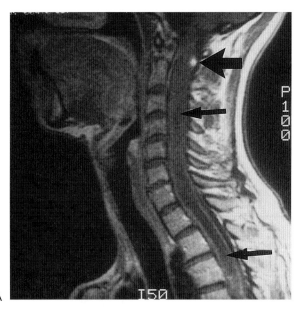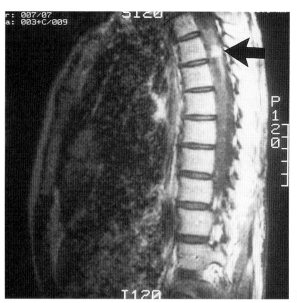

FIGURE 107.3. T1-weighted sagittal enhanced MRI of the spine demonstrates a large hemangioblastoma. The cystic component of the tumor extends from the medulla into the thoracic cord (*small arrows*). On the posterior wall of this cystic cavity, there are two enhancing mural nodules (*large arrows*), one between C1 and C2 (**A**) and the larger at T4 (**B**) .

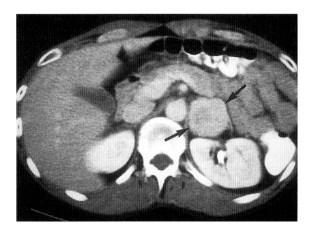

FIGURE 107.4. Postcontrast CT scan of the upper abdomen shows a 4-cm mass, a pheochromocytoma, in the left adrenal gland (*arrows*).

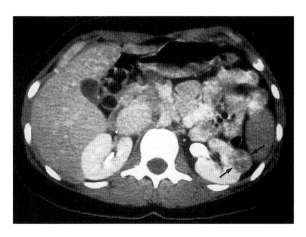

FIGURE 107.5. A 3-cm partially enhancing mass in the interpolar region of the left kidney (*arrows*) was found to be a clear cell carcinoma at laparotomy.

SUGGESTED READINGS

Hardwig PW. von Hippel-Lindau disease. In: Gold DH, Weingeist TA, eds. *The Eye in Systemic Disease.* Philadelphia: JB Lippincott; 1990:453–455.

Hardwig PW, Robertson DM. von Hippel-Lindau disease: A familial, often lethal, multi-system phakomatosis. *Ophthalmology* 1984;91:263–270.

Ridley M, Green J, Johnson G. Retinal angiomatosis: The ocular manifestations of von Hippel-Lindau disease. *Can J Ophthalmol* 1986;21:276–283.

von Hippel-Lindau disease (angiomatosis of the retina and cerebellum: central nervous system angiomatosis). In: Miller NR, ed. *Walsh and Hoyt's Clinical Neuro-Ophthalmology,* 4th ed, vol 3. Baltimore: Williams & Wilkins; 1988:1747–1827.

Chapter 108

WYBURN-MASON SYNDROME

Ahmad M. Mansour

I. GENERAL

1. Distinct clinical entity
   - Arteriovenous malformation (AVM) of the midbrain
   - AVM of the retina
   - Facial nevi occurring all on the same side
2. Mean age at presentation 25 years
   - The larger the AVM in the brain or in the retina, the earlier the age of onset of symptoms.
   - No sex predilection
3. Vascular malformations
   - Congenital but can undergo remodeling, spontaneous regression, and lead to complications such as bleeding and vasoocclusive disorders
   - Complications are the result of the highly turbulent flow from a direct communication of a high-pressure arterial system to a low-pressure venous system.
   - The area surrounding the AVM experiences the "steal phenomenon" with ischemia due to blood shunted to the area of the AVM.
4. The larger the retinal AVM, the higher the chance of having multiple systemic AVMs (small AVMs of the retina tend to be isolated), and the higher the chance of ocular complications.

II. SYSTEMIC MANIFESTATIONS

1. Central nervous system
   - Symptoms depend on location and size of AVM
     - Hemiparesis (pyramidal tract involvement)
     - Mental retardation
     - Seizures
     - Cerebellar dysfunction
     - Parinaud's syndrome
   - Rupture of AVM leads to ominous complications.
     - Intracerebral hemorrhage
     - Subarachnoid hemorrhage
2. Oronasopharynx
   - Epistaxis
   - Oral hemorrhage
3. Cutaneous
   - Facial vascular nevi

III. OCULAR MANIFESTATIONS

1. Ptosis
   - Secondary to lid involvement
2. Proptosis and orbital bruit
   - Secondary to orbit involvement
3. Dilated conjunctival vessels
4. Neovascular glaucoma
   - Secondary to ischemic retinal vein occlusion
5. Vitreous hemorrhage
6. Retina
   - Macular hemorrhage
   - Central retinal vein occlusion
   - Branch retinal vein occlusion
   - Central retinal artery occlusion
   - Retinal vascular tortuosity
7. Neuroophthalmologic
   - Secondary to involvement of central nervous system
   - Papilledema
   - Optic atrophy
   - Hemianopia (involvement of the visual pathways including the optic nerve and chiasm)
8. Ocular motor nerve palsy

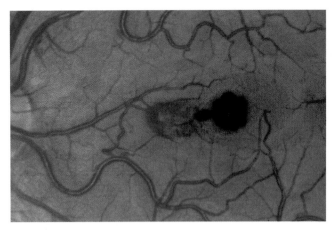

FIGURE 108.1 Macular hemorrhage from grade I macular arteriovenous anastomosis.

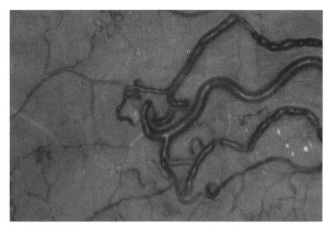

FIGURE 108.2 Branch retinal vein occlusion distal to the area of arteriovenous anastomosis grade II.

SUGGESTED READINGS

Mansour AM, Walsh JB, Henkind P. Arteriovenous anastomoses of the retina. *Ophthalmology* 1987;94:35–40.

Mansour AM, Wells CG, Jampol LM, et al. Ocular complications of arteriovenous communications of the retina. *Arch Ophthalmol* 1989;107:232–236.

Wyburn-Mason R. Arteriovenous aneurysm of mid-brain and retina, facial naevi and mental changes. *Brain* 1943;66:163–203.

PART 14. PHYSICAL AND CHEMICAL INJURY

Chapter 109

FETAL ALCOHOL SYNDROME

Marilyn T. Miller

I. GENERAL

1. A leading cause of mental retardation in the Western world and probably the most frequent *preventable* cause of mental retardation.
2. Less severe effects of alcohol result in a multiple array of anomalies and disabilities sometimes referred to as fetal alcohol effects (FAE).
3. Most cases of classical fetal alcohol syndrome (FAS) result from excessive alcohol intake (6–7 drinks/day), but absolute safe level of drinking in pregnancy is not known.
4. Incidence in the United States is estimated to be 2/1000 FAS; 6% children of women alcoholic in pregnancy.

II. SYSTEMIC MANIFESTATIONS

1. Criteria for diagnosis
   - Prenatal and postnatal deficiency (<10th percentile)
   - Pattern of characteristic facial anomalies that may include
     - Midface hypoplasia, flattened nasal bridge
     - Telecanthus
     - Long/smooth philtrum
     - Thin upper lip
   - Central nervous system (CNS) malformations such as microcephaly, delayed development, hyperactivity, mental retardation, seizures, etc.
   - Positive history of excessive alcohol intake during pregnancy
2. Other systemic anomalies such as
   - Cardiovascular system—murmurs, usually atrial or ventricular sextal defects; multiple other less frequent anomalies
   - CNS malformations—agenesis of corpus callosum, anomalies of the septum pellucidum, hypoplasia of other CNS structures
   - Skeletal/cutaneous anomalies—hemangiomas, aberrant palmar creases, pectus excavation
   - Facial—upturned nose, posterior rotated ears, joint anomalies, and others

III. OCULAR MANIFESTATIONS

1. Frequent (>25%)
   - Increased distance between medial canthi (telecanthus)
   - Strabismus (50%)
   - Optic nerve anomalies; often hypoplasia
   - Increased tortuously of retinal vessels
   - Epicanthus
2. Less frequent
   - Anterior segment anomalies (Peter's, Reiger, embryotoxon)
   - Microphthalmia
   - Long eyelashes
   - Ptosis, often asymmetrical
   - Nystagmus
   - Myopia
3. Other reported low-incidence anomalies
   - Cataract
   - Corneal opacity
   - Coloboma

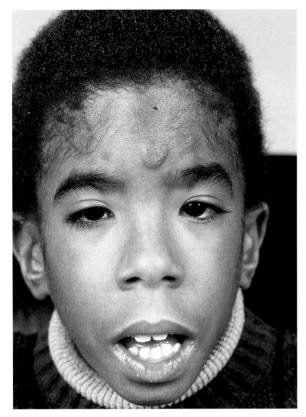

FIGURE 109.1. Note long flat philtrum, telecanthus, midface hypoplasia, mild ptosis.

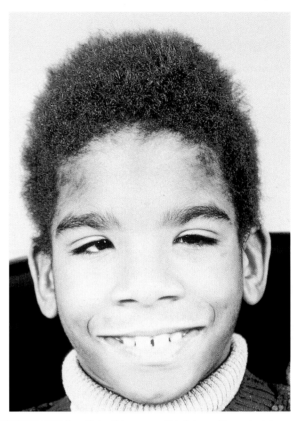

FIGURE 109.2. Note thin upper lid, telecanthus, strabismus.

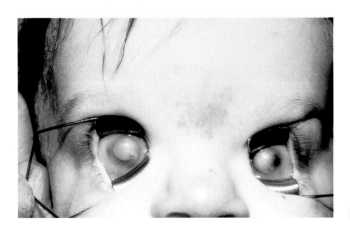

FIGURE 109.3. FAS with bilateral Peter's anomaly, telecanthus.

SUGGESTED READINGS

Gorlin RJ, Pindberg JJ, Cohen MM. *Syndromes of the Head and Neck,* 2nd ed. New York: McGraw-Hill; 1976;16–20.

Johnson VP, Swayze VW II, Sato Y, Anderasen NC. Fetal alcohol syndrome: Craniofacial and central nervous system malformations. *Am J Med Genetics* 1996;61:329–339.

Miller MT, Epstein, RJ, Sugar J, et al. Anterior segment anomalies associated with the fetal alcohol syndrome. *J Pediatr Ophthalmol Strabismus* 1984;21:8–18.

Strömland K. Ocular involvement in the fetal alcohol syndrome. *Surv Ophthalmol* 1987;3:277–284.

Chapter 110
CHILD ABUSE
Andrea Cibis Tongue

I. GENERAL

1. Type and extent of injury not compatible with alleged cause
2. Occurs in all socioeconomic and ethnic groups, higher risk in families with history of abuse, socioeconomic deprivation, dysfunctional family unit, poor employment record, and substance abuse
3. Ocular and vision damage most frequently associated with head injury in children under 3 years of age who are battered or shaken babies
4. Central nervous system (CNS) injuries usually result from rapid acceleration and deceleration, either by shaking infant in free space or hitting unsupported head against a surface.
5. Intracranial hemorrhage is a result of vessel rupture, leading to subdural, subarachnoid, parenchymal, and intraventricular bleeding.
6. Cerebral edema and elevated CNS pressure cause increasing neurologic impairment, respiratory, and cardiac arrest.
7. Retinal hemorrhages are frequently present in patients with head injuries.
8. Pathophysiology of retinal hemorrhages is not established but probably secondary to rapid increases in intracranial pressure and to changes in hemodynamics of retinal and cerebral circulation and ischemia. Local traction and shearing forces may also play a role.
9. Retinal hemorrhages in the absence of periocular or ocular damage or nervous system damage do not occur.
10. Acute ocular injury in children without CNS involvement is usually associated with signs of periorbital and periocular injury.
11. Multiorgan and multisystem injuries may be present.
12. Repetitive injury is common.

II. SYSTEMIC MANIFESTATIONS

1. Skin and subcutaneous tissue
   - Bruises, lacerations, abrasions, burns
     - Multiple, varying ages
     - Shape suggestive of outline of object used to inflict injury
     - Location usually not susceptible to accidental injury
     - Age-inappropriate injury
   - Adult human bite marks
2. Musculoskeletal
   - Fractures (multiple, varying stages of healing, age-inappropriate)
   - Rib fractures
   - Spiral fractures of long bones
   - Transverse fractures
   - Metaphyseal injury and epiphyseal dislocation
   - Periosteal hemorrhages
   - Skull fractures associated with intracranial injuries
3. Abdominal visceral injuries
   - Contusions
   - Lacerations
   - Hemorrhage
   - Abdominal distention
4. CNS injuries
   - Hemorrhages (subdural, subarachnoid, intraventricular, parenchymal)
   - Cerebral edema
   - Elevated intracranial pressure
   - Contusion injury (especially of frontal and occipital lobes)
   - Ischemia
   - Hydrocephalus
   - Seizures
   - Coma
   - Respiratory arrest
   - Cardiac arrest
   - Brain atrophy
   - Developmental delay
5. General
   - Failure to thrive
   - Irritable, fearful
   - Listless, unresponsive
   - Delayed medical care
   - Changing and inconsistent medical history
   - Shock

1. Periorbital
   - Ecchymosis, chemosis
   - Lacerations, abrasions, burns (thermal, chemical)
   - Fractures
   - Proptosis
2. Anterior segment
   - Chemical conjunctivitis, hemorrhage
   - Cornea
     - Abrasions
     - Keratitis
     - Vascularization
     - Opacification (usually inferior cornea)
     - Descemet's membrane tears
     - Laceration
   - Hyphema
   - Iris sphincter rupture, iridodialysis, angle recession
   - Iritis
3. Lens
   - Dislocation
   - Cataract
4. Vitreous
   - Hemorrhage
   - Veils
   - Strands
5. Retina/choroid
   - Hemorrhage in one or more layers (dome shaped, prehyaloid common)
   - Intraretinal demarcation line (fold) circumferential with disc
   - Retinoschisis, retinal detachment
   - Pigmentary changes, chorioretinal scars
   - Gliosis
   - Choroidal rupture
6. Optic nerve
   - Papilledema
   - Venous stasis
   - Hemorrhage
   - Optic atrophy
7. Other
   - Ruptured globe
   - Glaucoma
   - Visual field defect
   - Vision loss—ocular or cortical or both
   - Nystagmus
   - Amblyopia
   - Strabismus—paralytic and nonparalytic
   - Anisometropia

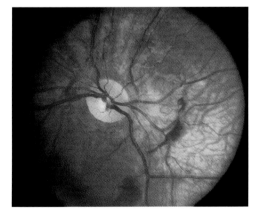

FIGURE 110.1. Retinal hemorrhages in posterior pole OD. Note varying sizes and small dome-shaped prehyaloid hemorrhage superior to disc (11 o'clock in picture).

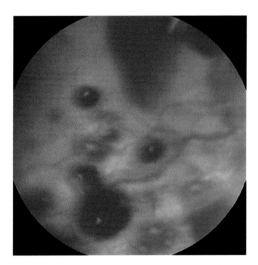

FIGURE 110.2. Unilateral and more peripherally located hemorrhages in another patient with head injury.

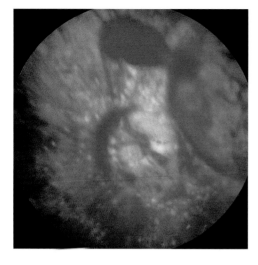

FIGURE 110.3. Hemorrhages involving all layers of retina and the choroid. Hemorrhage in vitreous superotemporal to disc is breakthrough from the dome-shaped prehyaloid hemorrhage in macular area. Note disc edema, venous stasis.

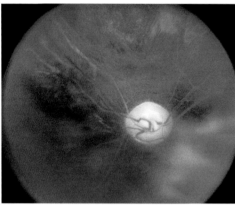

FIGURE 110.4. Optic atrophy, vitreous strands, occluded retinal vessels, chorioretinal atrophy and pigmentary changes in same patient as in Fig. 110.3.

SUGGESTED READINGS

Chadwick DL. Child abuse. In: Rudolph AM, Hoffman JIE, eds. *Pediatrics.* East Norwalk, CT: Appleton & Lange; 1987:760–769.

Duhaime AC, Alario AJ, Lewander WJ, et al. Head injury in very young children: Mechanisms, injury types, and ophthalmologic findings in 100 hospitalized patients younger than 2 years of age. *Pediatrics* 1991;90:179–185.

Gammon JA. Ophthalmic manifestations of child abuse. In: Ellerstein NS, ed. *Child Abuse and Neglect: A Medical Reference.* New York: John Wiley & Sons; 1987:121–139.

McNeese MC, Hebeler JR. The abused child, a clinical approach to identification and management. *Clin Symposia* 1977;29:2–36.

Tongue AC. Child abuse. In: Gold DH, Weingeist TA, eds. *The Eye in Systemic Disease.* Philadelphia: JB Lippincott; 1990:466–469.

Chapter 111
DECOMPRESSION SICKNESS
Frank K. Butler, Jr

I. GENERAL

1. Sudden reduction in the ambient pressure results in the formation of intravascular or extravascular gas bubbles.
2. May be seen in divers, pilots, aircrew, tenders in hyperbaric chambers, and tunnel workers
3. Variable presentation
4. Key to diagnosis is a history of exposure to a sudden decrease in pressure within 24 to 48 hours before onset of symptoms.
5. Requires emergent recompression therapy
6. Typically responds well to recompression and hyperbaric oxygen breathing

II. SYSTEMIC MANIFESTATIONS

1. Musculoskeletal or radicular pain
2. Hemiparesis or hemiplegia
3. Paraparesis or paraplegia
4. Sensory deficits
5. Paresthesias
6. Lymphadenopathy
7. Pulmonary edema
8. Unconsciousness
9. Vestibular symptoms
10. Cutaneous mottling

III. OCULAR MANIFESTATIONS

1. Nystagmus
2. Diplopia
3. Visual field defects
4. Scotomas
5. Homonymous hemianopia
6. Orbicularis oculi pain
7. Cortical blindness
8. Convergence insufficiency
9. Central retinal artery occlusion
10. Optic neuropathy

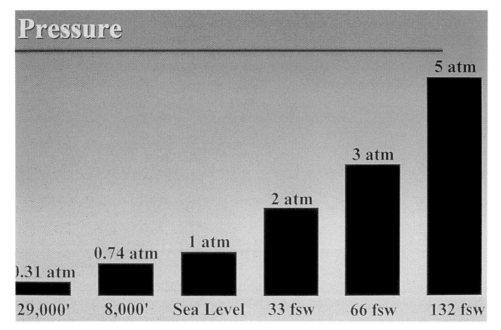

FIGURE 111.1. Ambient absolute pressures at different depths and altitudes. Courtesy of Richard Vann, MD.

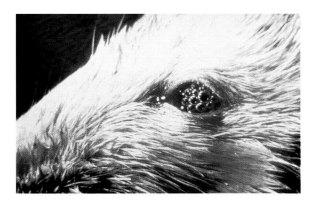

FIGURE 111.2. Gas bubbles in the eye of an experimental animal exposed to decompression stress. Courtesy of Richard Vann, MD.

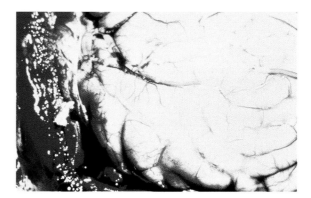

FIGURE 111.3. Intravascular gas bubbles in the cerebral circulation. Courtesy of Richard Vann, MD.

SUGGESTED READINGS

Bennett P, Elliott D. *The Physiology and Medicine of Diving,* 4th ed. London: WB Saunders; 1993;135–136.

Bove AA, Davis JC. *Diving Medicine,* 2nd ed. Philadelphia: WB Saunders; 1990:296.

Butler FK. Decompression sickness. In: Gold DH, Weingeist TA, eds. *The Eye in Systemic Disease.* Philadelphia: JB Lippincott; 1990:469–471.

Edmonds C, Lowry C, Pennefather J. *Diving and Subaquatic Medicine,* 3rd ed. Oxford: Butterworth-Heinemann, 1992.

U.S. Navy Diving Manual. Washington, DC: Commander Naval Sea Systems Command Publication 0994-LP-001-9010, Revision 3, 1993; vol 1, 2-23–2-25.

Chapter 112

ALTITUDE ILLNESS AND RETINOPATHY

Michael Wiedman

I. GENERAL

1. Altitude illness (AI) syndrome is composed of four related entities.
   - Acute mountain sickness (AMS)
   - High-altitude cerebral edema (HACE)
   - High-altitude pulmonary edema (HAPE)
   - High-altitude retinopathy (HAR)
2. AI is precipitated by rapid ascent without prior acclimatization.
3. Common physiologic alteration is hypoxia of altitude.
4. Comparative levels of pressures of inspired oxygen and arterial oxygen and hemoglobin saturations are critical.
   - Sea level
     - Baropressure—760 mmg Hg
     - Press insp O$_2$—150 mm Hg
     - Press Art sat—94 mm Hg
     - % Hb sat—98
   - Skiing at Vail, Zermatt, 11,000 to 12,000 feet
     - Baropressure—480 mm Hg
     - Press insp O$_2$—96 mm Hg
     - Press Art O$_2$—60 mm Hg
     - % Hb sat—89
   - Hiking Kilimanjaro, 19,347 feet
     - Baropressure—356 mm Hg
     - Press insp O$_2$—69 mm Hg
     - Press Art sat—39 mm Hg
     - % Hb sat—78
   - Climbing Mt. Everest, 29,028 feet
     - Baropressure—253 mm Hg
     - Press insp O$_2$—43 mm Hg
     - Press Art O$_2$—28 mm Hg
     - % Hb sat—70

II. SYSTEMIC MANIFESTATIONS

1. AMS—Generalized
   - Headache
   - Anorexia
   - Lethargy
   - Peripheral and facies edema
   - Insomnia
   - Cheyne-Stokes breathing
   - Nausea, emesis
   - Disorientation
2. HACE—Central nervous system (CNS)
   - Progressive, severe headache
   - Cerebral edema and petecheal hemorrhages
   - Cerebral vasodilation
   - Ataxia
   - Diplopia
   - Projectile vomiting
   - Memory and judgment loss
   - Irrationality
   - Depressed sensorium
   - Coma
   - Death
3. HAPE—Cardiopulmonary
   - Dry cough
   - Blood tinged sputum
   - Dyspnea
   - Hyperventilation
   - Tachycardia
   - Cyanosis
   - Pulmonary vasoconstriction and hypertension
   - Decreased lung perfusion
   - Moist bubbling rales
   - Respiratory failure
   - Death
4. HAR
   - Hypoxic endothelial vascular permeability factor

III. OCULAR MANIFESTATIONS

1. Retina
   - Hemorrhages, intraretinal and preretinal
   - Dilated retinal arterioles
   - Engorged retinal venules
   - Diffuse or macular hemorrhages
   - Ophthalmodynamometric retinal vascular hypertension
   - Decreased retinal circulation time
   - Increased light adaptation recovery time
   - Elevated rod and cone thresholds
2. Neuroophthalmologic
   - HAR is concomitant with CNS involvement.
   - Papilledema
   - Papillary hemorrhages
   - Visual field defect
   - Flicker fusion depression
   - Color vision defect
   - Visual evoked response delayed cortical conduction time
   - Diplopia
   - Paradoxical pupillary dilation to light
3. Accompaniment
   - HAR predicts HACE
   - Visual acuity loss
   - Entoptic symptoms
   - Vitreous hemorrhages

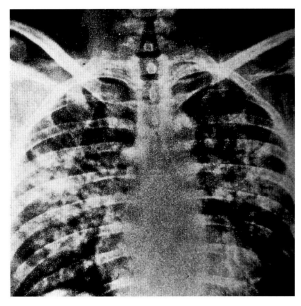

FIGURE 112.1. Chest x-ray, HAPE at 9000 feet. Note extensive, patchy infiltrate.

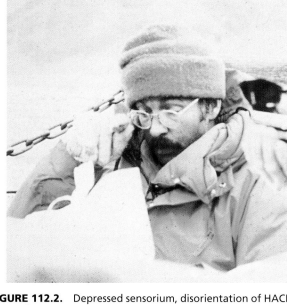

FIGURE 112.2. Depressed sensorium, disorientation of HACE at 17,000 feet.

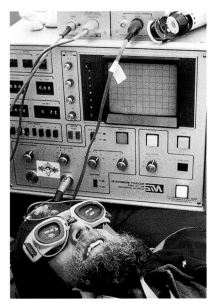

FIGURE 112.3. Visual evoked response at 21,300 feet, delayed cortical conduction time.

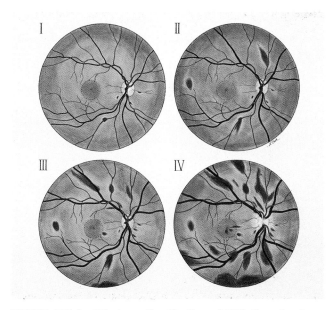

FIGURE 112.4. Wiedman Classification of HAR. One disc diameter hemorrhage increase per grade; vitreous, macular hemorrhages are grades III and IV, respectively.

SUGGESTED READINGS

Wiedman M. High altitude retinal hemorrhage. *Arch Ophthalmol* 1975;93:401–403.

Wiedman M. High altitude retinal hemorrhage: A classification. In: Henkind P, ed. *Acta XXIV International Congress of Ophthalmology.* Philadelphia: JB Lippincott, 1980;19:421–424. *A specific classification for comparing severity of HAR.*

Wiedman M. Nouvelle recherché oculaire au Mont Everest. *Bull Mem Soc Fr Ophtalmol* 1973;86:201–207. *International research aspects.*

West JB, Sukhamay L. *High Altitude and Man.* Bethesda, MD: American Physiologic Society; 1984. *A good review of the AI syndrome.*

Wiedman M, Tabin G. High altitude retinopathy and altitude illness. *Ophthal* 1999;106:1924–1927. *Documentation on Mt. Everset of HAR and neurological complications.*

Chapter 113

PURTSCHER'S RETINOPATHY

Elaine L. Chuang
Robert E. Kalina

I. GENERAL

1. Classic mechanism
   - Chest compression/trauma or head injury (for other causes of Purtscher's-like retinopathy see Systemic Manifestations)
   - Intravascular hydrostatic pressure wave travels via large veins.
   - "Shock wave" is transmitted via the valveless venous system of the head and neck.
   - Retinal vascular endothelial damage occurs at the level of peripapillary radial capillaries, retinal veins, and macular capillaries.
   - Head and neck position at time of injury, associated blood loss, shock, and other factors may modulate damage.
   - Possible role of autoregulation by retinal vasculature
2. Alternative hypotheses
   - "Lymphatic"/cerebrospinal fluid channels via optic nerve sheath (historic)
   - Posttraumatic fat embolism
   - Intraarterial air embolism
   - Leukoembolism via complement-activated pathway

II. SYSTEMIC MANIFESTATIONS

1. Acute pancreatitis (complement-mediated leukoembolism)
2. Complicated childbirth
3. Connective tissue diseases
4. Chronic renal failure

III. OCULAR MANIFESTATIONS

1. Retina
   - Nerve fiber layer infarcts (cotton-wool spots)
   - Preretinal and/or retinal (superficial) hemorrhages
   - Superficial ischemic retinal whitening
     - Peripapillary retina
     - Macula
   - Macular edema
   - Dilated retinal venous system
   - Late—retinal atrophy, central retinal pigment epithelium granularity
2. Optic nerve
   - Disc swelling
   - Late—optic disc pallor
3. Fluorescein angiography
   - Capillary nonperfusion
   - Arteriolar and venular closure
   - Late staining of vessel walls
   - Optic nerve staining
   - Normal choroidal perfusion

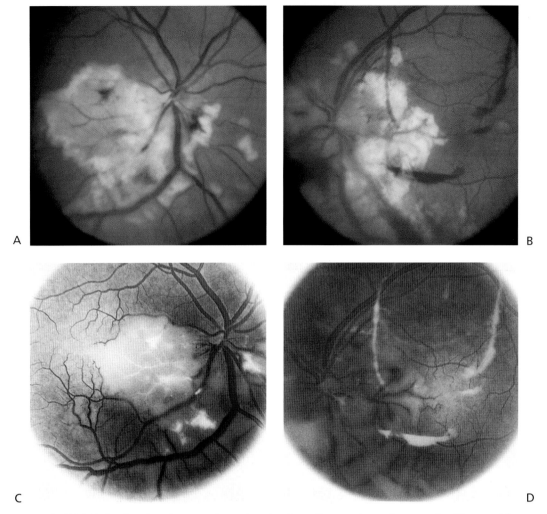

FIGURE 113.1. Fundus photographs and early phase fluorescein angiogram of a 39-year-old man with bilateral Purtscher's retinopathy several days following a motor vehicle accident. Note capillary nonperfusion and occlusion of retinal vasculature in peripapillary region and macula, both eyes, and preretinal hemorrhage, left eye. **(A)** Right eye (fundus photograph); **(B)** left eye (fundus photograph); **(C)** right eye (fluorescein angiogram); **(D)** left eye (fluorescein angiogram).

SUGGESTED READINGS

Archer DB. Richardson Cross Lecture: Traumatic retinal vasculopathy. *Trans Ophthalmol Soc U K* 1986;105:361–384.

Blodi BA, Johnson MW, Gass JDM, et al. Purtscher's-like retinopathy after childbirth. *Ophthalmology* 1990;97:1654–1659.

Jacob HS, Craddock PR, Hammerschmidt DE, Moldow CF. Complement-induced granulocyte aggregation. *N Engl J Med* 1980;302:7889–794. *Postulates the hypothesis that embolization by leukocytes occurs in the Purtscher's-like retinopathy of acute pancreatitis.*

Pratt MV, de Venecia G. Purtscher's retinopathy: A clinicopathological correlation. *Surv Ophthalmol* 1970;14:417–423.

Purtscher O. Angiopathia retinae traumatica. Lymphorrhagien des augengrundes. *Alb v Graef Arch Ophthalmol* 1912;82:347–371. *Of historic interest as first publication of this clinical entity; in German.*

Stoumbos VD, Klein ML, Goodman S. Purtscher's-like retinopathy in chronic renal failure. *Ophthalmology* 1992;99:1833–1839.

PART 15.   PREGNANCY

Chapter 114

PREGNANCY

Kathleen B. Digre
Michael Varner

I. GENERAL

1. Diabetes
   - Benign retinopathy may progress in pregnancy but regresses by 6 months postpartum.
   - Proliferative retinopathy progresses with pregnancy and should be treated.
2. Certain tumors increase in size.
   - Vascular tumors
   - Pituitary adenomas
   - Meningiomas
3. Pseudotumor cerebri
   - Pregnancy does not affect eventual visual outcome but careful serial evaluations are required.
4. Migraine
   - Can begin or worsen in the first half of pregnancy
   - Intensity and frequency generally decrease in the second half of pregnancy.

II. SYSTEMIC MANIFESTATIONS

Organ System	Normal Pregnancy	Severe Preeclampsia
Cardiac	30–50% increase in cardiac output	
Vascular	30–50% increase in blood volume and extracellular volume, midpregnancy decrease in blood pressure	Decreased blood volume due to arteriolar vasospasm
Pulmonary	20–30% increase in minute volume, increased respiratory rate	Possible pulmonary edema
Renal	30–50% increase in renal blood flow, decreased serum blood urea nitrogen and creatinine	Proteinuria
Gastrointestinal	Decreased motility, elevated alkaline phosphatase but no other elevated liver function tests	Increased transaminases
Neurologic	None	Seizures, scotomata, blindness, altered mental status, hyperreflexia
Hematologic	Decreased hematocrit, elevated leukocytes, decreased platelets	Hemoconcentration, thrombocytopenia
Mucocutaneous	Mucosal hyperemia, hyperpigmentation	
Nonspecific	Decreased serum osmolality with increased extracellular fluid	More common in women with first baby, concurrent microvascular disease, multiple pregnancy, positive family history of preeclampsia

Ocular System	Normal Pregnancy	Severe Pre-eclampsia	Magnesium Sulfate Therapy for Pre-eclampsia or Premature Labor
Lids	Hyperpigmentation, blepharoptosis	Edema	Ptosis
Cornea	Fluid retention Decreased sensitivity Refractory changes Contact lens intolerance Krukenberg spindles	None known	
Intraocular pressure	Decreased in late pregnancy		
Lens/ciliary body	Fluid retention Changes in accommodation		Decreased accommodation and near point of convergence
Retina	No changes with normal pregnancy	Segmental arteriolar vasospasm, cotton-wool spots, retinal hemorrhage, serous detachments, choroidal infarctions	
Optic nerves	No changes with normal pregnancy	Disc swelling	
Neuro-ophthalmologic	None	Seizures, coma, occipital blindness	
Ocular motility	None		Nonspecific dysfunction
Nonspecific	Bell's palsy more common during pregnancy Horner's reports after lumbar anesthesia	Abnormal Amsler grid	

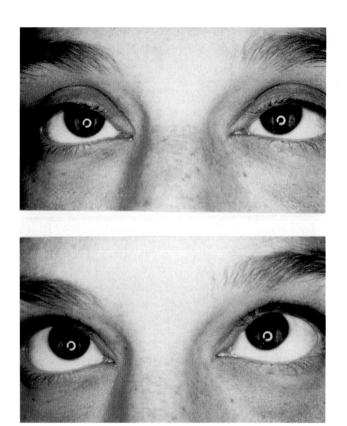

FIGURE 114.1. Ptosis with magnesium. (*Top*) On mag. (*Bottom*) Off mag.

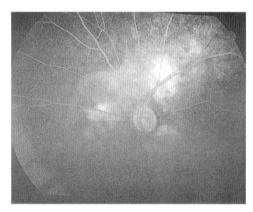

FIGURE 114.2. Serous detachment seen with fluorescein angiography.

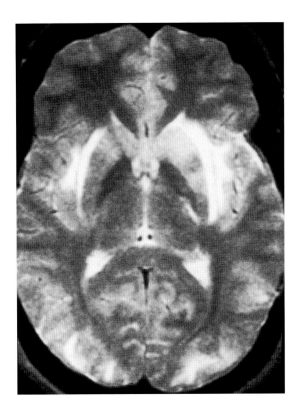

FIGURE 114.3. Magnetic resonance imaging in eclampsia.

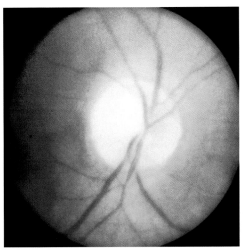

FIGURE 114.4. Segmental vasospasm.

SUGGESTED READINGS

Digre KB, Varner MW. The eye in pregnancy. In: Gold DH, Weingeist TA, eds. *The Eye in Systemic Disease*. Philadelphia: JB Lippincott; 1990:483–486.

Digre KB, Varner MW, Osborn AG, Crawford S. Cranial magnetic resonance imaging in severe pre-eclampsia versus eclampsia. *Arch Neurol* 1993;50:399–406.

Digre KB, Varner MW, Schiffman JS. Neuro-ophthalmologic effects of intravenous magnesium sulfate. *Am J Obstet Gynecol* 1990;163:1848–1852.

Jaffe G, Schatz H. Ocular manifestations of pre-eclampsia. *Am J Ophthalmol* 1987;103:309.

Sunness JS. The pregnant woman's eye. *Surv Ophthalmol* 1988;32:219–238.

Weinrub RN, Lu A, Key T. Maternal ocular adaptations during pregnancy. *Obstet Gynecol Surv* 1987;42:471–483.

PART 16. PULMONARY DISORDERS

Chapter 115
RESPIRATORY INSUFFICIENCY
Stephen H. Sinclair

I. GENERAL

1. Hypoxemia
   - Result in
     - Reduced arterial resistance
     - Increased cardiac output, vascular flow
     - Increased blood volume, hematocrit, viscosity
       - Clubbing (fingers or toes), plethoric faces
     - Increased pulmonary vascular resistance
       - Right heart failure, increased systemic venous pressure
             Peripheral edema
             Hepatomegaly
   - Causes
     - Hypoventilation
       - Injury to chest wall, splinting
       - Musculoskeletal weakness (polio, amyotrophic lateral sclerosis)
       - Decreased central drive
             Drug-induced
             Obesity-hypoventilation syndrome
             Central sleep apnea
     - Ventilation-perfusion mismatch
       - Chronic obstructive lung disease
       - Asthma
       - Mucous plugging (cystic fibrosis)
       - Pulmonary embolism
     - Shunt
       - Right to left intracardiac shunt
       - Pulmonary arteriovenous malformation
     - Diffusion impairment
       - Emphysema
       - Interstitial lung disease
       - Anemia
       - Carbon monoxide poisoning
2. Hypercapnia
   - Typically observed with hypoxemia
   - Results in
     - Tachypnea
     - Increased vascular resistance and flow
   - Causes
     - Ventilation-perfusion mismatch
       - Chronic obstructive lung disease
       - Asthma
       - Mucous plugging (cystic fibrosis)
       - Pulmonary embolism
     - Hypoventilation
       - Injury to chest wall, splinting
       - Musculoskeletal weakness (polio, amytrophic lateral sclerosis)
       - Decreased central drive
             Drug-induced
             Obesity-hypoventilation syndrome
             Central sleep apnea

II. SYSTEMIC MANIFESTATIONS

1. Chronic obstructive pulmonary disease/cystic fibrosis
   - Chronic bronchitis
     - Chronic/recurrent productive cough
     - Cyanosis
     - Edema
     - Wheezing
     - Hypercarbia
   - Emphysema
     - Dyspnea
     - Hyperinflated lungs
     - Exercise intolerance
     - Tachypnea
   - Cystic fibrosis
     - Recurrent pneumonia
     - Productive cough of thick, viscous sputum
     - Malabsorption
     - Infertility
2. Congenital cyanotic heart disease
   - Systemic manifestations
     - Cardiac murmur
     - Pulmonary hypertension
     - Clubbing
     - Cyanosis (if right-to-left shunt present)
   - Causes
     - Tetrology of Fallot
     - Ventricular septal defect
     - Atrial septal defect
     - Patent ductus arteriosus
3. High-altitude retinopathy
   - Cough and dyspnea
   - Pulmonary edema
   - Change in mental status/cerebral edema
4. Carbon monoxide poisoning
   - Headache, confusion, and change in mental status
   - Dyspnea
   - Cardiac arrhythmias
   - (Rare) cherry-red skin discoloration
5. Purtscher's retinopathy
   - Systemic manifestations
     - Adult respiratory distress syndrome
     - Hypoxia, dyspnea, tachypnea
     - Diffuse pulmonary edematous infiltrates
     - Petechial hemorrhages of chest, neck, and face
     - Cerebral symptoms, coma
   - Causes
     - Long, marrowed bone fracture
     - Acute pancreatitis
     - Postpartum

1. Chronic obstructive pulmonary disease/cystic fibrosis
   - Duskiness, dilation of conjunctival vessels
   - Dilation of major retinal arteries and veins
2. Congenital cyanotic heart disease
   - Duskiness, dilation of conjunctival vessels
   - Conjunctival edema
   - Dilation of major retinal arteries and veins
   - Optic disc edema
   - Striate retinal hemorrhages
3. High-altitude retinopathy
   - Intraretinal capillary hemorrhages
   - Dilation of major retinal arteries and veins
   - Rare optic disc edema
   - Rare vitreous hemorrhage
4. Carbon monoxide poisoning
   - Retinal vessels cherry-red color, not dusky
5. Purtscher's retinopathy
   - Conjunctival petechial hemorrhages
   - Multiple cotton-wool, nerve fiber layer infarcts
   - Occasional striate hemorrhages

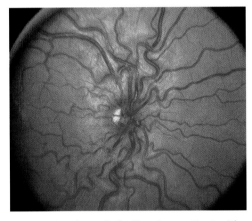

FIGURE 115.1. Funduscopic findings in a patient with congenital heart disease and cyanosis. Note dilated and tortuous retinal vessels.

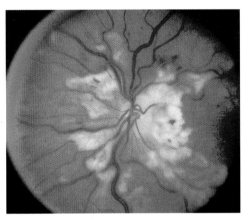

FIGURE 115.2. Purtscher's retinopathy in a patient with head trauma. Multiple nerve fiber layer infarcts are observed over and surrounding the optic nerve head.

SUGGESTED READINGS

Austen FK, Carmichael MW, Adams RD. Neurologic manifestations of chronic pulmonary insufficiency. *N Engl J Med* 1957;257:579.

Chuang EL, Miller FS, Kalina RE. Retinal lesions following long bone fractures. *Ophthalmology* 1985;92:370.

Ernst E, Hammerschmidt DE, Bagge U, et al. Leukocytes and the risk of ischemic diseases. *JAMA* 1987;257:2318.

Frayser R, Hickman JB. Retinal vascular response to breathing increased carbon dioxide and oxygen concentrations. *Invest Ophthalmol Vis Sci* 1964;3:427.

Frayser R, Houston CS, Gray G, et al. The response of the retinal circulation to altitude. *Arch Intern Med* 1971;127:708.

Grunwald JE, Riva CE, Petrig BL, et al. Effect of pure O_2 breathing on retinal blood flow in normals and in patients with background diabetic retinopathy. *Curr Eye Res* 1984;3:239–241.

Jacob HS, Goldstein IM, Shapiro I, et al. Sudden blindness in acute pancreatitis: possible role of complement-induced retinal leukoembolization. *Arch Intern Med* 1981;141:134.

Murray JF, Nadel JA, eds. *Textbook of Respiratory Medicine,* 2nd ed. Philadelphia: WB Saunders; 1994.

Shoemaker WC, Ayres S, Grenvik A, et al. *Textbook of Critical Care,* 2nd ed. Philadelphia: WB Saunders; 1989.

Shults WT, Swan KC. High altitude retinopathy in mountain climbers. *Arch Ophthalmol* 1975;93:404.

Spalter HF, Bruce GM. Ocular changes in pulmonary insufficiency. *Trans Am Acad Ophthalmol Otolaryngol* 1964;68:661.

PART 17. RENAL DISORDERS

Chapter 116
ALPORT SYNDROME
Karen M. Gehrs

I. GENERAL

1. Clinical triad of hereditary nephritis, sensorineural deafness, and ocular abnormalities
2. Inheritance pattern is generally X-linked dominant with incomplete penetrance although X-linked recessive, autosomal recessive, and autosomal dominant pedigrees have been reported. The gene frequency is estimated to be 1/5000.
3. Pathogenesis appears to involve a disorder of basement membranes specific to renal glomeruli, the cochlea, and the lens and retina.
4. A number of mutations in genes that encode for basement membrane (type IV) collagen have been identified in families with Alport syndrome. Mutations in a structural gene on the X chromosome, *COL4A5* at Xq22, have been identified in X-linked Alport kindreds. Mutations in *COL4A3* and *COL4A4* genes on chromosome 2 are associated with autosomal recessive Alport syndrome. Cotransmission of deletions in *COL4A5* and the adjacent *COL4A6* gene have been reported in families with leiomyomatosis associated with Alport syndrome.

It is unlikely that mutations or deletions in the *COL4A6* gene alone cause Alport syndrome.

5. The structural gene *COL4A5* codes for the alpha 5 chain of type IV collagen, a major structural component of glomerular basement membranes. The *COL4A3* and *COL4A4* genes encode, respectively, the alpha 3 and alpha 4 chains of type IV collagen, also major components of glomerular basement membranes. The alpha 3 and alpha 4 chains of collagen are found in the eye in Bowman's layer, Descemet's membrane, lens capsule, the internal limiting membrane, and Bruch's membrane. The location of these proteins in the cochlea has not been well characterized.
6. In both X-linked and autosomally inherited Alport syndrome the alpha 3, 4, and 5 chains of collagen have all been reported missing from glomerular basement membranes. This observation suggests that mutations in any one of the genes encoding for these proteins can interfere with the production of or integration of all three chains in the collagen IV molecule.

II. SYSTEMIC MANIFESTATIONS

1. Highly variable phenotypic expression of systemic manifestations
2. Renal
   - Hematuria—microscopic hematuria begins early in life
   - Glomerulonephritis
   - Renal failure
     - More likely in affected males in X-linked pedigrees
     - Males and females equally affected when autosomally inherited
     - Renal dialysis and renal transplantation often required by early adulthood.
   - Histologically see glomerular basement membrane thickening and splitting of the lamina densa.
3. Ear/nose/throat
   - Progressive high-frequency sensorineural hearing loss

4. Gastrointestinal/genitourinary/pulmonary
   - Diffuse leiomyomatosis, a benign smooth muscle proliferation in the esophagus, female genitalia, and trachea has been reported in association with X-linked Alport syndrome.
   - Associated leiomyomatosis is fully penetrant and completely expressed, even in females with only mild renal disease.
5. Skin
   - There are no clinical skin manifestations of Alport syndrome. However, X-linked Alport syndrome may be diagnosed by skin biopsy in affected males. Skin biopsy is not reliable in females because of mosaicism in females heterozygous for X-linked Alport syndrome.

1. General abnormalities
   - Highly variable phenotypic expression of ocular abnormalities
   - Ocular abnormalities reported in 15% to 20% of patients with Alport syndrome
   - Ocular abnormalities appear to increase in frequency and severity with age.
   - Normal ocular findings do not exclude Alport syndrome.
2. Cornea (rarely involved)
   - Corneal arcus
   - Posterior polymorphous dystrophy
   - Pigment dispersion syndrome
3. Lens
   - Anterior lenticonus
     - Most common anterior segment abnormality in Alport syndrome
     - Reported in 15% to 20% of patients with Alport syndrome
     - Almost pathognomonic of Alport syndrome (rarely reported in association with other disorders)

- Less common abnormalities
  - Spherophakia
  - Posterior subcapsular opacities
  - Cataract
3. Retina
   - Macular flecks
     - Classically spare the fovea
     - Located in the superficial retina
     - Large—about 70 to 130 μm in diameter
   - Midperipheral flecks
     - Located in the deep retina or retinal pigment epithelium
     - Small—less than 50 μm in diameter
   - Salt-and-pepper retinopathy in the midperipheral retina (rarely reported)
   - Normal electrophysiologic and psychophysical studies
   - Retinal flecks have no effect on visual function.

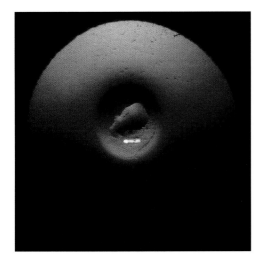

FIGURE 116.1. Slit-lamp photograph using retroillumination to demonstrate the characteristic oil-droplet reflex of anterior lenticonus. Reprinted with permission from Gehrs KM, Pollock SC, Zielkha G. Clinical features and pathogenesis of Alport retinopathy. *Retina* 1995;15:305–311.

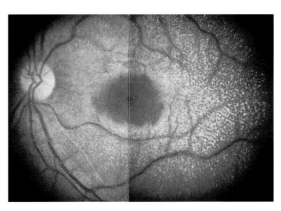

FIGURE 116.2. Fundus photograph demonstrating the classical appearance of macular flecks associated with Alport syndrome. Note that no flecks are present in the fovea or parafoveal region. Reprinted with permission from Gehrs KM, Pollock SC, Zilkha G. Clinical features and pathogenesis of Alport retinopathy. *Retina* 1995;15:305–311.

SUGGESTED READINGS

Cheong HI, Kashtan CE, Kleppel MM, Michael AF. Immunohistologic studies of type IV collagen in anterior lens capsules of patients with Alport syndrome. *Lab Invest* 1994;70:553–557.

Dahan K, Heidet L, Zhou J, et al. Smooth muscle tumors associated with X-linked Alport syndrome: Carrier detection in females. *Kidney Int* 1995;48:1900–1906.

Gehrs KM, Pollock SC, Zilkha G. Clinical features and pathogenesis of Alport retinopathy. *Retina* 1995;15:305–311.

Heiskari N, Zhang X, Zhou J, et al. Identification of 17 mutations in ten exons in the *COL4A5* collagen gene, but no mutations found in four exons in *COL4A6*: A study of 250 patients with hematuria and suspected of having Alport Syndrome. *J Am Soc Nephrol* 1996;7:702–709.

Jacobs M, Jeffrey B, Kriss A, et al. Ophthalmologic assessment of young patients with Alport syndrome. *Ophthalmology* 1992;99:1039–1044.

Kashtan CE. Clinical and molecular diagnosis of Alport syndrome. *Proceed Assoc Am Physicians* 1995;107:306–313.

Kashtan CE, Michael AF. Alport syndrome: From bedside to genome to bedside. *Am J Kidney Dis* 1993;22:627–640.

Lemmink HH, Mochizuki T, van den Heuel LP, et al. Mutations in the type IV collagen alpha 3 (*COL4A3*) gene in autosomal recessive Alport syndrome. *Hum Mol Genet* 1994;3:1269–1273.

Mochizuki T, Lemmink HH, Mariyama M, et al. Identification of mutations in the alpha 3 (IV) and alpha 4 (IV) collagen genes in autosomal recessive Alport syndrome. *Nat Genet* 1994;8:77–81.

Powell RG. Lenticonus in spina bifida. A case report. *Br J Ophthalmol* 1975;59:474–475.

Stevens PR. Anterior lenticonus and the Waardenburg syndrome. *Br J Ophthalmol* 1970;54:621–623.

Tryggvason K, Zhou J, Hostikka SL, Shows TB. Molecular genetics of Alport syndrome. *Kidney Int* 1993;43:38–44.

Weber M, Netzer KO, Pullig O. Molecular aspects of Alport's syndrome. *Clin Invest* 1992;70:809–815.

Zhang X, Zhou J, Reeders ST, Tryggvason K. Structure of the human type IV collagen *COL4A6* gene, which is mutated in Alport syndrome-associated leiomyomatosis. *Genomics* 1996;33:473–479.

Chapter 117

FAMILIAL JUVENILE NEPHRONOPHTHISIS

Ronald E. Carr

I. GENERAL: NONOCULAR

1. Heredity
   - Autosomal recessive or autosomal dominant
2. Symptoms
   - Presenting symptoms
     - Polydipsia
     - Polyuria
     - Nycturia, renal insufficiency later
     - Short stature

3. Histology
   - Small cystic kidneys
   - Diffuse interstitial fibrosis
4. Pathophysiology
   - Interstitial deposition of Tamm-Horsfall glyco-protein

II. SYSTEMIC MANIFESTATIONS

1. Congenital hepatic fibrosis (Boichis' syndrome)
2. Cerebellar ataxia
3. Mental retardation

4. Mitochondrial cytopathy
5. Asphyxiating thoracic dystrophy (Jeune's syndrome)
6. Cone-shaped epiphysis of the hands

III. OCULAR MANIFESTATIONS

1. Generalized retinal degeneration
   - Leber's congenital amaurosis—infantile onset, associated with poor central vision and nystagmus
   - Retinitis pigmentosa—later onset, good central vision initially, no nystagmus

2. All cases with retinal disease are inherited as autosomal recessive

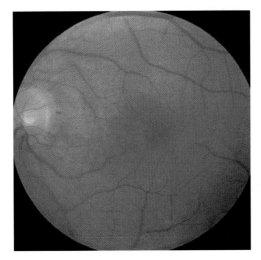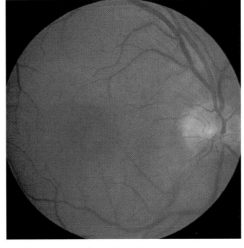

FIGURE 117.1. Fundus photographs of a 20-year-old patient with retinal degeneration associated with juvenile nephronophthisis. Note pigmentary changes at posterior pole.

SUGGESTED READINGS

Abraham FA, Yanko L, Licht A, et al. Electrophysiologic study of the visual system in familial juvenile nephronophthisis and tapetoretinal dystrophy. *Am J Ophthalmol* 1974;78:591.

Meier DA, Hass JW. Familial nephropathy with retinitis pigmentosa. *Am J Med* 1965;39:58.

Senior B, Freedman AF, Braudo JL. Juvenile familial nephropathy and tapetoretinal degeneration. A new oculorenal dystrophy. *Am J Ophthalmol* 1961;52:625.

Chapter 118
LOWE'S SYNDROME
Gerhard Wolfgang Cibis

I. GENERAL

1. Sex-linked recessive inheritance
   - Female carrier findings (cataract)
2. Exact biochemical defect is unknown; abnormalities in mucopolysaccharide and mitochondrial metabolism have been reported.
3. Gene has been isolated to the distal long arm of the X chromosome at Xq24-q26. A candidate gene has been identified. An inborn error of inositol phosphate metabolism is suspected.
4. Retardation with metabolic acidosis (renal Fanconi syndrome) and ocular findings are the main characteristics.

II. SYSTEMIC MANIFESTATIONS

1. Proximal tubular renal dysfunction develops by 3 months of age, not present at birth, creating diagnostic difficulties in newborns.
2. Sparse thin hair, frontal bossing, muscle laxity and yellow coloring are present.
3. Retardation can be minimized by vision, speech, and physical therapy intervention. Patients are functional in dressing, feeding, and personal hygiene, can work in sheltered environments and live in group homes, but are rarely able to be independent.
4. Osteoporosis and rickets require phosphate and vitamin D metabolite supplements.

III. OCULAR MANIFESTATIONS

1. Cornea
   - Keloids (Figure 118.1)
2. Lens (Figures 118.1 and 118.2)
   - Cataract—disciform, thin to absent posterior lens capsule, thickened anterior lens capsule, persistent nucleated lens fibers, integration of vitreous and lens. Carrier findings include posterior subcapsular plaques and multiple white cortical gray dots in a cuneiform pattern.
3. Nystagmus secondary to vision deprivation, strabismus
4. Congenitally anomalous chamber angle with glaucoma (60%). Onset is in the first few years of life, usually by six years; unlikely to occur later.
5. Miosis secondary to iris dilator muscle hypoplasia

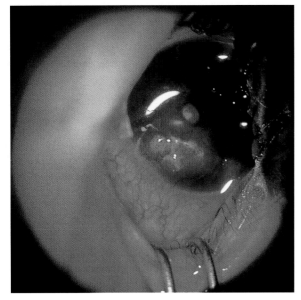

FIGURE 118.1. Pupil miosis (iris dilator hypoplasia), cataract, and corneal keloid.

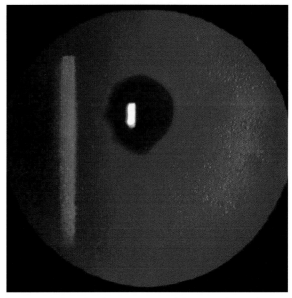

FIGURE 118.2. Carrier cataract with posterior subcapsular plaque and multiple gray white dotlike cortical changes at times in a cuneiform sectorial arrangement within the lens.

SUGGESTED READINGS

Atree O, Olivos IM, Okabe I, et al. The Lowe's oculocerbrorenal syndrome gene encodes a protein highly homologous to inositol polyphosphate-5-phosphatase. *Nature* 1992;358:239–342.

Cibis GW, Tripathi RC, Harris DJ. Corneal keloid in Lowe's syndrome. *Arch Ophthalmol* 1982;100:1795–1799.

Cibis GW, Waeltermann JM, Whitcraft CT, et al. Lenticular opacities in carriers of Lowe's syndrome. *Ophthalmology* 1986;93:1041–1045.

Kenworthy L, Park T, Charnas LR. Cognitive and behavioral profile of the oculocerebrorenal syndrome of Lowe. *Am J Med Genet* 1993;46:297–303.

Leahey AM, Charnas LR, Nussbau RL. Nonsense mutations in the OCRL-1 gene in patients with the oculocerebrorenal syndrome of Lowe. *Hum Mol Genet* 1993;2:461–463.

Chapter 119

WILMS' TUMOR (ANIRIDIA SYNDROME)

Neil J. Friedman
Richard Alan Lewis
Douglas D. Koch

I. GENERAL

1. Absence of the iris; usually, a small peripheral remnant exists.
2. Prevalence of 1/100,000 (estimated)
3. Almost always bilateral, but may be markedly asymmetrical
4. Hereditary or isolated
5. Three forms exist:
   - AN1 (85%)—autosomal dominant; only ocular findings.
   - AN2 (13%)—isolated; associated with deletion on chromosome 11p13, Wilms' tumor, genitourinary abnormalities, and mental retardation (WAGR complex, Miller syndrome)
   - AN3 (<2%)—autosomal recessive; associated with mental deficiency and ataxia (Gillespie syndrome)

II. SYSTEMIC MANIFESTATIONS

1. Renal
   - Wilms' tumor in isolated cases only
2. Genitourinary
   - Genitourinary malformations and abnormalities in WAGR complex
   - Renal agenesis in Gillespie syndrome
   - Gonadoblastoma
3. Neurologic
   - Mental retardation in WAGR complex and Gillespie syndrome
   - Cerebellar ataxia in Gillespie syndrome
4. Musculoskeletal
   - Absence of patella

III. OCULAR MANIFESTATIONS

1. Cornea
   - Corneal pannus (typically in AN1)
2. Intraocular pressure
   - Glaucoma in up to 50%
3. Uvea
   - Absence of iris; usually peripheral stump remains
4. Lens
   - Cataracts in up to 85%
   - Ectopia lentis uncommonly
   - Zonular weakness
5. Retina
   - Foveal hypoplasia
6. Optic nerve
   - Optic nerve hypoplasia
7. Ocular motility
   - Nystagmus
   - Strabismus
8. Nonspecific
   - Decreased visual acuity
   - Amblyopia
   - Photophobia

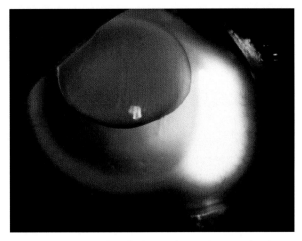

FIGURE 119.1. Aniridia. Slit-lamp photomicrography shows no visible iris tissue and superior subluxation of crystalline lens.

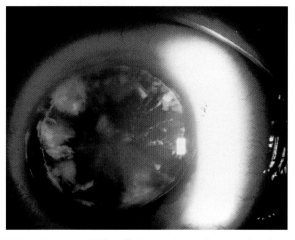

FIGURE 119.2. Aniridia. Slit-lamp photomicrography of autosomal dominant aniridia and cortical cataract.

SUGGESTED READINGS

American Academy of Ophthalmology Basic and Clinical Science Course. Section 2, pp. 134, 260; Section 4, p. 71; Section 11, p. 35. San Francisco: 1993.

Hittner HM, Riccardi VM, Francke U. Aniridia caused by a heritable chromosome 11 deletion. *Ophthalmology* 1979;86:1173.

Nelson LB, Spaeth GL, Nowinski TS, et al. Aniridia: A review. *Surv Ophthalmol* 1984;28:621.

Witting EO, Moreira CA, Freire-Maia N, Vianna-Morgante AM. Partial aniridia, cerebellar ataxia, and mental deficiency (Gillespie syndrome) in two brothers. *Am J Med Genet* 1988;30:703.

PART 18. SKELETAL DISORDERS

Section A. Cranial Deformity Syndromes

Chapter 120

CROUZON'S SYNDROME (CRANIOFACIAL DYSOSTOSIS)

David O. Magnante
John D. Bullock

I. GENERAL

1. No sex predisposition
2. Autosomal dominant
3. Sporadic mutations occur
4. Primary premature fusion of sphenoethmoidal synchondrosis
5. Hypoplasia and retrodisplacement of midface
6. Secondary premature fusion of sagittal, coronal, and lambdoidal sutures
7. Cranium often grows in horizontal direction.
8. Variation in rate, order, and severity of suture fusion determines diverse spectrum of cranial deformities.
9. Premature synostosis of cranial sutures may prevent normal brain maturation.

II. SYSTEMIC MANIFESTATIONS

1. Musculoskeletal
   - Brachycephaly most common (decreased anteroposterior skull diameter and wide lateral dimension)
   - Trigonocephaly and scaphocephaly may occur.
   - Hypoplastic maxillae
   - Malocclusion
   - Cleft palate
2. Ear/nose/throat
   - "Parrot-beak" nose
   - Short upper and drooping lower lip
   - Bifid uvula
   - Narrow nasopharynx
   - Oropharyngeal obstruction
   - Conductive hearing loss
3. Pulmonary
   - Upper respiratory infections
4. Central nervous system
   - Occasional mental impairment
   - Increased intracranial pressure

III. OCULAR MANIFESTATIONS

1. Orbit
   - Shallow orbits
   - Exophthalmos
   - Hypertelorism
   - Narrowed optic foramina
2. Optic nerve
   - Optic atrophy
   - Papilledema
3. Ocular motility
   - Exotropia
   - V pattern
   - Abnormal extraocular muscle origins and insertions
   - Nystagmus
4. Cornea
   - Keratoconus
   - Microcornea
5. Intraocular pressure
   - Glaucoma
6. Lens
   - Cataract
   - Ectopia lentis
7. Uvea
   - Aniridia
8. Neuroophthalmologic
   - Anisocoria
9. Retina
   - Medullated nerve fibers

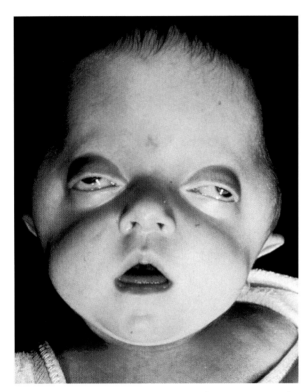

FIGURE 120.1. Characteristic facies of Crouzon's syndrome demonstrating exophthalmos, divergent strabismus, hypertelorism, and "parrot-beak" nose. Courtesy of Meinhard Robinow, MD.

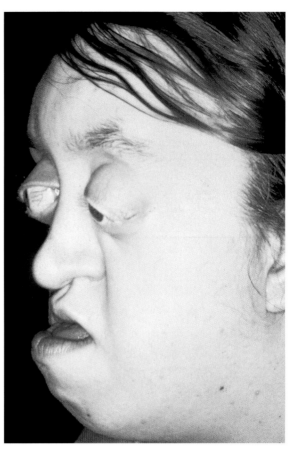

FIGURE 120.2. Side view of a patient with Crouzon's syndrome shows maxillary hypoplasia, mandibular prognathism, short upper lip, and drooping lower lip. Courtesy of Meinhard Robinow, MD.

SUGGESTED READINGS

Cohen MM Jr. An etiologic and nosologic overview of craniosynostosis syndromes. *Birth Defects* 1975;11(2):137.

Nelson LB, Ingoglia S, Breinin GM. Sensorimotor disturbances in craniostenosis. *J Pediatr Ophthalmol Strabismus* 1981;18:32.

Morax S. Oculo-motor disorders in craniofacial malformations. *J Maxillofac Surg* 1984;12:1.

Singh M, Hadi F, Aram GN, et al. Craniosynostosis—Crouzon's disease and Apert syndrome. *Indian Pediatr* 1983;20:608.

Wolter JR. Bilateral keratoconus in Crouzon's syndrome with unilateral acute hydrops. *J Pediatr Ophthalmol* 1977;14:141.

Section B.   Facial Malformation Syndromes

Chapter 121

MANDIBULOFACIAL DYSOSTOSIS (TREACHER-COLLINS SYNDROME)

Brian R. Wong
Steven J. Blackwell

I. GENERAL

1. Autosomal dominant with high penetrance
2. 1/10,000 live births
3. Genetic defect unknown
4. New mutations account for more than 50% of the cases
5. Defective development around the seventh fetal week when bony facial structures develop

II. SYSTEMIC MANIFESTATIONS

1. Musculoskeletal
   - Absence or severe hypoplasia of the zygomatic process of the temporal bone
   - Deformity, often with clefting, of the orbital rim
   - Deformity of the zygoma
   - Deformity of the mandible
   - Deformity of the medial pterygoid plates and hypoplasia of the medial pterygoid muscles
     - Causes a convex facial profile with a prominent nose and retrusive chin
   - Macrostomia with abnormal dentition and malocclusion
   - Skeletal and cranial synostosis
   - Syndactyly
   - Forearm and hand malformations
2. Cardiac
   - Congenital heart disease
3. Renal
   - Renal abnormalities
4. Gastrointestinal
   - Choanal atresia
   - Absence of the parotid gland
5. Genitourinary
   - Cryptorchidism
6. Neurologic
   - Mental retardation is unusual.
   - Hydrocephalus
   - Dolichocephaly
   - Small sella turcica
7. Mucocutaneous
   - Inferior extension of sideburns onto the upper cheek
8. Ear/nose/throat
   - Crumpled, misplaced pinna
   - Absent external auditory canal
   - Pretragal fistulae
   - Fusion or absence of one or more middle ear ossicles
   - Deafness
   - Sinus abnormalities
   - Nasal atresia
   - Cleft lip and palate

III. OCULAR MANIFESTATIONS

1. Lids
   - True colobomas (usually lateral lower lids)
   - Medial lower lid pseudocolobomas (tarsal plate reduced or absent, cilia absent)
   - Canthal dystopia (inferomedial displacement of the lateral canthus)
   - Absence of the lateral canthal tendon
   - Shortened horizontal palpebral fissure
   - Blepharoptosis
   - Ectropion
   - Entropion
   - Distichiasis
   - Trichiasis
2. Lacrimal system
   - Absence of lacrimal puncta (usually inferior)
   - Lacrimal duct atresia
3. Conjunctiva/sclera
   - Limbal dermoids
4. Cornea
   - Corneal guttata
5. Uvea
   - Pupil ectopia
   - Colobomas
6. Lens
   - Cataracts
7. Orbit
   - Inferolateral orbit defect
   - Superolateral orbit displaced caudally
   - Orbital lipodermoids
8. Motility
   - Esotropia
   - Exotropia
   - Duane's syndrome
   - Cranial nerve palsies
   - Overaction of oblique muscles
9. Nonspecific
   - Amblyopia caused by
     - Ametropia
     - Anisometropia
     - Strabismus
     - Blepharoptosis
   - Astigmatism
   - Microphthalmos
   - Anophthalmos

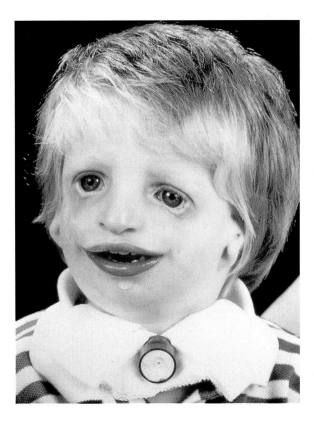

FIGURE 121.1. Mandibulofacial dysostosis. The face is small, but head size is normal. Antimongoloid slant of the palpebral fissures with underdeveloped or absent malar bones and zygomatic arch is evident. Lower eyelids show symmetrical colobomas in the outer one-third and sparse lashes medial to the eyelid notch defects. Ear deformities such as this symmetrical, microtia, and conduction deafness frequently accompanies these. Note the fish-mouth appearance, reflecting rudimentary macrostomia. The lower jaw is small and angled downward, giving an open bite malocclusion. This child required tracheostomy to manage severe airway problems caused by micrognathia and glossoptosis.

SUGGESTED READINGS

Bartley GB. Lacrimal drainage anomalies in mandibulofacial dysostosis. *Am J Ophthalmol* 1990;109:571–591.

Diamond G, Hollsten DA, Katowitz JA. Mandibulofacial dysostosis. In: Gold DH, Weingeist TA, eds. *The Eye in Systemic Disease.* Philadelphia: JB Lippincott; 1990:524–526.

Fries PD, Katowitz JA. Congenital craniofacial anomalies of ophthalmic importance. *Surv Ophthalmol* 1990;35:87–119.

Hertle RW, Ziylan S, Katowitz JA. Ophthalmic features and visual prognosis in the Treacher-Collins syndrome. *Br J Ophthalmol* 1993;77:642–645.

Wang FM, Millman AL, Sidoti PA, Goldberg RB. Ocular findings in Treacher Collins syndrome. *Am J Ophthalmol* 1990;110:280–286.

Chapter 122

OCULOAURICULOVERTEBRAL DYSPLASIA

Frederick M. Wang
Rosalie B. Goldberg

I. GENERAL

1. Congenital association of anomalies of the first and second brachial arches often with associated ocular and vertebral abnormalities
2. Large spectrum of severity from tiny ear tags and ocular dermoids to marked facial hypoplasia with clefts and sinuses
   - With ocular dermoids the condition is termed "Goldenhar's."
   - With unilateral hypoplasia of the face the condition is termed "hemifacial microsomia."
3. Anomalies, although frequently bilateral, are almost always significantly asymmetrical.
4. Usually sporadic
   - Rarely autosomal dominant, autosomal recessive, or multifactorial
   - Has been reported with a host of chromosomal abnormalities
5. Demographics
   - Sex—male predominance (3:2)
   - Race—no predispositions
   - Incidence—between 1/3000 to 1/26,500 births
6. Pathophysiology
   - Embryologic field defect
   - Sequence may be initiated by primary neural crest involvement or vascular disruption (hemorrhage) in developing first and second branchial arch region
   - More common in offspring of diabetic mothers
   - Thalidomide and retinoic acid have produced this sequence.

II. SYSTEMIC MANIFESTATIONS

1. Ear
   - Wide range of external anomalies from small preauricular tags to anotia; tags, preauricular sinuses, microtia most common (85%)
   - Hearing loss both sensorineural and conductive due to anomalies of external and internal structures especially ossicle hypoplasia (50%)
2. Facial
   - Soft tissue and bony (mandibular, maxillary, temporal, and malar) hypoplasia (80%)
   - Cleft lip or palate (7–15%)
   - Lateral, facial clefts (occasional)
   - Velopharyngeal insufficiency producing hypernasal speech
   - Facial nerve palsy usually from bony involvement in the facial canal (22%)
   - Parotid aplasia (occasional)
3. Skeletal
   - Vertebral abnormalities; cervical hemivertebrae and fusions
   - Klippel-Feil anomaly (occasional)
   - Scoliosis (occasional)
   - Limb defects including talipes equinovarus (20%) and radial anomalies (10%)
4. Central nervous system
   - Microcephaly (occasional)
   - Developmental delay/mental retardation (occasional)
5. Cardiac
   - Congenital heart disease (occasional)
6. Pulmonary
   - Lung hypoplasia (rare)
7. Renal
   - Absent or ectopic kidneys (rare)
   - Ureteral anomalies (rare)

III. OCULAR MANIFESTATIONS

1. Conjunctiva/sclera
   - Lipodermoids (33%)
   - Limbal dermoids (33%)
2. Cornea
   - Astigmatism induced by limbal dermoids
3. Orbit
   - Asymmetry (common)
4. Lids
   - Ptosis (12%)
   - Coloboma of the upper or lower (11%)
5. Lacrimal system
   - Obstruction (10%)
   - Fistula and sinuses (occasional)
   - Ectopic puncta (occasional)
6. Ocular motility
   - Esotropia (10%)
   - Exotropia (5%)
   - Duane's syndrome (occasional)
7. Uvea
   - Iris and chorioretinal coloboma (occasional)
8. Retina
   - Tortuous vessels (occasional)
   - Macular hypoplasia (occasional)
9. Optic nerve
   - Hypoplasia (occasional)
10. Nonspecific
    - Microphthalmia (occasional)

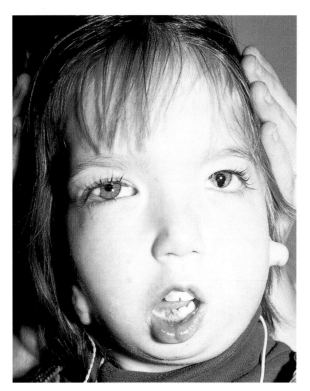

FIGURE 122.1. Goldenhar-Gorlin syndrome. Note right-sided limbal dermoid, right-sided inferotemporal lipodermoid, left iris coloboma, bilateral grade III microtia, and facial asymmetry with mandibular deficiency and dental malocclusion.

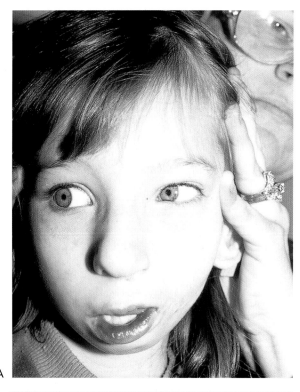

A

FIGURE 122.2. Goldenhar-Gorlin syndrome. Left-sided Duane's syndrome type I with left-sided hemifacial microsomia. Bilateral hearing aids for mixed sensorineural and conductive loss. (**A**) Right gaze. (**B**) Primary position. (**C**) Left gaze.

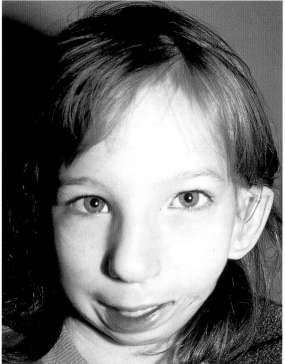

B

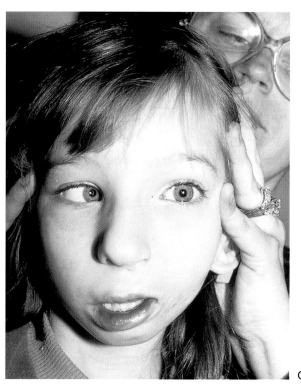

C

SUGGESTED READINGS

Johnston MC, Bronsky PT. Animal models for human craniofacial malformations. *J Craniofac Genet Dev Biol* 1991;22:227–291. *A good review of normal and variant facial development.*

Mansour AM, Wang FM, Henkind P, et al. Ocular findings in the facioauriculovertebral sequence (Goldenhar-Gorlin syndrome). *Am J Ophthalmol* 1973;75:250–257. *A large series describing ophthalmic features.*

Rollnick BR, Goldberg RB. Oculoauriculovertebral spectrum (hemifacial microsomia, Goldenhar syndrome). In: Gorlin RJ, Cohen MM Jr, Levin SL, eds. *Syndromes of the Head and Neck.* New York: Oxford University Press, 1990:641–649. *A good review of the spectrum of anomalies.*

Chapter 123

OCULOMANDIBULODYSCEPHALY (HALLERMAN-STREIFF SYNDROME)

Johane Robitaille
Ronald V. Keech

I. GENERAL

1. Congenital disorder of unknown etiology
2. Majority are sporadic, some familial cases have been reported.
3. No sex predilection
4. Belongs to the branchial arch syndromes and ectodermal dysplasias, affecting the cranial and facial bones, skin, hair, teeth enamel, and lens
5. Difficulty breathing and failure to thrive due to narrow upper airways
6. Death in infancy or childhood may occur from respiratory or feeding difficulties.
7. Possible development of cardiopulmonary disease if presence of obstructive airway disease

II. SYSTEMIC MANIFESTATIONS

1. Skeletal
   - Facial and skull
     - Mandibular hypoplasia
     - Thin tapered nose with hypoplastic alae nasi
     - Bird- or parrotlike facies
     - Microstomia
     - Narrow, high arched palate
     - Double chin with central cleft
     - Brachycephaly, (rarely scaphocephaly, microcephaly)
     - Anteriorly displaced temporomandibular joint
     - Hypoplastic paranasal sinuses
     - Delayed closure of fontanelles with widening of longitudinal and lamboidal sutures
     - Occasional malar hypoplasia
   - Other
     - Proportionate short stature
     - Poorly mineralized bone
     - Winging of scapula
     - Scoliosis
     - Spina bifida
     - Syndactyly
2. Dental
   - Natal or neonatal teeth
   - Absent, malformed, or supernumary teeth
   - Premature caries
3. Integument
   - Cutaneous atrophy, especially scalp and nose
   - Multiple telangiectasias
   - Hypotrichosis, especially scalp, eyebrows, and eyelashes
   - Fine, hypopigmented hair
4. Respiratory
   - Obstructive sleep apnea
   - Chronic snoring
   - Recurrent upper/lower respiratory tract infections
5. Nonspecific
   - Possible mental retardation
   - Failure to thrive
   - Feeding difficulties
6. Cardiovascular
   - Pulmonary hypertension
   - Right heart failure
   - Pulmonary stenosis, ventricular septal defect, atrial septal defect, patent ductus arteriosus, and tetralogy of Fallot
7. Genitourinary
   - Hypogenitalism

III. OCULAR MANIFESTATIONS

1. Lens
   - Bilateral congenital cataracts, total or partial
2. Nonspecific
   - Bilateral microphthalmos (varying degrees)
   - Intraocular inflammation (in cases of degenerating cataracts)
   - Enophthalmos
3. Intraocular pressure
   - Glaucoma secondary to
     - Peripheral anterior and posterior synechiae from intraocular inflammation
     - Congenitally anomalous angle
4. Optic nerve
   - Coloboma
   - Dysplasia
5. Lids
   - Antimongoloid fissures
   - Hypotrichosis
   - Hypotelorism
   - Epicanthal folds
   - Ptosis
   - Hypoplastic lacrimal puncta

6. Retina/uvea
   - Retinal folds
   - Chorioretinal scars
   - Intraocular inflammation (in cases of degenerating cataracts)
   - Iris atrophy
   - Iris/choroidal colobomas
   - Persistent pupillary membrane
7. Neuroophthalmologic
   - Nystagmus
8. Ocular motility
   - Strabismus
9. Sclera
   - Blue sclera
10. Others
    - Conjunctival defects
    - Vitreous degeneration
    - Epibulbar tumors

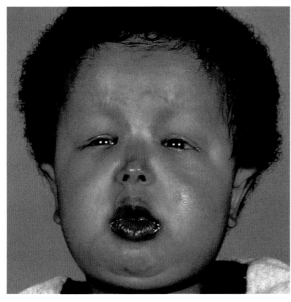 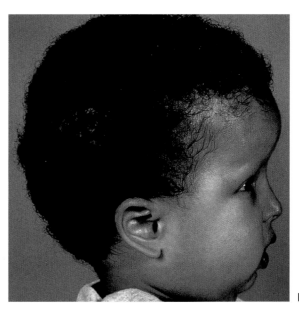

A   B

FIGURE 123.1. Hallermann-Streiff syndrome. **(A)** Frontal view. **(B)** Side view.

Oculomandibulodyscephaly (Hallerman-Streiff Syndrome)   **491**

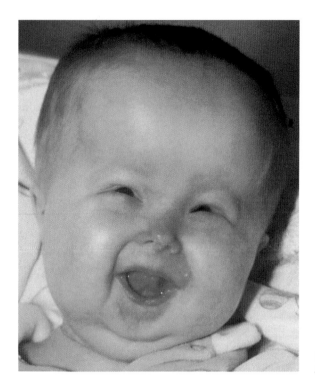

FIGURE 123.2. Hellerman-Streiff syndrome, frontal view. Courtesy of Alex Levin, MD.

SUGGESTED READINGS

Barrucand D, Benradi C, Schmitt J. Le syndrome de Francois: a propos de deux cas. *Oto-Neuro-Ophthalmol* 1978;50:305–326.

Bitoun P, Timsit JC, Trang H, Benady R. A new look at the management of oculo-mandibulo-facial syndrome. *Ophthal Paediatr Genet* 1992;13:19–26.

Gorlin JR, Cohen MM, Levin LS, eds. *Syndromes of the Head and Neck.* New York: Oxford University Press; 1990:306–309.

Keech RV. Oculomandibulodyscephaly, Hallerman-Streiff syndrome. In: Gold DH, Weingeist TA, eds. *The Eye in Systemic Disease.* Philadelphia: JB Lippincott; 1990:530–532.

Chapter 124

PIERRE-ROBIN SEQUENCE

Brian R. Wong
Steven J. Blackwell

I. GENERAL

1. Usually sporadic but also reported in dominant and recessive inheritance patterns
2. Defect in development of the first branchial arch, mandibular portion, occurring prior to 9 weeks' gestation

II. SYSTEMIC MANIFESTATIONS

1. Musculoskeletal
   - Micrognathia (hypoplasia of the mandible)—improves with age
   - Cleft palate
   - Glossoptosis
     - Causes respiratory difficulties
   - Hand and foot anomalies—syndactyly, club feet
2. Cardiac
   - Congenital heart defects—patent ductus arteriosus, atrial septal defect, coarctation of the aorta
3. Gastrointestinal
   - Choanal atresia
4. Neurologic
   - Microcephaly
   - Hydrocephalus
   - May be mentally retarded
5. Ear/nose/throat
   - Low-set ears

III. OCULAR MANIFESTATIONS

1. Lacrimal system
   - Nasolacrimal duct obstruction
2. Intraocular pressure
   - Glaucoma
3. Lens
   - Cataracts
4. Retina
   - Retinal detachment
   - Maculopathy
5. Motility
   - Strabismus
6. Nonspecific
   - Myopia
   - Micropthalmos
   - Associated with Stickler syndrome

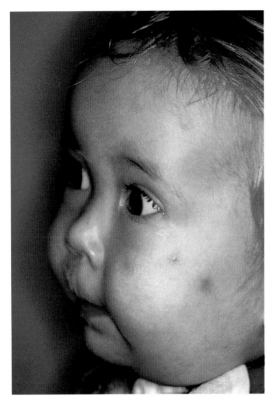

FIGURE 124.1. The small, undershot chin and mandible give a birdlike facial appearance. The resultant inspiratory ball valve airway obstruction caused by glossoptosis within these tiny jaw confines made tracheostomy necessary.

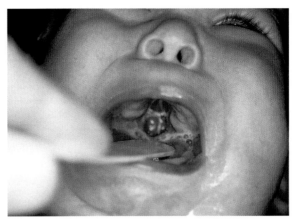

FIGURE 124.2. Isolated cleft palate is noted with this condition.

SUGGESTED READINGS

Cosman B, Keyser JJ. Eye abnormalities and skeletal deformities in the Pierre Robin syndrome: A balanced evaluation. *Cleft Palate J* 1974;11:404–411.

McKusker S, Kushner BJ. Pierre Robin sequence. In: Gold DH, Weingeist TA, eds. *The Eye in Systemic Disease.* Philadelphia: JB Lippincott; 1990:532–533.

Rogers NK, Strachan IM. Pierre Robin anomalad, maculopathy, and autolytic cataract. *J Pediatr Ophthalmol Strabismus,* 1995;32:391–392.

Smith JL, Stowe FR. The Pierre Robin syndrome (glossoptosis, micrognathia, cleft palate): A review of 39 cases with emphasis on associated ocular lesions. *Paediatrics* 1961;26:128–133.

Chapter 125

WAARDENBURG SYNDROME

Andrea L. Lusk
Ronald V. Keech

I. GENERAL

1. First described in 1951 by Johannes Waardenburg
2. Autosomal dominant inheritance
3. Variable penetrance
4. Three types
   - Type I (WS1) with dystopia canthorum
   - Type II (WS2) without dystopia canthorum
   - Type III (WS3) with limb anomalies
5. Mapped to *PAX3* gene on chromosome 2q (WS1)
6. WS1 genetically heterogeneous—more than one genotype associated with the typical features of the syndrome
7. Abnormality of neural crest development or migration has been suggested.

II. SYSTEMIC MANIFESTATIONS

1. Cutancous
   - Hair
     - Synophrys (growing together of the eyebrows with hypertrichiasis of their medial portions)
     - White forelock
     - White eyelashes
     - White eyebrows
     - Premature graying
   - Skin
     - Dystopia canthorum (telecanthus)—lateral displacement of the medial canthi (WS1)
     - Partial albinism
2. Cochlear
   - Congenital hearing loss (unilateral or bilateral)
   - Accounts for approximately 2% of congenital hearing loss
3. Musculoskeletal
   - Hypoplastic lower lateral cartilages (narrow lower third of nose)
   - Prominent broad nasal bridge
   - Spina bifida (rare)
   - Cleft palate or lip (rare)
   - Limb defects (rare)
4. Gastrointestinal
   - Hirschsprung disease (rare)

III. OCULAR MANIFESTATIONS

1. Iris
   - Heterochromia totalis
   - Heterochromia partialis
   - Hypopigmentation
2. Inner canthi
   - Dystopia canthorum
3. Fundus
   - Hypopigmentation of choroid
4. Pigmentation
   - Iris heterochromia
   - White eyelashes
   - White eyebrows

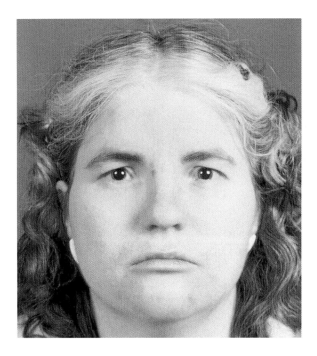

FIGURE 125.1. White forelock (bilateral profound hearing loss).

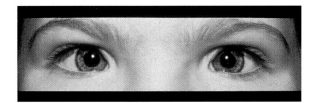

FIGURE 125.2. Dystopia canthorum.

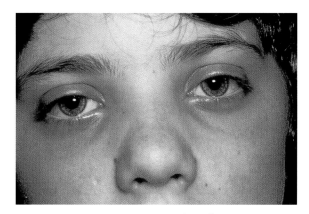

FIGURE 125.4. Broad nasal root.

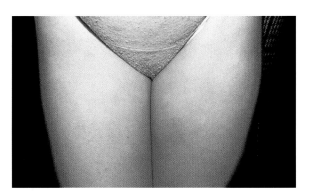

FIGURE 125.3. Skin hypopigmentation.

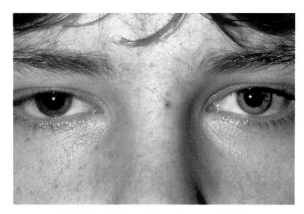

FIGURE 125.5. Heterochromia totalis.

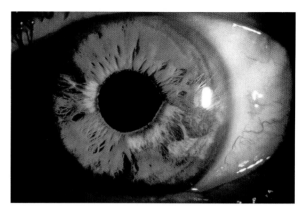

FIGURE 125.6. Heterochromia partialis.

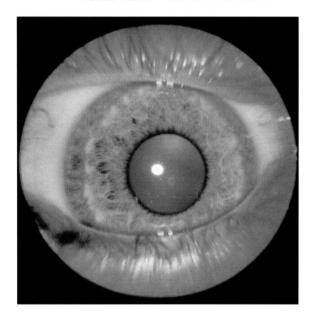

FIGURE 125.7. Hypopigmented iris.

SUGGESTED READINGS

Arias S. Genetic heterogeneity in the Waardenburg syndrome. *Birth Defects: Original Article Series* 1971;7:87–101.

Bard LA. Heterogeneity in Waardenburg's syndrome. Report of a family with ocular albinism. *Arch Ophthalmol* 1978;96:1193–1198.

Bloom KE. Advances in inherited disorders of hypopigmentation; comparisons of mice and men. *Curr Opin Pediatr* 1993;5:458–463.

Delleman JW, Hageman MJ. Ophthalmological findings in 34 patients with Waardenburg's syndrome. *J Pediatr Ophthalmol Strabismus* 1978;15:341–345.

Goldberg MF. Waardenburg's syndrome with fundus and other anomalies. *Arch Ophthalmol* 1966;76:797–810.

Grundfast KM, Agustin TB. Finding the gene(s) for Waardenburg syndrome(s). *Otolaryngol Clin North Am* 1992;25:935–951.

Hageman MI, Delleman JW. Heterogeneity in the Waardenburg syndrome. *Am J Hum Genet* 1977;29:468–485.

Liu XZ. Waardenburg syndrome II: Phenotypic findings and diagnostic criteria. *Am J Med Genet* 1995;55:95–100.

Liu X, Newton V, Read A. Hearing loss and pigmentary disturbances in Waardenburg syndrome with references to WS type II. *J Laryngol Otol* 1995;109:96–100.

Waardenburg PJ. A new syndrome combining anomalies of the eyelids, eyebrows, and nose root with pigmentary defects of the iris and head hair and with congenital deafness. *Am J Hum Genet* 1951;3:195–255.

Section C. Generalized Skeletal Disorders

Chapter 126

APERT'S SYNDROME (ACROCEPHALOSYNDACTYLY)

David O. Magnante
John D. Bullock

I. GENERAL

1. No sex or racial predisposition
2. Possible correlation between incidence and increased paternal age
3. Autosomal dominant
4. Sporadic mutations
5. Malformation initiated between 29th and 35th days of embryonic life
6. Original malformation at base of skull
7. Secondary premature fusion of cranial sutures, particularly coronal suture
8. Cranium grows in a vertical direction.
9. Premature closure of cranial sutures may prevent normal brain development.

II. SYSTEMIC MANIFESTATIONS

1. Musculoskeletal
   - Oxycephaly ("tower skull")
   - Syndactyly of hands and feet—partial to complete
   - Hypoplastic maxillae
   - Malocclusion
   - Cleft palate
   - Aplasia and ankylosis of shoulders, hips, elbows, and cervical spine
2. Ear/nose/throat
   - "Parrot-beak" nose
   - Bifid uvula
3. Cardiac
   - Ventricular septal defects
4. Central nervous system
   - Agenesis of corpus callosum
   - Variable mental impairment
   - Increased intracranial pressure
5. Renal
   - Polycystic kidneys
6. Gastrointestinal
   - Ectopic anus
   - Pyloric stenosis

III. OCULAR MANIFESTATIONS

1. Orbit
   - Shallow orbits
   - Exophthalmos
   - Hypertelorism
   - Antimongoloid slanting of palpebral fissures
   - Narrowed optic foramina
2. Optic nerve
   - Optic atrophy
   - Papilledema
3. Ocular motility
   - Vertical deviation more common than horizontal
   - Exotropia more frequent than esotropia
   - V pattern
   - Inferior oblique overaction
   - Abnormal extraocular muscle origins and insertions
   - Mechanical restriction of ocular motility
   - Nystagmus
4. Cornea
   - Exposure keratitis
   - Keratoconus
   - Megalocornea
5. Lens
   - Congenital cataract
   - Subluxation of lens
6. Uvea
   - Iris coloboma
7. Lids
   - Ptosis
8. Retina
   - Retinal detachment
   - Medullated nerve fibers
9. Nonspecific
   - Axial shortening of globe
   - Refractive errors (hyperopia most common)

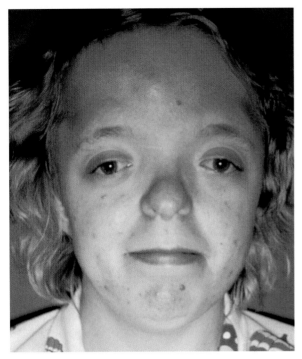

FIGURE 126.1. Typical facies of Apert's syndrome. Note anti-mongoloid slanting of the palpebral fissures, exophthalmos, hypertelorism, oxycephaly, and midfacial hypoplasia. Courtesy of Meinhard Robinow, MD.

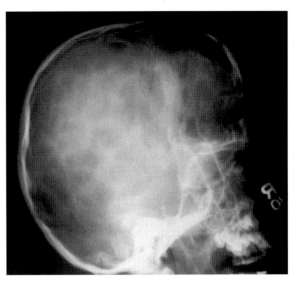

FIGURE 126.2. Skull x-ray shows characteristic changes of oxycephaly and prominent digital impressions. Courtesy of Meinhard Robinow, MD.

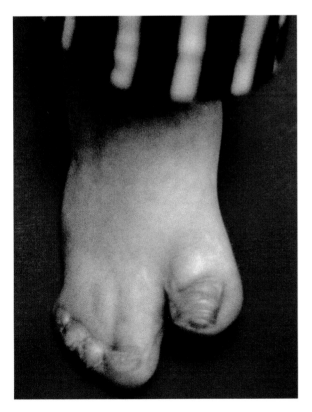

FIGURE 126.3. Left foot shows marked syndactyly and a central nail mass. Courtesy of Meinhard Robinow, MD.

SUGGESTED READINGS

Blank CE. Apert's syndrome (a type of acrocephalosyndactyly)—Observations on a British series of thirty-nine cases. *Ann Hum Genet* 1960;24:151.

Krueger JL, Ide CH. Acrocephalosyndactyly (Apert's syndrome). *Ann Ophthalmol* 1974;6:787.

Morax S. Oculo-motor disorders in craniofacial malformations. *J Maxillofac Surg* 1984;12:1.

Seelenfreund M, Gartner S. Acrocephalosyndactyly (Apert's syndrome). *Arch Ophthalmol* 1967;78:8.

Stewart RE, Dixon G, Cohen A. The pathogenesis of premature craniosynostosis in acrocephalosyndactyly (Apert's syndrome). *Plast Reconstr Surg* 1977;59:699.

Chapter 127

HYPOPHOSPHATASIA

Stuart T. D. Roxburgh

I. GENERAL

1. Extremely rare inherited metabolic bone disease characterized by defective bone mineralization. Three types
  - Infantile autosomal recessive (most severe, often fatal)
  - Childhood autosomal recessive or autosomal dominant
  - Adult autosomal dominant inheritance with variable penetrance (least severe)

2. In hypophosphatasia there is a deficiency of alkaline phosphatase activity. Osteoblasts cannot incorporate calcium into otherwise normal bone matrix preventing bone maturation. Patients present with ricketslike symptoms in childhood and osteomalacia in adulthood.

II. SYSTEMIC MANIFESTATIONS

1. Renal nephrocalcinosis
2. Skeletal ricketslike changes (joint pains and swelling valgus deformities, costochondral beading)
  - Craniostenosis
  - Premature loss of teeth

3. Neurologic craniostenosis leading to raised intracranial pressure and nerve palsies

III. OCULAR MANIFESTATIONS

1. Blue sclera
2. Conjunctival calcification
3. Band keratopathy
4. Cataracts
5. Optic atrophy
6. Retinitis pigmentosa
7. Shallow orbits, proptosis

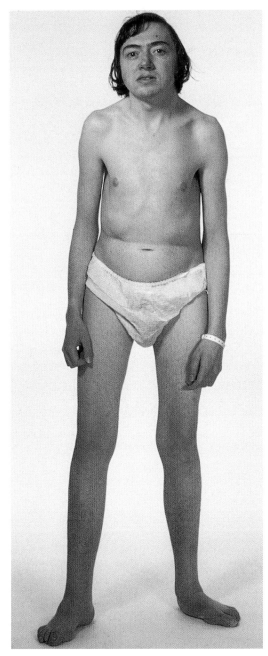

FIGURE 127.1. A case of childhood hypophosphatasia (patient now 26 years old). Note the rachitic features with costochondral beading and valgus deformities. This patient had craniostenosis, optic atrophy, and retinitis pigmentosa.

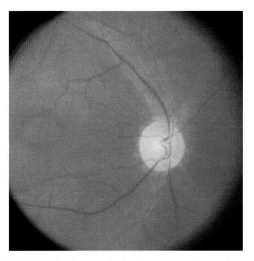

FIGURE 127.2. Optic atrophy in the same patient who also had atypical retinitis pigmentosa with marked attenuation of the arterioles and fine pigmentary changes.

SUGGESTED READINGS

Brenner TL, Smith J, Cleveland WW, et al. Eye signs in hypophosphatasia. *Arch Ophthalmol* 1964;71:497–499.

Fraser D. Hypophosphatasia. *Am J Med* 1957;22:730–745.

Roxburgh STD. In: Gold DH, Weingeist TA, eds. *The Eye In Systemic Diseases.* Philadelphia: JB. Lippincott; 1990:545–547.

Chapter 128

MARFAN SYNDROME

Neil J. Friedman
Richard Alan Lewis
Douglas D. Koch

I. GENERAL

1. Connective tissue disorder with ocular, cardiovascular, and skeletal abnormalities
2. Prevalence of approximately 1/15,000
3. Hereditary (autosomal dominant)
   - New mutations associated with increased paternal age
   - New mutations tend to have a more severe phenotype than inherited cases.
4. Variable expressivity
5. Defect in *fibrillin 1* gene on chromosome 15
6. Mean age of death in early forties due to aortic complications (dissecting thoracic or thoracoabdominal aneurysms)

II. SYSTEMIC MANIFESTATIONS

1. Cardiac
   - Degeneration of heart valves and chordae tendineae
   - Mitral valve prolapse
   - Mitral regurgitation
   - Tricuspid regurgitation
   - Aortic valve insufficiency
   - Arrhythmias
2. Vascular
   - Aortic dilation (aortic root and ascending aorta)
   - Aortic aneurysm, dissection, and rupture
   - Pulmonary artery dilation
3. Pulmonary
   - Lung cysts
   - Spontaneous pneumothorax
   - Emphysema
4. Musculoskeletal
   - Tall stature (though classic, not universal)
   - Long limbs (arm span exceeds height)
   - Arachnodactyly
   - Kyphoscoliosis
   - Pectus deformities (excavatum and carinatum)
   - Joint laxity
   - Flat feet
   - Hernias
   - High-arched palate

III. OCULAR MANIFESTATIONS

1. Uvea
   - Iridodonesis
   - Incomplete development of angle structures and ciliary body
   - Prominent iris processes
2. Lens
   - Ectopia lentis (usually bilateral and superotemporal in direction)
3. Retina
   - Retinal detachment (due to myopia and aphakia)
4. Nonspecific
   - Axial myopia

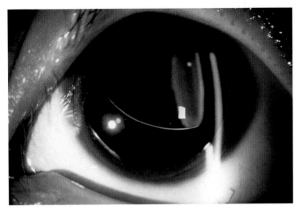

FIGURE 128.1. Marfan syndrome. Slit-lamp photomicrography shows ectopia lentis with typical pattern of superior subluxation.

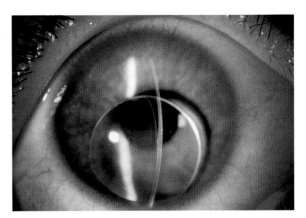

FIGURE 128.2. Marfan syndrome. Slit-lamp photomicrography shows ectopia lentis with microspherophakia; the lens is completely luxated into the anterior chamber, predisposing to pupillary block glaucoma.

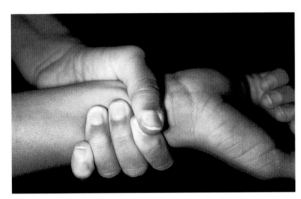

FIGURE 128.3. Evidence of the disproportionate finger length and lean extremity is the ability to wrap fingers around the wrist and overlap the digits.

SUGGESTED READINGS

Allen RA, Straatsma BR, Hall MO. Ocular manifestations of the Marfan syndrome. *Trans Am Acad Ophthalmol Otol* 1967;71:18.

Berkow R. *Merck Manual,* 16th ed. Rahway, NJ: Merck; 1992:2251–2252.

Maumenee IH. The eye in the Marfan syndrome. *Trans Am Ophthalmol Soc* 1981;79:684.

Pyeritz RE, McKusick VA. The Marfan syndrome: Diagnosis and management. *N Engl J Med* 1979;300:772.

Wyngaarden JB, Smith LH Jr, eds. *Cecil Textbook of Medicine.* Philadelphia: WB Saunders, 1988;148, 371–373, 1177–1178.

Chapter 129

STICKLER SYNDROME

Scott R. Sneed
David M. Brown
Thomas A. Weingeist

I. GENERAL

1. Autosomal dominant inheritance with variable penetrance

2. Connective tissue disorder (mutation in type II collagen gene found in 50% of families)

II. SYSTEMIC MANIFESTATIONS

1. Cardiac
  - Mitral valve prolapse
2. Musculoskeletal
  - Epiphyseal dysplasia (tibia, distal femur, distal radius)
  - Anterior wedging of vertebral bodies
  - Joint laxity and hyperextensibility
  - Bony enlargement (ankles, knees, wrists)
  - Pronounced arthralgias/degenerative arthritis
3. Ear/nose/throat
  - Sensorineural or mixed hearing loss
  - Cleft palate
  - Submucous cleft
  - Highly arched palate
  - Bifid uvula
  - Dental anomalies (maleruption, natal teeth, enamel hypoplasia, noneruption)
4. Nonspecific
  - Midfacial "flattening"
  - Flat nasal bridge
  - Epicanthus
  - Long philtrum
  - Pierre-Robin anomaly

III. OCULAR MANIFESTATIONS

1. Lens
  - Posterior subcapsular cataracts
  - Progressive presenile nuclear sclerotic cataracts
  - Stationary peripheral cortical opacities
2. Vitreous
  - Pronounced vitreous syneresis
  - Optically empty vitreous
  - Vitreous membranes
3. Retina
  - Complicated retinal detachments
  - Giant retinal tears
  - Multiple and posterior retinal breaks
  - Latticelike degeneration
  - Choroidal hypopigmentation
  - Perivascular pigmentary changes
  - Peripheral vascular sheathing, attenuation, nonperfusion
4. Nonspecific
  - Axial myopia
  - Abnormal anterior chamber vessels
  - Fine membranes over the trabecular meshwork
  - Atrophic patches of the iris root with absent iris processes
  - Long, thick iris processes

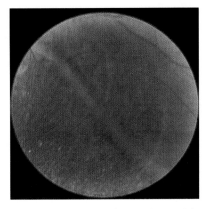

FIGURE 129.1. Vitreous band in a patient with Stickler syndrome. The retinal pigment epithelium is atrophic.

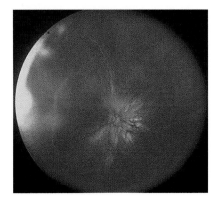

FIGURE 129.2. Multiple areas of radial and circumferential lattice in a patient with Stickler syndrome.

SUGGESTED READINGS

Brown DM, Nickols BE, Weingeist TA, et al. Procollagen II gene mutation in Stickler syndrome. *Arch Ophthalmol* 1992;110:1589–93. *A reference describing ocular findings as well as the molecular basis of the defect in this family with procollagen II mutation.*

Liberfarb R, Goldblatt A. Prevalence of mitral valve prolapse in the Stickler's syndrome. *Am J Hum Genet* 1986;24:387–392.

Weingeist TA, Hermsen V, Hanson JW, et al. Ocular and systemic manifestations of Stickler syndrome: A preliminary report. In: Cotlier E, Maumene JH, Berman ER. *Genetic Eye Diseases, Retinitis Pigmentosa and Other Inherited Eye Disorders.* Proceedings of the International Symposium on Genetics in Ophthalmology. New York: Allen R. Liss; 1982:539–560.

Section D. Miscellaneous Developmental Disorders

Chapter 130

BARDET-BIEDL SYNDROME

Elise Héon
Val C. Sheffield
Edwin M. Stone

I. GENERAL

1. Rare autosomal recessive, multisystemic disorder with no racial or sexual predilection
2. Cardinal signs are retinal dystrophy, obesity, dysmorphic extremities, kidney anomalies, mental retardation, and hypogonadism.
3. Consanguinity present in 25% of families
4. Retinal dystrophy is usually diagnosed in childhood; 70% are legally blind by the age of 20.
5. Kidney involvement may be life-threatening and can be detected with renal ultrasound, blood pressure, and urine osmolarity measurements.
6. Digit anomaly may be subtle and a radiologic assessment may be required for its identification. (Most often, all four extremities are involved.)
7. Often confused with Laurence-Moon syndrome where spastic paraplegia is common but obesity and polydactyly are not.
8. Differential diagnosis: Biemond syndrome (iris coloboma, polydactyly, mental retardation, obesity) and Alström syndrome (severe retinal dystrophy, obesity, deafness, kidney anomalies, diabetes, acanthosis nigricans)

II. SYSTEMIC MANIFESTATIONS

1. Interfamilial and intrafamilial variability
2. Kidney
   - Persistence of fetal lobulation or cortical cyst/diverticula(detected by ultrasound)
   - Hypertension
   - Chronic glomerulonephritis
   - Renal failure
3. Dysmorphic extremities
   - Polydactyly (postaxial, extra digit often amputated at birth)
   - Syndactyly and/or brachydactyly
4. Genital
   - Hypogonadism is most notable in males (small penis and small testis).
   - Female may show menstrual abnormalities, lowered estrogen levels, and reproductive difficulties.
   - Vaginal and uterine anomalies may be present but are more difficult to detect.
5. Weight
   - Obesity usually involves the trunk.
   - Variable with age
6. Intellect
   - Mental retardation variable, most often mild
   - 30% within normal limits
7. Genetics
   - Genetic heterogeneity
   - Linkage identified to chromosomes 16, 11, 3, 15
   - No phenotype-genotype correlation
   - No gene yet identified
8. Other
   - Diabetes type II
   - Hepatic fibrosis
   - Cardiac anomalies

III. OCULAR MANIFESTATIONS

1. Retina
   - Early rod-cone dystrophy: severe, bilateral, and diffuse
   - Often "sine pigmento" but the amount of bone spiculing is very variable
   - Frequent and early macular involvement
   - Early and severe visual field constriction
   - Interfamilial variability
2. Anterior segment
   - Early cataracts
3. Refraction
   - Variable
   - Rarely emmetrope (myopic refractive error being most frequent)
4. Neuroophthalmologic
   - Nystagmus
   - Optic atrophy
5. Others
   - Strabismus
   - Papilledema

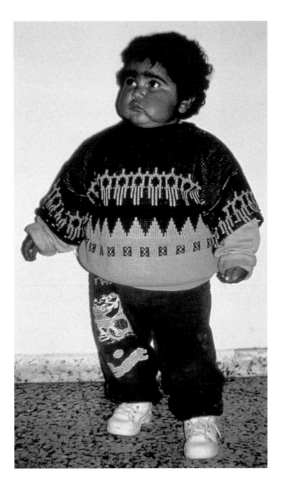

FIGURE 130.1. Child affected with the Bardet-Biedl syndrome and early-onset obesity. Courtesy of Rivca Carmi, MD.

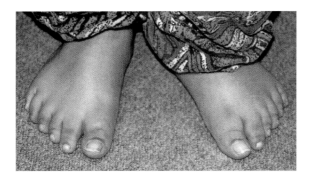

FIGURE 130.2. Postaxial polydactyly involving the toes.

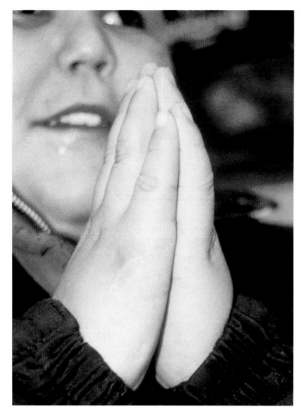

FIGURE 130.3. Scar following amputation of the extra digit at birth.

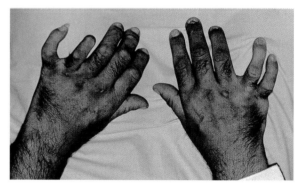

FIGURE 130.4. Clinodactyly of the fourth and fifth digits. Courtesy of Rivca Carmi, MD.

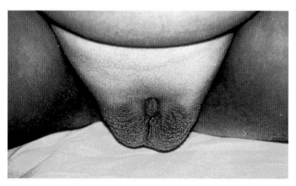

FIGURE 130.5. Male hypogonadism. Courtesy of Rivca Carmi, MD.

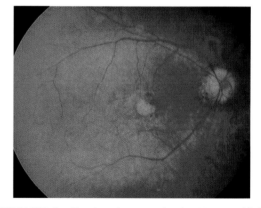

FIGURE 130.6. Fundus photograph of a 14-year-old child with Bardet Biedl syndrome. Note vessel attenuation, macular and retinal pigmented epithelium changes and the absence of "bone spiculing."

SUGGESTED READINGS

Carmi R, Rokhlina T, Kwitek-Black A, et al. Use of a DNA pooling strategy to identify a human obesity syndrome locus (Bardet-Biedl) on chromosome 15. *Hum Mol Genet* 1995;4:9–13.

Green JS, Parfrey PS, Harnett JD, et al. The cardinal manifestations of Bardet-Biedl syndrome, a form of Laurence-Moon-Biedl syndrome. *N Engl J Med* 1989;321:1002–1009.

Harnett JD, Green JS, Cramer BC, et al. The spectrum of renal disease in Laurence-Moon-Biedl syndrome. *N Engl J Med* 1988;319:615–618.

Jacobson SG, Borruat FX, Apathy PP. Patterns of rod and cone dysfunction in Bardet-Biedl syndrome. *Am J Ophthalmol* 1990;109:676–688.

Riise R. Visual function in Laurence-Moon-Bardet-Biedl syndrome. A survey of 26 cases. *Acta Ophthalmol Suppl* 1987;182:128–131.

Chapter 131

CARPENTER'S SYNDROME

Andrew E. Choy

1. Premature closure of sutures leading to cranial, orbital, and skeletal deformities
   - Part of the craniosynostosis syndromes.
2. Acrocephaly with peculiar facies and shallow orbits
3. Preaxial polysyndactyly of the feet
4. Variable syndactyly of the hands
5. Hypogonadism
6. Obesity
7. May be misidentified as Lawrence-Moon-Biedl syndrome or Apert's syndrome
8. Mental delay is not a constant finding.
9. No biochemical, hormonal, or chromosomal abnormality has been discovered to date.
   - A presumed autosomal recessive
10. Fine motor dysfunction secondary to digit anomalies
11. Eustachian tube dysfunction secondary to short cranial base
12. Speech problems from articulation errors may be due to difficulty in performing rapid alternating movements of lips and tongue.

II. SYSTEMIC MANIFESTATIONS

1. Musculoskeletal
   - Skull
     - Brachycephaly
     - Variable synostosis of
       - Coronal suture
       - Lambdoidal suture
       - Sagittal suture
     - Kleeblattschädel skull may result.
   - Feet
     - Preaxial polydactyly
     - Partial syndactyly
   - Hands
     - Brachydactyly with clinodactyly (short and angulated)
     - Partial syndactyly
     - Camptodactyly (bent and curved)
     - Single flexion crease
     - Subluxation distal interphalangeal joints
   - Knees
     - Angulation deformities
   - Occasional
     - Postaxial polydactyly
     - Second thumb phalanx duplication
     - Metatarsus varus
     - Flat acetabulum
     - Pelvic flare
     - Genu valgum
     - Patella—lateral displacement
     - Scoliosis
     - Coxa valga
     - Spina bifida
2. Ear/nose/throat
   - Flattened nasal bridge
   - Low-set auricles
   - Preauricular pits
   - Recurrent otitis media from short cranial base and abnormal middle ear anatomy
   - Conductive and neurosensory hearing loss
   - High-arched palate
   - Dental abnormalities
3. Endocrine
   - Hypogonadism
   - Short stature
   - Occasional
     - Empty sella
     - Precocious growth
4. Nonspecific
   - Obesity
5. Cardiac
   - Congenital heart defects in approximately one-third of patients (patent ductus arteriosus, ventricular septal defect, pulmonic stenosis, transposition of the great vessels, atrial septal defect)
6. Neurologic
   - Delayed to normal intellectual performance
7. Genitourinary
   - Pilonidal dimple
   - Renal anomalies
8. Gastrointestinal
   - Accessory spleen
   - Abdominal hernias or omphalocele

III. OCULAR MANIFESTATIONS

1. Orbit
   - Shallow
   - Shallow supraorbital ridges
2. Lids
   - Lateral displacement of medial canthi
   - Variable presence of epicanthal folds
   - Antimongoloid slant of the palpebral fissures
3. Cornea
   - Proptosis
   - Exposure keratopathy
   - Corneal opacity
   - Microcornea
4. Optic nerve
   - Papilledema
   - Optic nerve atrophy
5. Strabismus
   - Exotropia
   - Hypertropia
   - Esotropia
6. Occasional
   - Coloboma of the iris and choroid
   - Congenital cataract
   - Lens subluxation
   - Retinal detachment
   - Nystagmus

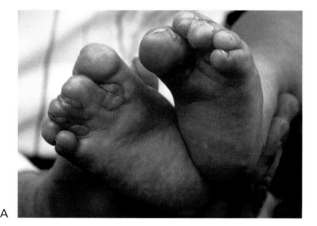 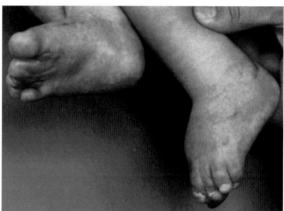

A   B

FIGURE 131.1. Partial syndactyly and polydactyly.

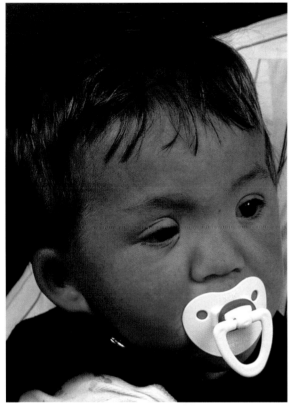
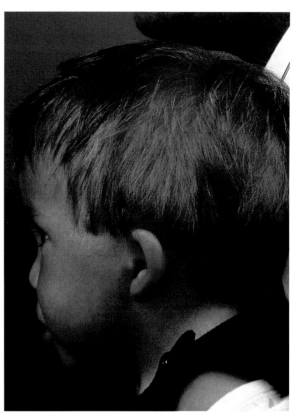

FIGURE 131.2. Telecanthus, epicanthus, depressed nasal bridge, and low-set ears.

FIGURE 131.3. Brachycephally, shallow orbits, and low-set ears.

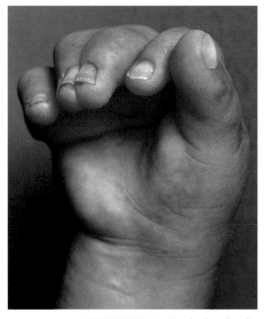
A

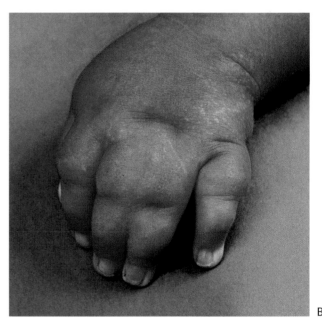
B

FIGURE 131.4. Brachydactyly, clinodactyly, partial syndactyly, and camptodactyly.

SUGGESTED READINGS

Carpenter G. Two sisters showing malformations of the skull and other congenital abnormalities. *Rep Soc Study Dis Child Lond* 1901;1:110–118.

Cohen DM, Green JG, Miller J, et al. Acrocephalopolysyndactyly type II—Carpenter syndrome: Clinical spectrum and an attempt of unification with Goodman and Summit syndromes. *Am J Med Genet* 1987;28:311–324. *A review of Carpenter syndrome and possible linkage with two variants.*

Frias JL, Felman AH, Rosenbloom AL, et al. Normal intelligence in two children with Carpenter syndrome. *Am J Med Genet* 1978;2:191–199. *First report mental retardation is not an obligate feature of Carpenter syndrome.*

Newman SA. Ophthalmic features of craniosynostosis. *Neurosurg Clin North Am* 1991;2:587–610.

Temtamy SA. Carpenter's syndrome: Acrocephalopolysyndactyly. An autosomal recessive syndrome. *J Pediatr* 1966;69:111–120. *A report and literature review to 1966 with the suggestion of possible autosomal recessive inheritance.*

Chapter 132

COHEN'S SYNDROME

Reijo Norio
Christina Raitta

I. GENERAL

1. An autosomal recessive disorder with mental retardation, typical facies and other structural abnormalities, chorioretinal dystrophy, and granulocytopenia

2. Gene mapped in chromosome 8

3. Pathophysiologic mechanism unknown

II. SYSTEMIC MANIFESTATIONS

1. Central nervous system
   - Mental retardation, moderate, nonprogressive
   - Microcephaly
   - Motor clumsiness
   - Brisk tendon reflexes
   - High-pitched voice
   - Active, cheerful disposition
2. Developmental
   - Short stature, moderate
   - Truncal obesity in some
   - Floppiness
3. Facial
   - Prominent root of nose
   - Short philtrum
   - Prominent upper central incisors
   - Open-mouthed appearance
   - Hypoplastic ear lobuli
   - Abundant hair, eyebrows, eyelashes

4. Musculoskeletal
   - Narrow palate
   - Micrognathia
   - Maxillar hypoplasia
   - Slender hands and feet
   - Gap between toes 1 and 2
   - Hypermobility of joints
     - Pes planovalgus
     - Genu valgum
     - Kyphosis
5. Cardiac
   - Heart murmur in some
   - (Floppy mitral valve?)
6. Nonspecific
   - Leukopenia, intermittent
   - Granulocytopenia, intermittent

III. OCULAR MANIFESTATIONS

1. Lids
   - High arched, wave shaped
2. Refraction
   - Myopia
3. Lens
   - Presenile cataract
4. Retina
   - Chorioretinal dystrophy

   - Bull's-eye macula
   - Peripheral pigment dystrophy, pigment deposits
5. Neuroophthalmologic
   - Decreased visual acuity, progression slow
   - Hemeralopia
   - Narrowing visual fields
   - Abolished electroretinography

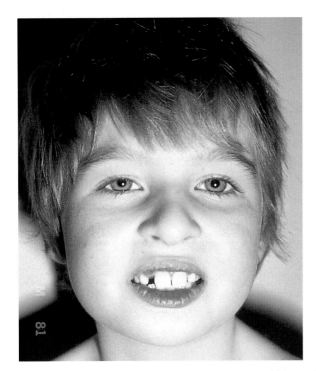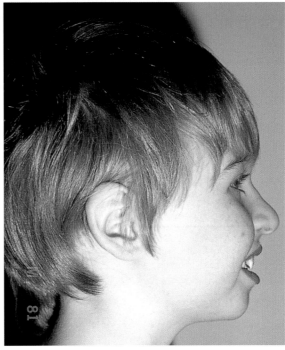

FIGURE 132.1 and 132.2. A 7-year-old boy with the Cohen syndrome. Note beautiful, wave-shaped eyelids, prominent root of nose, short philtrum, prominent upper central incisors, open-mouth appearance, thick hair and eyebrows, and long eyelashes.

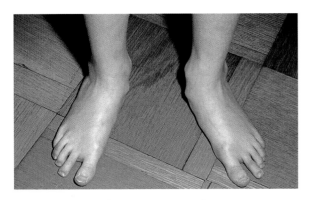

FIGURE 132.3. Slender feet with pes planus and gap between toes 1 and 2.

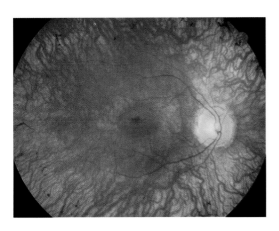

FIGURE 132.4. Chorioretinal dystrophy, bull's-eye macula and some peripheral pigment deposits in the ocular fundus of a 20-year-old man with the Cohen syndrome.

SUGGESTED READINGS

Cohen MM Jr. A new syndrome with hypotonia, obesity, deficiency, and facial, oral, ocular, and limb anomalies. *J Pediatr* 1973;83:280–284. *The first publication on the syndrome.*

Norio R, Raitta C, Lindahl E. Further delineation of the Cohen syndrome; report on chorioretinal dystrophy, leukopenia and consanguinity. *Clin Genet* 1984;25:1–14. *An extensive review with plenty of patient photographs.*

Raitta C, Norio R. Cohen's syndrome. In: Gold DH, Weingeist TA, eds. *The Eye in Systemic Disease.* Philadelphia: JB Lippincott; 1990:565–568. *A review of ocular manifestations of the syndrome.*

Tahvanainen E, Norio R, Karila E, et al. Cohen syndrome gene assigned to the long arm of chromosome 8 by linkage analysis. *Nat Genet* 1994;7:201–204.

Warburg M, Pedersen SA, Horlyk H. The Cohen syndrome; retinal lesions and granulocytopenia. *Ophthalmic Paediatr Genet* 1990;11:7–13. *A non-Finnish patient with typical ocular and haematologic findings.*

Chapter 133

PRADER-LABHART-WILLI SYNDROME

Richard Alan Lewis

I. GENERAL

1. First recognized in 1956 (although first description by Landgon Down, 1887); frequency estimated at $^{1}/_{25,000}$ births.
2. Characteristics include hypotonia, failure to thrive in infancy, small hands and feet, hypogonadism, mental retardation, and marked hyperphagia and obesity.
3. Majority (70–80%) of cases are associated with isolated de novo cytogenetic interstitial deletions of chromosome 15q11-q13.
4. Deletions occur exclusively in the paternal chromosome 15.
5. Maternal uniparental disomy with normal karyotype occurs in the vast majority of patients with no detectable deletion.
6. Presumably, only paternal alleles of genes at the PWS locus are active.
7. Molecular diagnosis is highly reliable with fluorescent in situ hybridization.
8. If no deletion is detected, the absence of a paternal contribution by short tandem repeat polymorphisms indicates maternal uniparental disomy.

II. SYSTEMIC MANIFESTATIONS

Because of the difficulty in the diagnosis of Prader-Willi Syndrome (PWS), a list of major and minor diagnostic criteria and supportive findings has been espoused. Each major criterion is valued at 1 point, each minor criterion ½ point, and each supportive criterion zero value. To establish PWS in a child 3 years old or younger, a total score of 5 (at least 4 major points) is needed; for an individual over 3 years old, a total score of 8 (at least 5 major points) is required.*

1. Major criteria (1 point each)
   - Hypotonia in neonatal period
   - Failure to thrive in infancy and early childhood
   - Rapid weight gain after 1 year old
   - Characteristic facies
   - Hypogonadism
     - Male: small penis, cryptorchidism
     - Female: delayed gonadarche
   - Developmental delay
   - Hyperphagia; aggressive food-seeking behavior
   - Deletion of chromosome 15q11-q13 or evidence of maternal 15 disomy
2. Minor criteria (½ point each)
   - Diminished in utero movement
   - Behavioral stereotypes: tantrums, violent outbursts; obsessive-compulsive, rigid, argumentative, oppositional, stubborn, lying (5 or more required)
   - Sleep disturbances/apnea
   - Short stature
   - Hypopigmentation of skin, hair, eyes (fundus)
   - Small hands/feet
   - Narrow hands
   - Esotropia; myopia
   - Viscous saliva
   - Difficulty with articulation
   - Skin picking
3. Supportive features (0 points)
   - High pain threshold
   - Decreased vomiting
   - Temperature instability
   - Kyphosis/scoliosis (second decade)
   - Early adrenarche
   - Osteopenia
   - Skilled at jigsaw puzzles
   - Normal neuromuscular studies

III. OCULAR MANIFESTATIONS

1. Skin and adnexa
   - Blond to albinotic hair
   - Type I or type II skin
2. Motility
   - Increased frequency of nonaccommodative esotropia nystagmus, rarely
3. Iris
   - Blue color predominates
   - Punctate iris transillumination
4. Retina
   - Hypopigmentation (compared to siblings, parents)
   - Occasional foveal hypoplasia

*Revised from Holm VA, Cassidy SB, Butler MG, et al. Prader-Willi syndrome: Consensus diagnostic criteria. *Pediatrics,* 1993;91:398–402.

SUGGESTED READINGS

American Society of Human Genetics/American College of Medical Genetics Test and Technology Transfer Committee. Diagnostic testing for Prader-Willi and Angelman syndromes. *Am J Hum Genet* 1996;58:1085–1088.

Cassidy SB. Prader-Willi syndrome. *J Med Genet* 1997;34:917–923.

Cassidy SB, Schwartz S. Prader-Willi and Angelman syndromes: Disorders of genomic imprinting. *Medicine* 1998;77:140–151.

Holm VA, Cassidy SB, Butler MG, et al. Prader-Willi syndrome: Consensus diagnostic criteria. *Pediatrics* 1993;91:398–402.

Lee ST, Nicholls RD, Bundey S, et al. Mutations of the *P* gene in oculocutaneous albinism, ocular albinism, and Prader-Willi syndrome plus albinism. *N Engl J Med* 1994;330:529–534.

Wevrick R, Francke U. Diagnostic test for the Prader-Willi syndrome by SNRPN expression in blood. *Lancet* 1996;348:1068–1069.

PART 19. SKIN AND MUCOUS MEMBRANE DISORDERS

Section A. Benign Proliferative and Neoplastic Disorders

Chapter 134

BASAL CELL NEVUS SYNDROME

David T. Tse

I. GENERAL

1. An uncommon, autosomal dominant, multisystem disorder with high penetrance and variable expressivity
2. A defective gene may be responsible for the disorder. However, chromosome abnormalities have been found in only a small number of patients.
3. Males and females are affected with equal frequency, and the condition is most commonly found in whites.
4. This hereditary disease complex involves organs and systems of both ectodermal and mesodermal origin.
5. The syndrome is characterized by multiple nevoid basal cell carcinomas (BCCs), adontogenic keratocysts of the jaw, congenital skeletal anomalies, palmar and plantar pits, and ectopic calcification.
6. A diagnosis may be established by the presence of any two of these characteristics and a positive family history.
7. The typical facies of a patient with basal cell nevoid syndrome demonstrates orbital hypertelorism, broad nasal bridge, frontoparietal bone bossing with prominent supraorbital ridges, mandibular prognathism, and multiple cutaneous basal cell carcinomas.
8. In most cases the BCCs appear in the second and third decade. Diagnosis may be suggested by the presence of BCCs in unexposed areas of the body.
9. Treatment of BCC with ionizing radiation is contraindicated because of the potential of radiation-induced malignant sarcomatous degeneration.

II. SYSTEMIC MANIFESTATIONS

1. Cardiac
   - Fibromas of the myocardium
   - Mitral valve prolapse
2. Gastrointestinal
   - Lymphomesenteric cysts
   - Gastrointestinal polyposis
3. Genitourinary
   - Female—Ovarian fibroma with calcification, ovarian cyst, bicornuate uterus, theca cell tumor, uterine lymphoma, fibrocystic diseases of the breasts
   - Male—Hypogonadism (cryptorchidism or absent testes), hydrocele, infantile external genitalia, a female pubic hair pattern, scanty facial hair, gynecomastia
4. Central nervous system
   - Calcification of dura, falx cerebri, tentorium, choroid plexus, petroclinoid ligament
   - Bridging of sella turcica
   - Medulloblastoma, meningioma
   - Mental retardation, variable schizophrenia
   - Nonspecific electroencephalographic changes
   - Partial agenesis of corpus callosum
   - Congenital communicating hydrocephalus
5. Endocrine
   - Male hypogonadism
   - Hyporesponsiveness to parathyroid hormone
   - Gynecomastia
6. Musculoskeletal
   - Ribs
     - Bifurcation
     - Splaying
     - Synostosis
     - Partial agenesis
     - Rudimentary cervical ribs
     - Pectus excavatum
   - Vertebrae
     - Kyphoscoliosis
     - Cervical or upper thoracic fusion
     - Hemivertebrae
     - Spina bifida occulta
   - Extremity
     - Long bone cysts
     - Brachymetacarpalism (shortened fourth metacarpals)
     - Hallux valgus
     - Fibromas
     - Lipomas
   - Cranium
     - Frontal and temporoparietal bossing
     - Bridging of sella turcica
     - Broad nasal root
     - Prominent supraorbital ridge
   - Dental
     - Multiple jaw cysts
     - Fibrosarcoma of the palate or maxillary antrum
     - Ameloblastoma
     - Mandibular prognathism
     - Defective dentition
     - Bifid uvula
     - Submucous cleft
     - Cleft palate
7. Mucocutaneous
   - Multiple basal cell carcinomas with calcification or bone or osteoid formation
   - Pits (dyskeratosis) of palms and soles
   - Milia
   - Epithelial and sebaceous cysts, lipomas
8. Ear/nose/throat
   - Bilateral ear anomalies
9. Nonspecific
   - Low plasma α-globulins
   - Severe bradycardia and hypotension during induction of general anesthesia

III. OCULAR MANIFESTATIONS

1. Lids
   - Dystopia canthorum
   - Meibomian cysts
   - Lid malposition
2. Cornea
   - Opacities
3. Intraocular pressure
   - Glaucoma
4. Uvea
   - Coloboma
5. Lens
   - Cataract
6. Retina
   - Unilateral or bilateral myelinated nerve fibers

7. Optic nerve
   - Coloboma, optic atrophy
8. Orbit
   - Hypertelorism
   - Prominent supraorbital ridges
   - Frontoparietal bossing
9. Neuroophthalmologic
   - Nystagmus
   - Facial nerve palsies
10. Ocular motility
    - Strabismus (esodeviation, exodeviation)
11. Nonspecific
    - Congenital blindness (coloboma of choroid and optic nerve, corneal opacities, cataracts, glaucoma)

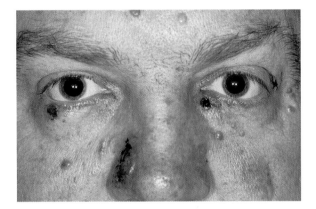

FIGURE 134.1. The typical facies of a patient with basal cell nevus syndrome demonstrates orbital hypertelorism, prominent supraorbital ridges, a broad nasal root, and multiple cutaneous BCCs.

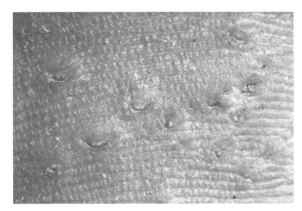

FIGURE 134.2. Close-up view of palmar pits.

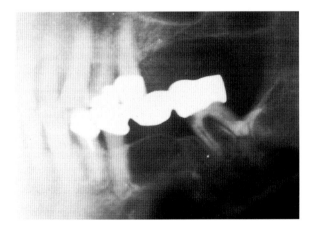

FIGURE 134.3. Panoramic radiograph showing a radiolucent mandibular cyst displacing the lower canine tooth.

SUGGESTED READINGS

Clendenning WE, Block JB, Radde IC. Basal cell nevus syndrome. *Arch Dermatol* 1964;90:38–53.

Gorlin RJ, Vickers RA, Kelly E, Williamson JJ. The multiple basal-cell nevi syndrome. *Cancer* 1965;18:89–103.

Southwick GJ, Schwartz RA. The basal cell nevus syndrome: Disasters occurring among a series of 36 patients. *Cancer* 1979;44:2294–2305.

Chapter 135

HEMANGIOMAS

Gregory S. Carroll
Barrett G. Haik

I. GENERAL

1. Benign neoplasm as a result of vasoformative tissue proliferation
2. Most common childhood orbital tumor
3. 3:2 female/male ratio; no racial predilection
4. Two predominant growth stages
   - Proliferative stage
     - Explosive growth within 3 to 6 months of diagnosis
     - Rapid multiplication of endothelial cells forming small, irregular vascular spaces
     - Vascular spaces become more defined with decreased endothelial cellularity.
   - Involutional stage
     - 1 to 5 years in length
     - Fibrofatty deposits around blood vessels with atrophy and collapse of vascular spaces

II. SYSTEMIC MANIFESTATIONS

1. Cardiac
   - High output congestive heart failure
2. Vascular
   - Uncontrolled hemorrhage
   - Compression of critical structures (neurovascular bundles)
3. Hematologic
   - Kassabach Merritt syndrome—platelet/fibrin consumption
   - Thrombocytopenia
   - Decreased factors V, VIII, fibrinogen levels
   - Microangiopathic hemolytic anemia
4. Gastrointestinal
   - Melena, gastrointestinal bleeding
   - Compression of esophagus with reflux
5. Dermatologic
   - Superficial ulceration with possible sepsis
   - Crepe–paper–like superficial skin following regression
6. Ear/nose/throat
   - Subglottic/paratracheal lesions with compression, respiratory distress
   - Respiratory arrest from nasal hemangioma
   - Hemorrhage during intubation
7. Neurologic
   - Oculomotor nerve palsy
   - Cerebellar hypoplasia
   - Agenesis of corpus callosum
   - Dandy-Walker cyst
8. Pulmonary
   - Hemoptysis

III. OCULAR MANIFESTATIONS

1. Lids
   - Classic superficial strawberry nevus
   - Dark blue or purple subcutaneous mass
   - May involve tarsus
   - Blepharoptosis, occlusion of visual axis
2. Conjunctiva
   - Subconjunctival mass
   - Telangiectatic vessels
3. Intraocular pressure
   - May be elevated with severe compression or sudden intralesional hemorrhage
4. Optic nerve
   - Compressive neuropathy
5. Orbit
   - Proptosis
   - Expansion of orbital volume
6. Neuroophthalmologic
   - Amblyopia—derivational, anisometropic
7. Ocular motility
   - Cranial nerve palsies
   - Restrictive motility disturbances
8. Uvea
   - Choroidal folds
9. Cornea
   - Induced astigmatism
10. Sclera
    - Deformation/compression

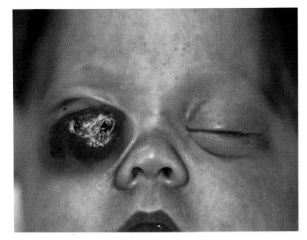

FIGURE 135.1. Four-month-old infant with capillary hemangioma of right lower eyelid demonstrating superficial ulceration.

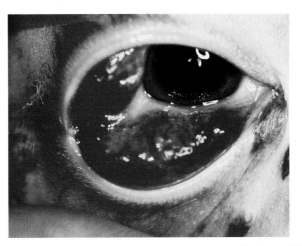

FIGURE 135.2. Capillary hemangioma involving both eyelids with subconjunctival involvement.

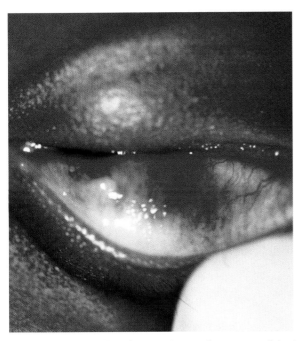

FIGURE 135.3. Capillary hemangioma of upper eyelid with tarsal conjunctival involvement.

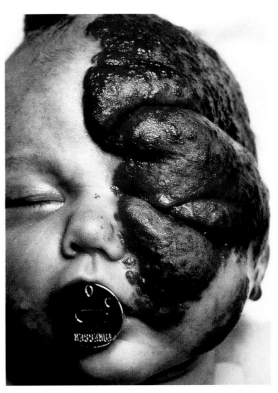

FIGURE 135.4. Extensive facial and periorbital involvement with occlusion of visual axis.

SUGGESTED READINGS

Bilyk JR, Adamis AP, Mulliken JB. Treatment options for periorbital hemangioma of infancy. In: Shore JW, ed. *Orbital Disease,* vol 32, number 3. Boston: Little, Brown; 1992:95–109.

Haik BG, Karcioglu ZA, Gordon RA, et al. Capillary hemangioma (infantile periocular hemangioma). *Surv Ophthalmol* 1994;38:399–426. *An excellent review of capillary hemangioma and its treatment.*

Mulliken JB, Young AE. *Vascular Birthmarks: Hemangiomas and Malformations.* Philadelphia: WB Saunders; 1988. *Comprehensive review of congenital vascular tumors.*

Chapter 136
JUVENILE XANTHOGRANULOMA

Jacob Pe'er

I. GENERAL

1. A benign, idiopathic, usually asymptomatic histiocytic inflammatory cutaneous disorder, that shows spontaneous regression in most cases
2. A disorder of infants and young children; adults rarely are affected. It appears within the first year of life in 80% of patients.
3. Infants commonly have multiple lesions, whereas adults have a solitary lesion.
4. No sexual or racial predilection
5. Ocular involvement is the most common extracutaneous involvement. Visceral and central nervous system (CNS) involvement is rare.
6. Café-au-lait spots of neurofibromatosis are occasionally seen.
7. Histologically the lesions are composed of foamy histiocytes, foreign body giant cells, Touton giant cells, lymphocytes, eosinophils, and neutrophils.

II. SYSTEMIC MANIFESTATIONS

1. Mucocutaneous
   - Papular form
     - Numerous, firm hemispheric lesions, 1 to 5 mm in diameter
     - Pink-red-brown color at first and turns to yellowish throughout the skin, but mainly on the upper part of the body.
     - Mucous membranes are seldom involved.
   - Nodular form
     - Less common
     - One or a few lesions
     - Round lesions, 10 to 20 mm in diameter.
     - Translucent, red or yellowish, may show telangiectasis
     - Mucous membrane lesions are more common.
2. Visceral lesions
   - Lungs
   - Bones
   - Kidneys
   - Pericardium
   - Colon
   - Ovaries
   - Testes
3. CNS involvement is rare.

III. OCULAR MANIFESTATIONS

1. Uveal mass
   - Iris
     - Most common
     - Solitary diffuse or nodular mass
     - Heterochromia iridis—congenital or acquired
     - Spontaneous hemorrhage—hyphema
       - Secondary glaucoma
       - Large and cloudy cornea
   - Uveitis
     - Redness of the eye
   - Ciliary body
   - Choroid—exceedingly rare
2. Eyelid mass
3. Epibulbar mass
   - Sclera
   - Conjunctiva
   - Cornea
   - Limbus
4. Orbital mass—proptosis
     - Orbital bone
     - Extraocular muscle
5. Retina—exceedingly rare

FIGURE 136.1. A pink-yellow skin papule in a patient with juvenile xanthogranuloma (JXG).

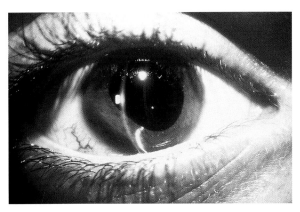

FIGURE 136.2. A pink-brown iris-base mass in a child with JXG.

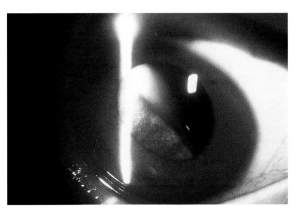

FIGURE 136.3. A ciliochoroidal mass in the inferotemporal quadrant is seen through the dilated pupil in a patient with JXG.

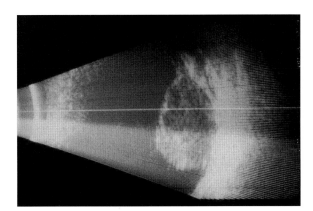

FIGURE 136.4. B-scan ultrasonography of the lesion seen in Fig. 136.3 shows a solid elongated dome-shaped ciliochoroidal mass.

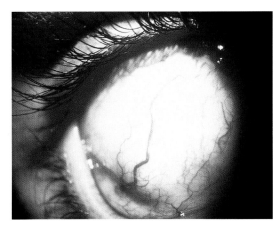

FIGURE 136.5. An episcleral xanthogranuloma mass under congested conjunctiva in the inferotemporal fornix area of an eye of a patient with JXG.

SUGGESTED READINGS

DeBarge LR, Chan CC, Greenberg SC, et al. Chorioretinal, iris and ciliary body infiltration by juvenile xanthogranuloma masquerading as uveitis. *Surv Ophthalmol* 1994;39:65–71.

Sanders TE. Intraocular juvenile xanthogranuloma (nevoxanthogranuloma): A survey of 20 cases. *Trans Am Ophthalmol Soc* 1960;58:58–69.

Sonoda T, Hashimoto H, Enjoji M. Juvenile xanthogranuloma. Clinical analysis and immunohistochemical study of 57 cases. *Cancer* 1985;56:2280–2286.

Zimmerman LE. Ocular lesions of juvenile xanthogranuloma. *Am J Ophthalmol* 1965;60:1011–1035.

Chapter 137
XERODERMA PIGMENTOSUM

Jacob Pe'er

I. GENERAL

1. Xeroderma pigmentosum means pigmented dry skin.
2. An uncommon inherited, usually autosomal recessive disease (consanguinity in about 30%)
3. Characterized by clinical and cellular hypersensitivity to ultraviolet radiation, with defective repair of DNA damage caused by short-wavelength radiation, and certain chemicals
4. Occurs in all races worldwide in approximately 1/250,000 births. (In the United States, the estimated frequency is 1:1,000,000.) No sex predilection is apparent.
5. Genetic heterogeneity of the molecular defect: 9 different complementation groups
6. Patients experience sun-induced cutaneous and ocular abnormalities, including neoplasia. Some patients have, in addition, progressive neurologic degeneration.
7. The median age at onset of cutaneous symptoms is between 1 and 2 years. The median age at onset of first cutaneous neoplasm is 8 years.

II. SYSTEMIC MANIFESTATIONS

1. Mucocutaneous
   - Acute sunburn reaction on minimal UV exposure
   - Numerous freckle-like hyperpigmented macules
   - Skin abnormalities are strikingly limited to sun-exposed areas.
   - Dry, scaly, atrophic, and hyperpigmented skin
   - Telangiectasia and areas of hypopigmentation
   - Premalignant actinic keratosis and verrucous papules
   - Multiple primary cutaneous neoplasms
   - Under 20 years of age: greater than 1000-fold increased risk of skin neoplasia
   - Basal cell carcinoma
   - Squamous cell carcinoma
   - Melanoma
   - Soft tissue tumors—rare
2. Central nervous system (Desanctis-Cocchione syndrome) in approximately 30% of patients (early or delayed, mild or severe)
   - Hyporeflexia or areflexia
   - Sensorineural deafness
   - Spasticity
   - Low intelligence
   - Choreoathetosis
   - Ataxia
   - Quadriparesis
   - Progressive mental retardation
   - Microencephaly
   - Retarded growth
   - Loss (or absence) of neurons in the cerebrum and cerebellum
3. Nonspecific
   - Oral cavity neoplasma (tip of tongue)
   - 10- to 20-fold increase in internal neoplasm
   - Immature sexual development
   - Early death due to metastatic disease, infection, or other causes

III. OCULAR MANIFESTATIONS

(limited to portions of the eye exposed to UV radiation)

1. Lids
- Skin damage—erythema, pigmentation, atrophy
- Madarosis
- Ectropion, entropion
- Lid tissue loss
- Symblepharon, ankyloblepharon
- Benign lesions—papillomas
- Neoplasms
  - Basal cell carcinoma
  - Squamous cell carcinoma
  - Melanoma
  - Soft tissue tumors

2. Conjunctiva/limbus
- Hyperemia
- Conjunctivitis with serous or mucopurulent discharge
- Xerosis
- Epidermalization, keratinization
- Melanosis
- Benign lesions
  - Pinguecula
  - Phlyctenulas
  - Pseudopterygium
- Neoplasms
  - Squamous cell carcinoma
  - Basal cell carcinoma
  - Melanoma
  - Soft tissue tumors
- Under 20 years of age—about 2000-fold increased risk of neoplasms of the anterior eye

3. Cornea
- Exposure keratitis
- Xerosis
- Ulceration
- Opacification
- Vascularization
- Band-shaped nodular dystrophy
- Neoplasms

4. Iris
- Iritis
- Iris atrophy
- Synechiae

5. Symptoms
- Photophobia
- Lacrimation
- Blepharospasm
- Impaired vision

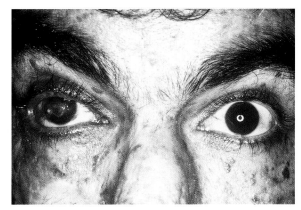

FIGURE 137.1. A 36-year-old patient with xeroderma pigmentosum showing multiple freckles and pigmented and nonpigmented facial cutaneous lesions. The right cornea is opaque.

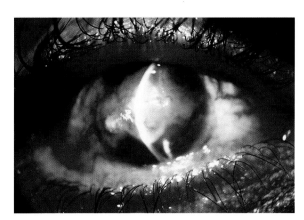

FIGURE 137.2. The patient shown in Figure 137.1 with opacification and vascularization of the right cornea.

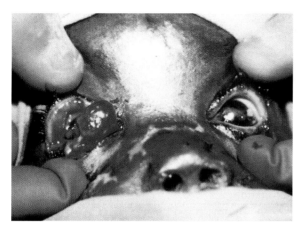

FIGURE 137.3. A 3-year-old African-American child with xeroderma pigmentosum showing a protruding neoplasm of the conjunctiva in his right eye.

SUGGESTED READINGS

El-Hifnawi H, Mortada A. Ocular manifestations of xeroderma pigmentosum. *Br J Dermatol* 1965;77:261–276.

Kraemer KH, Lee MM, Andrews AD, Lambert WC. The role of sunlight and DNA repair in melanoma and nonmelanoma skin cancer. The xeroderma pigmentosum paradigm. *Arch Dermatol* 1994;130:1018–1021.

Kraemer KH, Lee MM, Scotto J. Xeroderma pigmentosum. Cutaneous, ocular and neurologic abnormalities in 830 published cases. *Arch Dermatol* 1987;123:241–250.

Newsome DA, Kraemer KH, Robbins JH. Repair of DNA in xeroderma pigmentosum conjunctiva. *Arch Ophthalmol* 1975;93:660–662.

Pe'er J, Levinger S, Chirambo M, et al. Malignant fibrous histiocytoma of the skin and the conjunctiva in xeroderma pigmentosum. *Arch Pathol Lab Med* 1991;115:910–914.

Section B.   Disorders of Connective Tissue

Chapter 138

EHLERS-DANLOS SYNDROME

Darlene Skow Johnson
Glenn Kolansky
Duane C. Whitaker

Category	Type	Mode of Inheritance	Biochemical Defect	Diagnostic Features
EDS I	Gravis type	AD	Unknown	Soft, hyperextensible skin Easy bruising and thin atrophic "cigarette paper" healing of cutaneous wounds Molluscoid pseudotumors Hypermobile joints Mitral valve prolapse Premature rupture of fetal membranes
EDS II	Mitis type	AD	Unknown	Similar to EDS I but less severe
EDS III	Familial Hypermobile type	AD	Unknown	Marked hypermobility of joints Minimal skin laxity
EDS IV	Arterial type	AD	Type III collagen gene deletion point mutation	Rupture of arteries, bowel, and uterus Thin, translucent skin with visible veins Easy bruising Lack of skin extensibility or joint hypermobility
EDS V	X-linked type	XLR	Unknown	Similar to EDS II with minimal skin extensibility and joint hypermobility Female carriers asymptomatic
EDS VI	Ocular-scoliotic type	AR	Lysyl-hydroxylase deficiency	Hyperextensibile skin and joint laxity Scoliosis Increased bleeding tendency Hypotonia and muscular weakness Ocular fragility: rupture of sclera/cornea, keratoconus, microcornea, glaucoma
EDS VII	Arthrochalasis Multiplex congenita	AD	Exon deletions from type I collagen genes that encode the amino-terminal propeptide cleavage sites	Minimal skin findings with normal scarring Severe joint laxity with congenital hip dislocations, short stature Micrognathia
EDS VIII	Periodontal type	AD	Unknown	Cutaneous fragility with pretibial scarring Periodontitis, gingival recession, and premature tooth loss
EDS IX		XLR	Abnormal copper utilization resulting in a defect of lysl oxidase	Skeletal abnormalities: occipital horns, broad clavicles, short humeri, limited pronation/suppination Lax, soft skin Bladder diverticula
EDS X		AR	Fibronectin abnormality	Similar to EDS II Abnormal platelet adhesion

AD, autosomal dominant; AR, autosomal recessive; EDS, Ehlers-Danlos syndrome; XLR, X-linked recessive.

II. SYSTEMIC MANIFESTATIONS

1. Cardiac
   - Mitral valve prolapse
   - Papillary muscle dysfunction
   - Aneurysm of membranous ventricular septum
2. Vascular
   - Rupture of aorta and other large arteries
   - Multiple aneurysms and dissecting aneurysm of aorta
3. Pulmonary
   - Tracheobronchiomegaly (Mounier-Kuhn syndrome)
   - Spontaneous pneumothorax
   - Fibrous pseudotumors
4. Renal
   - Polycystic kidneys
5. Gastrointestinal
   - Megaesophagus, megacolon
   - Torsion of the stomach
   - Diverticula of the stomach, duodenum, colon, bile duct
   - Bowel perforation (colon > small intestine)
   - Ectasia of the colon
   - Rectal prolapse
6. Genitourinary
   - Diverticula of the bladder
   - Anomalies of the ureteropelvic junction
7. Hematologic
   - Platelet aggregation abnormalities (tendency to clump)
8. Musculoskeletal
   - Hypermobile joints
   - Congenital and recurrent dislocations
   - Ectopic bone formation
   - Spondylolisthesis and spinal malalignment (rare cord compression)
   - Scoliosis
   - Short stature
   - Hypotonicity, muscle soreness, and easy fatigability
9. Mucocutaneous
   - Hyperextensibility of skin and mucous membranes
   - Skin fragility and decreased tensil strength with poor wound healing
   - "Cigarette paper" scars after trauma or surgery
   - Hyperpigmentation and atrophy of skin over extensor surfaces
   - Decreased subcutaneous fat
   - Subcutaneous nodules of calcification or adpose tissue
   - Molluscoid pseudotumors (organization of superficial hematomas) at pressure points
   - Redundant skin of palms, soles, knees, and elbows
10. Ear/nose/throat
    - Chronic temporomandibular joint subluxation
    - Maldeveloped, irregularly positioned, and easily fracturing teeth
    - Gingival fragility and recurrent periodontitis
11. Nonspecific
    - Premature rupture of fetal membranes

III. OCULAR MANIFESTATIONS

1. Lids
   - Redundant skin of eyelids and easily inverted lids (Metenire's sign)
   - Epicanthal folds
   - Telecanthus
2. Conjunctiva/sclera
   - Ocular fragility
   - Blue sclera secondary to thinning
3. Cornea
   - Microcornea
   - Keratoconus (localized corneal thinning) and stromal scarring
   - Keratoglobus (bilateral general thinning and anterior protrusion of the cornea)
   - Corneal rupture
   - Corneal edema (acute hydrops) due to spontaneous central breaks in Descemet's membrane
   - Absent Bowman's layer
   - Irregular astigmatism of the cornea
   - Amblopia due to corneal curvature
4. Intraocular pressure
   - Glaucoma
5. Lens
   - Lens dislocation
   - Ectopic lentis
   - Myopia
6. Retina
   - Retinal detachment (type two)
   - Angioid streaks
   - Depigmentation in the preequatorial region of the fundus
   - Retinitis proliferans
7. Neuroophthalmologic
   - Strabismus

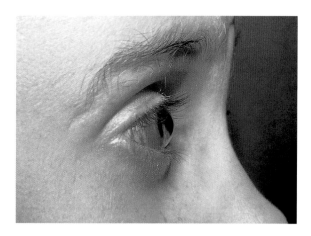

FIGURE 138.1. Keratoglobus demonstrating protuding, spherical cornea, accompanied by central and peripheral corneal thinning. Courtesy of *Archives of Opthalmology* 1976;94:1489–1491.

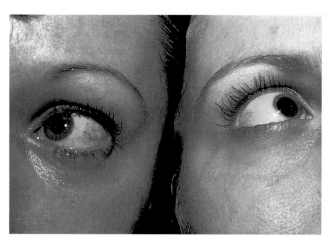

FIGURE 138.2. Characteristic blue sclera in a patient with Ehlers-Danlos syndrome (normal patient on right for comparison). Thinning of the sclera allows the underlying choroid to cast a blue hue on the sclera. Courtesy of F. Judisch, MD.

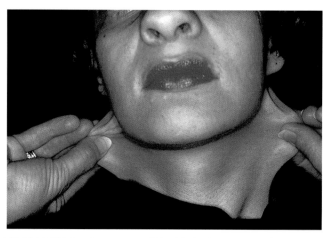

FIGURE 138.3. Hyperextensible skin is demonstrated. Courtesy of G. Seafield, MD.

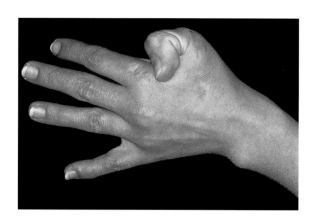

FIGURE 138.4. Joint hypermobility. Courtesy of G. Seafield, MD.

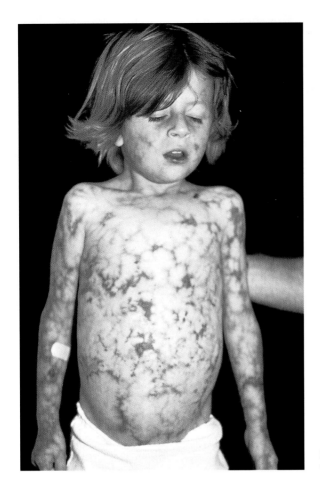

FIGURE 138.5. Ehlers-Danlos type IV (ecchymotic variant) associated with thin skin with visible veins.

SUGGESTED READINGS

Cameron JA. Corneal abnormalities in Ehlers-Danlos type IV. *Cornea* 1993;12:54–59.

Tucker LB. Heritable disorders of connective tissue and disability and chronic disease in childhood. *Curr Opin Rheumatol* 1992;4:731–740.

Wenstrup RJ, Murad S, Pinnell SR. Collagen. In: Goldsmith LA, ed. *Physiology, Biochemistry, and Molecular Biology of the Skin*. New York: Oxford University Press; 1991:494–497.

Chapter 139

PSEUDOXANTHOMA ELASTICUM

Darlene Skow Johnson
Glenn Kolansky
Jeffrey A. Nerad

I. GENERAL

1. Production of abnormal elastic fibers and secondary calcification
2. Principle sites of involvement are the skin, eye, and blood vessels.
3. Criteria for the diagnosis of pseudoxanthoma elasticum (PXE)
   - Major criteria
     - A. Characteristic skin plaques
     - B. Characteristic histopathology of plaques
     - C. Ocular involvement in patient 20 years old and older (not required in children due to late onset)
   - Minor criteria
     - D. Characteristic histopathology on nonlesional skin
     - E. Family history of PXE in first-degree relative
4. Classification of PXE based on major and minor criteria
   - Category I: A, B, C (not required in children)
   - Category IIa: C, D, E
   - Category IIb: C, D
   - Category IIc: C, E
   - Category IId: D, E
5. Characteristic skin biopsy shows fragmentation and clumping of elastin fibers in the middle and lower dermis on hematoxylin and eosin, with elastic fiber calcification demonstrated with von Kossa stain.
6. Hallmark of PXE ocular involvement is angioid streaks.
7. Arterial involvement is manifested by calcification of the internal elastic laminae, with surrounding reaction and swelling resulting in occlusion of the lumen.
8. Prevalence is 1/100,000 to 160,000
   - 1 in 200 people carry the gene for PXE
   - Average age of onset is 13

II. SYSTEMIC MANIFESTATIONS

1. Cardiac
   - Premature coronary atherosclerosis
   - Mitral valve prolapse (70% of patients)
   - Fibrous thickening of the endocardium and atrioventricular valves
   - Restrictive cardiomyopathy
2. Vascular
   - Vascular calcification
   - Peripheral vascular disease by age 30, manifest by intermittent claudication and angina
   - Aneurysms of medium-sized vessels
   - Hemorrhage
   - Hypertention due to renal artery narrowing
3. Gastrointestinal
   - Hemorrhage
4. Genitourinary
   - Hemorrhage
5. Neurologic
   - Intracranial calcifications of the dura mater, falx cerebri, pineal gland, and choroid plexus
   - Lacunar infarcts
   - Cortical atrophy
   - Subarachnoid and intracerebral hemorrhage
6. Musculoskeletal
   - Ligamentous calcifications
   - Hyperextensible joints
   - Frontal and parietal hyperostosis
   - Fibro-osseous dysplasia of the long bones and vertebrae
7. Mucocutaneous
   - Redundant folds of soft, wrinkled, and lax skin
   - Xanthomatous, coalescing *peau d'orange* plaques of skin folds (sides of neck, axilla, antecubital and inguinal areas)
   - Mucosal *peau d'orange* plaques (lower lip, rectum, vagina)
   - Soft tissue calcifications in juxtaarticular areas
8. Nonspecific
   - Increased risk of first trimester miscarriages

1. Retina
   - Angioid streaks
     - Bilateral, asymmetrical, clinically manifest cracks in an abnormal Bruch's membrane (at the choroidal-retinal interface)
     - Histopathology shows calcification and basophilia of Bruch's membrane
     - Associated with fibrous or fibrovascular proliferation of underlying choroid into the subretinal space, accompanied by serous and hemorrhagic detachment of the retina
     - Form an incomplete ring around the optic disc, radiating and tapering anteriorly; following lines of force of extraocular muscles
     - Vary in color from red-brown to dark brown
     - Number increase with age
     - Delineated by fluorescein angiography
   - *Peau d'orange,* mottled appearance of the fundus
   - Diminished visual acuity, loss of central vision (70% of affected patients) secondary to macular hemorrhage and scaring
   - Choroiditis

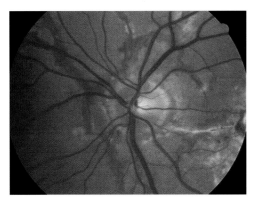

FIGURE 139.1. Typical angioid streaks in fundus of patient with PXE.

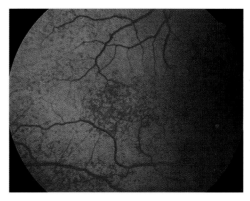

FIGURE 139.2. Mottled appearance of macula (same patient as in Fig. 139.1).

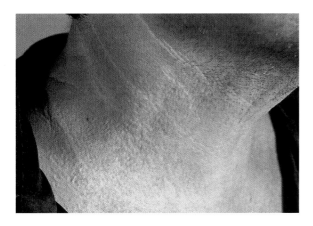

FIGURE 139.3. *Peau d'orange* plaques are visible on the skin.

SUGGESTED READINGS

Hacker SM, et al. Juvenile pseudoxanthoma elasticum: Recognition and management. *Pediatr Dermatol* 1993;10:19–25.

Legwohl M, et al. Classification of pseudoxanthoma elasticum: Report of a consensus conference. *J Am Acad Dermatol* 1994;30:103–107.

Nerad JA, Whitaker DC. Pseudoxanthoma elasticum. In: Gold DH, Weingeist TA, eds. *The Eye in Systemic Disease.* Philadelphia: JB Lippincott; 1990:596–598.

Orlow SJ, et al. Continuing medical education: Skin and bones I. *J Am Acad Dermatol* 1991;25:205–221.

Section C.   Hyperkeratotic Disorders

Chapter 140

PSORIASIS

Alan Sugar

I. GENERAL

1. Common chronic skin disease affecting about 2% of world population
2. Onset any age, peaks in young adulthood and older middle age
3. Decreased incidence in African-Americans
4. Strong genetic predisposition, association with HLA-B27, Cw6, DR7
5. Most common form is chronic plaque psoriasis
6. Other forms include guttate, pustular, and arthritic psoriasis
7. Hyperproliferation of the epidermis and inflammation in dermis and epidermis
8. T-cell–mediated immune reaction.
9. May be initiated or exacerbated by β-blocking drugs, rarely including topical ophthalmic preparations

II. SYSTEMIC MANIFESTATIONS

1. Skin
   - Multiple large red plaques with overlying silvery scales
   - Flexor surfaces, scalp, sites of trauma (Koebner phenomenon)
   - Ridges, pits, separation of finger and toenails
   - Pustular form—pustules around plaques
   - Guttate form—papules in children
2. Musculoskeletal
   - Arthritis in 5% to 7%
   - Most often oligoarthritis, digits most affected
   - May resemble rheumatoid arthritis
   - Associated with ankylosing spondylitis and Reiter syndrome
   - Seronegative arthritis
3. Gastrointestinal
   - Association with Crohn's disease and ulcerative colitis
4. Nonspecific
   - Exacerbation and possible increased incidence in acquired immunodeficiency syndrome

III. OCULAR MANIFESTATIONS

1. Lids
   - Plaques on lids and periocular skin
   - Blepharitis and lash loss
   - Lid thickening
2. Conjunctiva
   - Conjunctivitis
   - Irritation and lacrimation
   - Dry eye
   - Trichiasis
   - Conjunctival plaque
   - Symblepharon
3. Cornea
   - Punctate epithelial keratopathy
   - Peripheral infiltrates
   - Peripheral ulceration, thinning, vascularization
   - Dellen
   - Filamentary keratitis
4. Uvea
   - Iridocyclitis, usually in arthritic form
5. Retina
   - Vasculitis (rare)
6. Lens
   - Potential for cataract from steroid or psoralen and UV light (PUVA) therapy

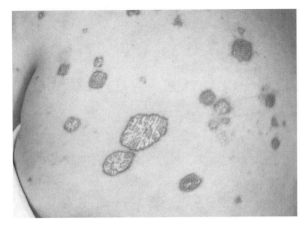

FIGURE 140.1. Typical lesions of plaque psoriasis on skin of the back.

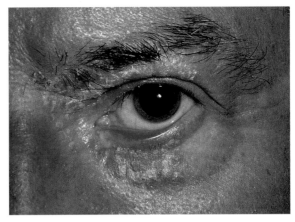

FIGURE 140.2. Plaque lesions of lower lid, scaling of upper lid, ectropion, and chronic conjunctivitis in a middle-aged man with plaque psoriasis.

SUGGESTED READINGS

Camisa C. *Psoriasis.* Boston: Blackwell Scientific; 1994. *A comprehensive clinical text with emphasis on treatment.*

Catsarou-Catsari A, Katsambas A, Theodoropoulos P, Stratigos J. Ophthalmological manifestations in patients with psoriasis. *Acta Dermatol Venereol (Stockh)* 1984;64:557–559. *Results of ophthalmic examination of 101 psoriasis patients.*

Eustace P, Pierse D. Ocular psoriasis. *Br J Ophthalmol* 1970;54:810–813. *Well-illustrated description of corneal involvement in psoriasis.*

Sousa LB, Bass LJ. Psoriasis. In: Mannis MJ, Macsai MS, Huntley AC, eds. *Eye and Skin Disease.* Philadelphia: Lippincott-Raven; 1996;319–325. *A well-illustrated clinical review.*

Section D.   Miscellaneous Skin Disorders

Chapter 141

ACNE ROSACEA

Michael A. Lemp

I. GENERAL

1. Occurrence
- Age 20 to 60
- Both sexes
- Occurs predominantly in fair-skinned individuals

2. Signs
- Telangiectasis
- Vascular dilation with perivascular inflammation
- Sebaceous gland hypertrophy

II. SYSTEMIC MANIFESTATIONS

1. Skin
- Erythema
- Telangiectases

- Papules
- Pustules
- Sebaceous gland hypertrophy

III. OCULAR MANIFESTATIONS

1. Recurrent or chronic blepharitis
2. Meibomitis
3. Styes
4. Chalazia
5. Papillary conjunctivitis

6. Nodular conjunctivitis
7. Episcleritis
8. Superficial punctate keratitis
9. Infiltrative keratitis
10. Ulcerative keratitis

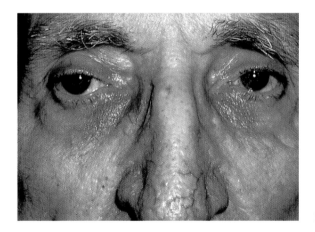

FIGURE 141.1. Full-face view of a patient with rosacea.

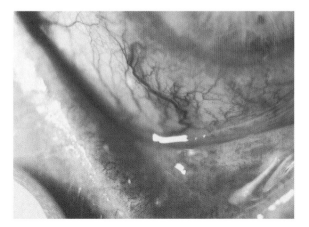

FIGURE 141.2. Chronic meibomitis with papillary conjunctivitis.

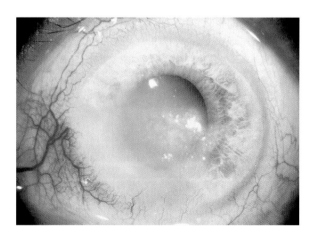

FIGURE 141.3. Rosacea infiltrative keratitis.

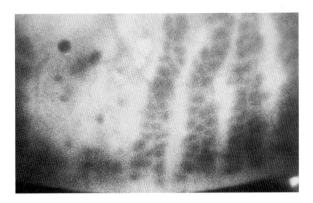

FIGURE 141.4. Infrared meibography showing obliteration of meibomian glands.

SUGGESTED READINGS

Browning DJ, Proia AD. Ocular rosacea. *Surv Ophthalmol* 1986;31:145.

Frucht-Pery J, Chayet AS, Feldman ST, et al. The effect of doxycycline on ocular rosacea. *Am J Ophthalmol* 1989;107:434.

Goldsmith AJB. The ocular manifestations of rosacea. *Br J Dermatol* 1953;65:448.

Solamon SM. Tetracycline in ophthalmology. *Surv Ophthalmol* 1985;29:263.

Chapter 142
ATOPIC DERMATITIS

Fiaz Zaman
Stefan D. Trocme

I. GENERAL

1. The onset of disease is usually late teens to adulthood and may persist for years.
2. There is no sex or race predilection.
3. The pathophysiology is not known but it is most likely a combination of immune hypersensitivity reaction types I and IV.
4. It appears to have a genetic basis.

II. SYSTEMIC MANIFESTATIONS

1. Skin
   - Erythematous, papular, excoriated, crusted skin lesions
   - Lichenification
   - Pruritis (*sine qua non* of atopic dermitis)
2. Neurologic
   - Migraine headaches
3. Ear/nose/throat
   - Rhinitis
4. Pulmonary
   - Associated with asthmatic patients
5. Nonspecific
   - Urticaria
   - Hay fever

III. OCULAR MANIFESTATIONS

1. Lids
   - Trichiasis
   - Entropion
   - Eyelid margin is thickened, injected, and crusted
   - Dennie-Morgan sign (infraorbital folds in eyelids)
   - Susceptible to secondary lid infections (mainly from staph or herpes simplex)
2. Lacrimal system
   - Epiphora
3. Conjunctiva
   - Papillary reaction
   - Trantas' dots at limbus
   - Acute reaction has hyperemia/chemosis
   - Chronic reaction has pale conjunctiva with scarring/contracture
   - Symblepharon (inferior fornix, palprebal conjuctiva)
4. Cornea
   - Acute reaction is punctate epithelial erosions
   - Chronic reaction shows superficial and deep vascularization
   - Stromal scarring
   - Thinning
   - Marginal ulceration
5. Lens
   - Anterior subcapsular cataract or posterior pole cataract

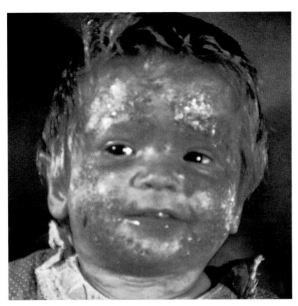

FIGURE 142.1. Exudative papules of infantile atopic dermatitis. Courtesy of Derek Cripps, MD.

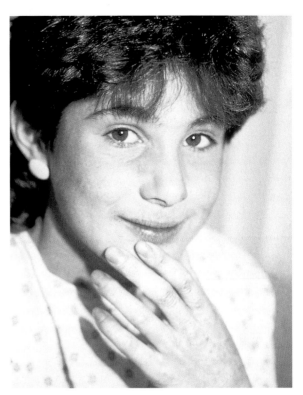

FIGURE 142.2. Lichenification of the face, neck, and hands in adolescent/adult atopic dermatitis. Courtesy of Derek Cripps, MD.

SUGGESTED READINGS

Arffa R. *Grayson's Disease of the Cornea*. St. Louis: CV Mosby; 1997:167–171.

Smolin G. *The Cornea*. Boston: Little, Brown; 1994:352–354.

Trocme SD, Raizman MB, Bartley GB. Medical therapy for ocular allergy. *Mayo Clin Proc* 1992;67:557–565.

Chapter 143

MALIGNANT ATROPHIC PAPULOSIS

David A. Lee
W. P. Daniel Su

I. GENERAL

1. Cause and pathogenesis are still unknown.
2. Very rare condition
3. Males may be more often affected than females and males may have a worse prognosis.
4. No apparent age predilection
5. Multiple organ systems involved
6. Generally regarded as a fatal disease, but may have a chronic, benign variant of the syndrome
7. Characteristically lymphocyte-mediated necrotizing vasculitis that affects the entire cutaneous microvasculature
8. Vasculitis with lymphocytes as the predominant inflammatory cells
9. Obliterating arteriolitis or endovasculitis with secondary thrombosis and slow tissue necrosis
10. Disturbance of endothelial function leads to impairment of the normal fibrinolytic activity, causing slow occlusion of arterioles.
11. Possible viral cause
12. Various immunologic tests usually are negative.
13. Analogous to the generalized vasculitis in systemic lupus erythematosus

II. SYSTEMIC MANIFESTATIONS

1. Skin
   - Asymptomatic papular cutaneous eruption on the trunk and extremities that later evolves into lesions with atrophic porcelain-white centers surrounded by an erythematous telangiectatic rim varying from 2 to 10 mm in diameter.
   - Episodic occurrence and often the first sign of the disease
   - Isolated, noncontiguous lesions pass through progressive stages from small, pink-gray-yellow papules that later become umbilicated and centrally depressed.
   - The lesions are not painful and are usually located on the trunk and upper body, sparing the head and peripheral extremities.
2. Gastrointestinal
   - Generally the most pronounced and tends to occur shortly after the skin lesions develop
   - Vague abdominal discomfort
   - Abdominal distention
   - Alternating diarrhea and constipation
   - Multiple "white infarcts" may be found throughout the small intestine with an intact mucosa.
   - Characteristically death results from an episode of violent intestinal bleeding.
3. Central and peripheral nervous system
   - Usually affected after several bouts of the skin disease
   - Multiple foci may be involved with vascular thrombosis, giving a wide array of neurologic signs.
   - Meningoencephalitis
   - Cranial nerve involvement
   - Hemiparesis
   - Motor or sensory nerve abnormalities
   - Death may occur from cerebral infarction and hemorrhage within a few years after onset of the skin disease.
4. Less frequently involved organ systems
   - Cardiovascular
   - Pulmonary
   - Genitourinary

III. OCULAR MANIFESTATIONS

1. Lids
   - Cutaneous papules
2. Conjunctiva
   - Telangiectatic lesions
3. Retina
   - Vascular tortuosity
   - Infarction
4. Choroid
   - Infarction
5. Neuroophthalmologic
   - Secondary to central nervous system involvement
6. Diplopia
   - Visual field defects
   - Ophthalmoplegia
   - Ptosis
   - Papilledema
   - Optic atrophy

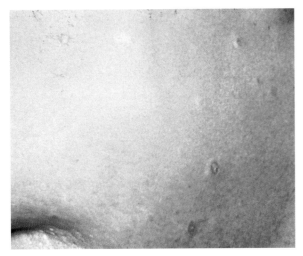

FIGURE 143.1. The porcelain-white depressed centers and erythematous borders of the skin lesions in malignant atrophic papulosis.

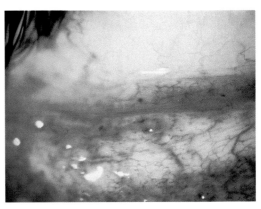

FIGURE 143.2. A telangiectatic conjunctival lesion seen in malignant atrophic papulosis.

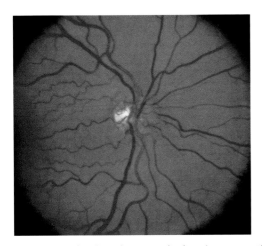

FIGURE 143.3. A fundus photograph showing an optic disc with vascular tortuosity and cilioretinal arteries anastomosing to retinal arteries at the optic disc with optic disc pallor inferotemporally.

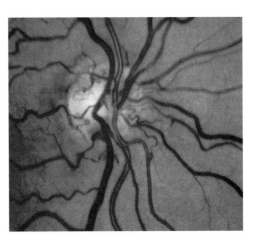

FIGURE 143.4. A magnified view of Fig. 143.3.

SUGGESTED READINGS

Degos R, Delort J, Triot R. Dermatite papulo-squameuse atrophiante. *Bull Soc Fr Dermatol Syphiligr* 1942;49:148–150.

Henkind P, Clark WE II. Ocular pathology in malignant atrophic papulosis: Degos' disease. *Am J Ophthalmol* 1968;65:164–169.

Kohlmeier W. Multiple Hautnekrosen bei Thrombangiitis obliterans. *Arch Dermatol Syphilol* 1941;181:783–792.

Lee DA, Su WPD, Liesegang TJ. Ophthalmic changes of Degos' disease (malignant atrophic papulosis). *Ophthalmology* 1984;91:295–299.

Su WPD, Schroeter AL, Lee DA, et al. Clinical and histologic findings in Degos' syndrome (malignant atrophic papulosis). *Cutis* 1985;35:131–138.

Chapter 144

LINEAR NEVUS SEBACEUS SYNDROME

H. Michael Lambert

I. GENERAL

1. Considered one of the phakomatoses
2. Classic triad consisted of
   - Linear nevus sebaceous of Jadassohn
   - Seizures
   - Mental retardation
3. Updated triad
   - Linear nevus sebaceous of Jadassohn
   - Neurologic abnormalities
   - Ophthalmologic abnormalities
4. No age, sex, or familial predilection

II. SYSTEMIC MANIFESTATIONS

1. Neurologic
   - Arachnoid cysts
   - Ipsilateral dilated cerebral ventricles
   - Cerebral hypoplasia
   - Cerebellar hypoplasia
   - Electroencephalographic abnormalities
   - Unilateral cortical atrophy
   - Hydrocephalus
   - Unilateral extremity atrophy
   - Seizures
     - Apneic spells
     - Myoclonic seizures
     - Psychomotor seizures
     - Jacksonian seizures
     - Grand mal seizures
   - Mental retardation
   - Hemimegalencephaly
   - Heterotopic gray matter
   - Agenesis of corpus callosum
   - Dandy-Walker malformation
2. Cutaneous
   - Midline facial linear nevus of Jadasson
     - Smooth to verrucous pale yellow plaque
     - One side to midline
   - Malignant transformation of nevus possible
     - Basal cell carcinoma most common
   - Alopecia in area of nevus
3. Musculoskeletal
   - Unilateral extremity atrophy
   - Vitamin D–resistant rickets
4. Cardiac abnormalities

III. OCULAR MANIFESTATIONS

1. Ptosis
2. Strabismus
3. Amblyopia
4. Lid coloboma
5. Conjunctival complex choristoma
6. Iris coloboma
7. Lens coloboma
8. Choroidal coloboma
9. Disc coloboma
10. Choroidal osseous choristoma
11. Intrascleral calcification
12. Subretinal neovascularization
13. May be bilateral despite localized nevus of Jadassohn

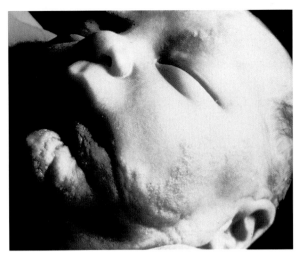

FIGURE 144.1. Typical unilateral linear nevus sebaceous of Jadassohn.

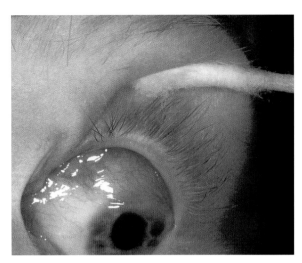

FIGURE 144.2. Superior conjunctival lipodermoid of left eye.

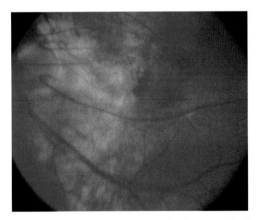

FIGURE 144.3. Fundus photograph of left eye with choroidal osseous choristoma and overlying subretinal neovascular membrane.

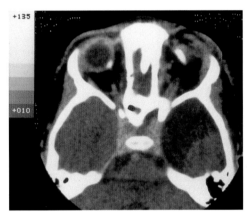

FIGURE 144.4. Computed tomography scan illustrating bilateral osseous choristomas and atrophy of left hemisphere of brain.

SUGGESTED READINGS

Dodge NN, Dobyns WB. Agenesis of the corpus callosum and Dandy-Walker malformation associated with hemimegalencephaly in the sebaceous nevus syndrome. *Am J Med Genet* 1995;56:147–150.

Feuerstein RC, Mims LC. Linear nevus sebaceous with convulsions and mental retardation. *Am J Dis Child* 1962;104:675–679. *Original description of the syndrome with classic triad.*

Lambert HM, Sipperley JO, Shore JW, et al. Linear nevus sebaceous syndrome. *Ophthalmology* 1987;94:278–282. *Updated triad delineating oculoneurocutaneous components.*

Section E.   Pigmentary Disorders

Chapter 145

CHEDIAK-HIGASHI SYNDROME

Raymond G. Watts
Frederick J. Elsas

I. GENERAL

1. Syndrome of partial oculocutaneous albinism, immune dysfunction, and pathognomonic large lysosomal granules in granulocytes and other cells
2. Autosomal recessive inheritance
3. Onset in childhood with recurrent infections
4. Pathophysiology is understood as abnormal granule membrane function and fusion of uncertain etiology. Presence of abnormal granules in cells is associated with cellular malfunction.
5. Immunodeficiency is due to combined functional granulocyte abnormalities and impaired lymphocyte cell-mediated immunity.
6. Some patients experience an "accelerated phase" characterized by aggressive mononuclear cell infiltration of organs resulting in death.
7. Deaths are due to infection or hemorrhage.
8. Bone marrow transplantation is curative for hematologic manifestions.

II. SYSTEMIC MANIFESTATIONS

1. Hematologic
   - Neutrophil functional defects
   - Platelet granule functional defects
   - Prolonged bleeding time
   - Impaired lymphocyte function
   - Neutropenia
   - Pancytopenia in the accelerated phase
2. Dermatologic
   - Partial oculocutaneous albinism (skin, hair, or eyes)
   - Nevi and lentigines
3. Central and peripheral nervous system
   - Mental retardation (20%)
   - Peripheral neuritis or neuropathy
   - Seizures
4. Gastrointestinal
   - Hepatosplenomegaly and hypersplenism in accelerated phase
5. Nonspecific
   - Fever
   - Recurrent bacterial infections
   - Gingivitis, stomatitis

III. OCULAR MANIFESTATIONS

1. Uvea
   - Variable pigmentation
   - Irises may transilluminate
2. Optic nerve
   - Papilledema and infiltration with leukocytes in accelerated phase
3. Orbit
   - Cellulitis secondary to immune system dysfunction
4. Neuroophthalmologic
   - Nystagmus
5. Nonspecific
   - Photophobia

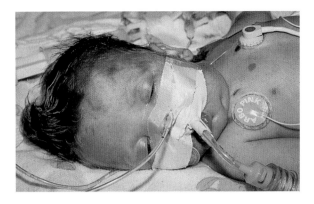

FIGURE 145.1. Six-week-old patient with Chediak-Higashi syndrome.

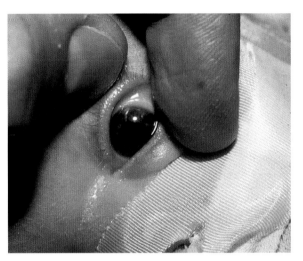

FIGURE 145.2. Anterior segment in patient with Chediak-Higashi syndrome. The iris transilluminates.

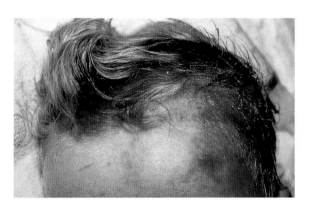

FIGURE 145.3. Typical silver pigmentation of hair in Chediak-Higashi syndrome.

SUGGESTED READINGS

Ben Ezra D, Mengistu F, Cividalli G, et al. Chediak-Higashi syndrome: Ocular findings. *J Pediatr Ophthalmol Strabismus* 1980;17:68. *Report of case with diminished visual evoked response and electroretinography.*

Blume RS, Wolff SM. The Chediak-Higashi syndrome: Studies in four patients and a review of the literature. *Medicine* 1972;51:247–280. *An excellent clinical review of all published cases to 1972.*

Filipovich AH, Shapiro RS, Ramsay NK, et al. Unrelated donor bone marrow transplantation for correction of lethal congenital immunodeficiencies. *Blood* 1992;80:270–276.

Spencer WH, Hogan MJ. Ocular manifestations of Chediak-Higashi syndrome. *Am J Ophthalmol* 1960;50:1197.

Watts RG, Howard TH. Functional disorder of granulocytes and monocytes. In: Bick RL, ed. *Hematology: Clinical and Laboratory Practice.* St. Louis: CV Mosby; 1993:1106–1107. *Details hematologic manifestations and pathophysiology.*

Chapter 146

INCONTINENTIA PIGMENTI (BLOCH-SULZBERGER SYNDROME)

Stephen R. Russell

I. GENERAL

1. Incontinentia pigmenti (IP; Bloch-Sulzberger syndrome) is an uncommon inherited ectodermal dysplasia that affects the skin, dentition, hair, eyes, central nervous system, and in rare cases, the heart.
2. The disorder is inherited in an X-linked dominant fashion, with male lethality. Two distinct genetic loci, IP1 at Xp11.21 and IP2 at Xq28, have been identified by positional cloning. Most affected males have Kleinfelter syndrome (XXY), which provides for one unaffected X chromosome. Less common genetic defects such as a half chromatid mutation or somatic mutation in early development may explain other affected males. Prenatal diagnosis can be made by trophoblast biopsy.
3. Peripheral retinal vascular anomalies and recent magnetic resonance imaging and proton spectroscopic imaging data from IP patients with neurologic defects suggests that the pathogenesis involves a small vessel occlusive phenomenon associated with developing ectoderm.
4. The disorder is named for the absence of pigmentation in the dermal basal epithelium found in stage 3 skin lesions (these cells are "incontinent of pigment").
5. The ophthalmic clinical presentation in an adolescent or adult patient with IP typically includes an unexplained vitreous hemorrhage or (vaso) proliferative retinopathy.

II. SYSTEMIC MANIFESTATIONS

1. Skin—characteristic clinical and histopathologic dermatosis begins at or shortly after birth, evolves through four stages
   - Stage 1
     - Erythematous macules, papules, and bullae randomly distributed
     - Biopsy shows intraepithelial vesicles filled with eosinophils, seen in 90% of affected individuals.
   - Stage 2
     - Verrucous lesions, random, often overlooked in progression to stage 3
   - Stage 3
     - Hyperpigmented whorls and streaks, often found in a linear distribution along the thorax (nevus lines of Blascko)
     - Present in 98%
     - Fade in childhood
   - Stage 4
     - Hypopigmented patches and streaks
     - May be difficult to detect in adulthood
2. Central nervous system (30% of patients)
   - Cerebral edema
   - Cerebral hemorrhagic necrosis
   - Cerebral atrophy
   - Hydrocephalus, may include mental retardation, spastic parasis, seizures
   - Cortical blindness
   - Gyral dysplasia
3. Dental
   - Hypodontia
4. Hair
   - Alopecia
5. Cardiac
   - Patent ductus arteriosis

III. OCULAR MANIFESTATIONS

1. Retina and vitreous
   - Peripheral retinal avascular area
   - Tortuous, irregular vessels with arborizing arteriovenous anastomoses at juncture of avascular and vascularized retina
   - Aneurysmal dilation and aneurisms, telangectasia
   - Retinal exudate
   - Foveal hypoplasia
   - Retinal neovascularization
   - Vitreous hemorrhage
   - Preretinal fibrosis
   - Retinal detachment
   - Retinal pigment epithelial (RPE) mottling, granularity
   - RPE hypopigmentation, coloboma
2. Strabismus and oculomotor disorders
   - Esotropia
   - Nystagmus
3. Conjunctival pigmentation
4. Cataract
5. Optic atrophy
6. End stage
   - Phthisis

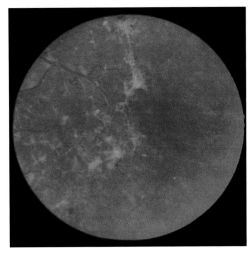

FIGURE 146.1. Fundus photograph of peripheral retinal avascularity, telangectasia, and neovascularization.

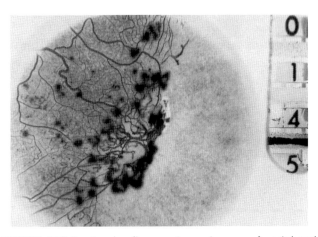

FIGURE 146.2. Fundus fluorescein angiogram of peripheral vascular dysplasia, telangectasia, and neovascularization.

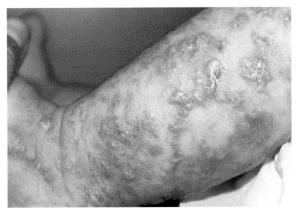

FIGURE 146.3. Verrucous dermatosis (stage 2 lesion). Courtesy of Mary Stone, MD.

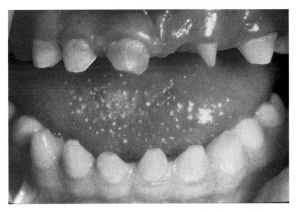

FIGURE 146.4. Hypodontia. Courtesy of Gilbert Lilly, DDS.

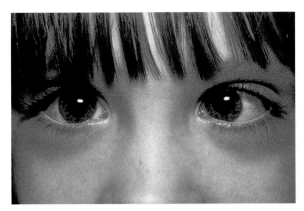

FIGURE 146.5. Esotropia (strabismus).

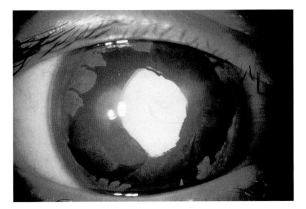

FIGURE 146.6. Intumescent cataract and posterior senechia.

SUGGESTED READINGS

Friedman WF, Child JS. In: Isselbacher KJ, Braunwald E, Wilson JD, et al. eds. *Harrison's Textbook of Internal Medicine,* 13th ed. New York: McGraw-Hill; 1994:1038. *Identifies cardiac abnormalities.*

Gass JDM. *Stereoscopic Atlas of Macular Diseases: Diagnosis and Treatment.* St. Louis: CV Mosby; 1987;420–421.

Goldberg MF, Custis PH. Retinal and other manifestations of incontinentia pigmenti (Bloch-Sulzberger syndrome). *Ophthalmology* 1993;100:1645–1654. *Identifies foveal hypoplasia as frequent finding in this condition.*

Gorski JL, Burright EN. The molecular genetics of incontinentia pigmenti. *Semin Dermatol* 1993;12:255–265. *Review article, comprehensive discussion of the molecular genetics of this disorder.*

Lee AG, Goldberg MF, Gillard JH, et al. Intracranial assessment of incontinentia pigmenti using magnetic resonance imaging, angiography, and spectroscopic imaging. *Arch Pediatr Adolesc Med* 1995;149:573–580. *Advances the concept that vasooclusive phenomena is the unifying pathogenesis.*

Rosenfeld SI, Smith ME. Ocular findings in incontinentia pigmenti. *Ophthalmology* 1985;92:543–546. *Clinicopathologic correlation.*

Watzke RC, Stevens TS, Carney RG Jr. Retinal vascular changes of incontinentia pigmenti. *Arch Ophthalmol* 1976;94:743–746.

Chapter 147

OCULODERMAL MELANOCYTOSIS

James R. Patrinely

I. GENERAL

1. Also known as nevus of Ota.
2. Involves skin in distribution of first and second (rarely third) divisions of fifth cranial nerve; may include ipsilateral nasal and oral mucosa, tympanic membrane, and external auditory canal; rarely occurs bilaterally.
3. Changes in size and color may be noted with age, trauma, puberty, menarche, menses, menopause, and pregnancy.
4. Bimodal presentation. Majority are apparent at birth with second peak in second to third decades.
5. Two to five times more common in females, but this may represent a presentation bias
6. Most commonly reported among Asians. All darkly pigmented races probably at increased risk for the nevus and at decreased risk for malignant transformation.
7. Whites may have a 30-fold risk of developing an uveal (choroid, ciliary body, or iris), cutaneous, orbital, or intracranial malignancy at a mean age of 50 years.
8. Associated with higher risk for increased intraocular pressure and glaucoma, unrelated to degree of angle pigmentation
9. Very rarely associated with other developmental abnormalities (spinocerebellar degeneration and Duane's retraction syndrome) and hamartomatous syndromes (Sturge-Weber, Klippel-Trenaunay-Weber, and neurofibromatosis)
10. Typically sporadic, although rarely reported in successive generations

II. SYSTEMIC MANIFESTATIONS

1. Mucocutaneous
   - Local pigmented malignancies (malignant melanoma, rarely basal cell carcinoma)
   - Bilateral cases associated with persistent Mongolian spots
   - Rarely associated with nevus of Ito (pigmentation of deltoid, supraclavicular, and scapular regions)
2. Central nervous system
   - Pigmented malignancies of dura and leptomeninges

III. OCULAR MANIFESTATIONS

1. Lids
   - Dermis
   - Orbicularis oculi
   - Tarsus
2. Conjunctiva
3. Episclera
4. Sclera
5. Cornea
   - Epithelium
   - Stroma
   - Pigmented cells on endothelium
6. Trabecular meshwork
7. Lens
   - Pigmented cells on anterior capsule surface
8. Uvea
   - Choroid
   - Ciliary body
   - Iris
9. Optic nerve
   - Nerve head
   - Dural sheath
10. Orbit
    - Fat
    - Long posterior ciliary arteries
    - Periorbita
    - Orbital bone
    - Meninges (dura) of the optic nerve

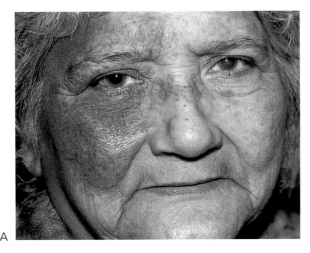

A

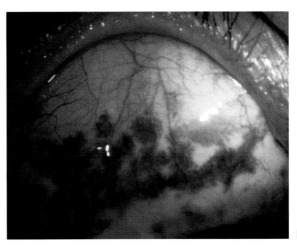

B

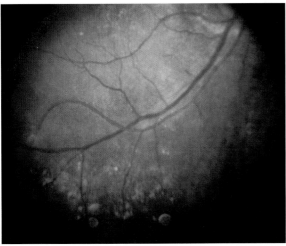

C

FIGURE 147.1. Oculodermal melanocytosis. Slate gray to deep brown, macular hyperpigmentation of the skin (**A**) and mucous membranes is classically seen in the distribution of the first and second divisions of the fifth cranial nerve. A patchy blue-gray appearance to the conjunctiva and sclera is common (**B**). Associated choroidal pigmentary changes may also ocur (**C**).

SUGGESTED READINGS

Dutton JJ, Anderson RL, Schelper RL, et al. Orbital malignant melanoma and oculodermal melanocytosis: Report of two cases and review of the literature. *Ophthalmology* 1984;91:497–507. *An excellent review of the spectrum of malignancies associated with oculodermal melanocytosis up to 1983, including the age at presentation.*

Kopf AW, Weidman AI. Nevus of Ota. *Arch Dermatol* 1962;85:75–88. *A discussion of the histopathology and pathophysiology of oculodermal melanocytosis and related skin lesions.*

Ota M. Naevus fusco-caeruleus ophthalmomaxillaris. *Jpn J Dermatol* 1939;46:369–372. *Ota's original report.*

Teekhasaenee C, Ritch R, Rutnin U, Leelawongs N. Ocular findings in oculodermal melanocytosis. *Arch Ophthalmol* 1990;108:1114–1120. *A careful and complete presentation of the ocular tissues involved in a Thai population.*

Teekhasaenee C, Ritch R, Rutnin U, Leelawongs N. Glaucoma in oculodermal melanocytosis. *Ophthalmology* 1990;97:562–570. *An evaluation of the risks of glaucoma and increased intraocular pressure in oculodermal melanocytosis in a Thai population.*

Theunissen P, Spincemaille G, Pannebakker M, Lambers J. Meningeal melanoma associated with nevus of Ota: Case report and review. *Clin Neuropathol* 1993;12:125–129. *A review of intracranial malignancies associated with oculodermal melanocytosis and an insightful discussion regarding the dural versus leptomeningeal origin of these lesions.*

Velazquez N, Jones IS. Ocular and oculodermal melanocytosis associated with uveal melanoma. *Ophthalmology* 1983;90:1472–1476. *Estimation of the risk of uveal melanoma associated with the nevi.*

Chapter 148

VITILIGO

Daniel M. Albert

I. GENERAL

1. Equal racial and gender distribution
2. Family history in 30% to 40%; inheritance may be polygenic or by autosomal dominant gene of variable penetrance.
3. 50% of cases develop by age 20 years
4. Etiology
   - Destruction of melanocytes
   - Autoimmune hypothesis
     - High incidence of organ-specific autoantibodies (thyroid, gastric parietal cells, adrenal tissue)
     - Serum antibodies to normal human melanocytes
   - Neurogenic hypothesis (little support)
     - Compound released at peripheral nerve endings that is toxic to melanocytes
   - Self-destruct theory of Lerner
     - Defect of protective mechanism that removes toxic melanin precursors

II. SYSTEMIC MANIFESTATIONS

1. Halo nevi
   - Frequently seen, antedate vitiligo, in patients with malignant melanoma
2. Other associated conditions
   - Thyroid disease (hyperthyroidism and hypothyroidism)
   - Hypoparathyroidism
   - Pernicious enemia
   - Addison's disease
   - Myasthenia gravis
   - Alopecia areata
   - Morphea and lichen sclerosus
   - Malignant melanomas
   - Severe food and drug allergies

III. OCULAR MANIFESTATIONS

1. External
   - Depigmentation of lid
   - Poliosis
   - Whitening of brow
2. Uveal tract
   - Discrete areas of depigmentation
   - Active uveitis
   - Atrophy of iris pigment epithelium
   - Atrophy of retinal pigment epithelium
   - Pigment clumping in perphery
   - Severe symptoms of night blindness
3. Optic nerve
   - Optic atrophy
   - Papilledema

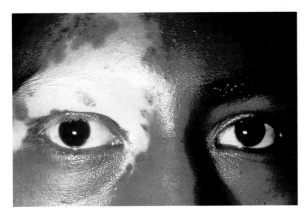

FIGURE 148.1. Area of depigmentation of skin surrounding the eye in a patient with vitiligo associated with severe iritis. From Wagoner MD, Albert DM, Lerner AB, et al. New observations on vitiligo and ocular disease. *Am J Ophthalmol* 1983;96:16–23.

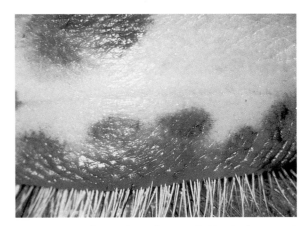

FIGURE 148.2. Closer view of area of skin depigmentation. Note associated whitening of lashes (poliosis).

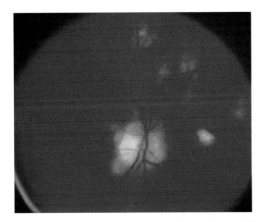

FIGURE 148.3. Left eye of patient with complete vitiligo and active uveitis. There was a strong family history of retinitis pigmentosa (brother, two neices). From Albert DM, Nordlund JJ, Lerner AB. Ocular abnormalities occurring with vitiligo. *Ophthalmology* 1979;86:1145–1158.

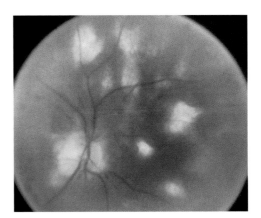

FIGURE 148.4. Progression of uveitis in left eye two years later in patient in Figure 148.3. From Albert DM, Nordlund JJ, Lerner AB. Ocular abnormalities occurring with vitiligo. *Ophthalmology* 1979;86:1145–1158.

SUGGESTED READINGS

Albert DM, Nordlund JJ, Lerner AB. Ocular abnormalities occurring with vitiligo. *Ophthalmology* 1979;86:1145–1158.

Albert DM, Wagoner MD, Pruett RC, et al. Vitiligo and disorders of the retinal pigment epithelium. *Br J Ophthalmol* 1983;67:153–156.

Bleehen SS, Ebling FJG, Chamption RH. Disorders of skin color. In: Champion RH, Burton JL, Ebling FJG, eds. *Textbook of Dermatology,* 5th ed. Oxford: Blackwell Scientific; 1992:1608–1611.

Lerner AB, Nordlund JJ. Vitiligo. What is it? Is it important? *JAMA* 1978;239:1183–1187.

Wagoner MD, Albert DM, Lerner AB, et al. New observations on vitiligo and ocular disease. *Am J Ophthalmol* 1983;96:16–26.

Section F. Vesiculobullous Disorders

Chapter 149
CICATRICIAL PEMPHIGOID

Melvin I. Roat

I. GENERAL

1. Affects women almost twice as often as men
2. Usually presents in the fifth or sixth decade of life, but may begin in the third decade
3. The lesions of cicatricial pemphigoid are believed to result from an antibody-mediated cytotoxic response (type II hypersensitivity response), with abnormal production of a circulating autoantibody, the cicatricial pemphigoid antibody; and binding of this autoantibody to the cicatricial pemphigoid antigen. Possibilities for the cicatricial pemphigoid antigen include beta 4 or laminin 5, both components of the lamina lucida of the stratified squamous epithelial basement membrane.
4. Complement fixation occurs and an inflammatory infiltrate consisting of polymorphonuclear neutrophils, acute, or mononuclear cells, chronically, forms in the subepithelial tissue.
5. Complement, and proteolytic enzymes, reactive oxygen species, monokines, and lymphokines (*eg*, transforming growth factor –beta 1 and 3) from effector cells and other products of inflammation result in
   - Disruption of the lamina lucida of the basement membrane, which leads to subepithelial bullae formation
   - Epithelial hypermitosis, which results in abnormal epithelium differentiation with epithelial decreased goblet cell frequency
   - Abnormal fibroblast activation, fibroblast hyperproliferation, and abnormal extracellular matrix production leading to subepithelial fibrosis resulting in abnormal scarring and contracture
   - Damage and failure of the corneal stem cells, which reside at the limbus, leading to inadequate repopulation of central corneal epithelium
   - Direct central corneal epithelial cell damage

II. SYSTEMIC MANIFESTATIONS

1. Pulmonary
   - Larynx stricture
2. Gastrointestinal
   - Esophageal stricture
   - Anal stricture
3. Genitourinary
   - Vaginal stricture
   - Urethral stricture
4. Cutaneous
   - Recurrent, nonscarring, generalized, tense bullous eruption
   - Localized erythematous plaque, with recurrent bullae, which scar
5. Ear/nose/throat
   - Diffuse or patchy gingivitis, which desquamates leaving ulcerated area
     - Oral bullae with peripheral erythema, which rupture resulting in large areas of denuded epithelium
   - The gingival disease leads to periodontal disease and oral bone loss resulting in dental extractions.
   - Nasal mucosal ulceration and scarring
   - Pharynx stricture

III. OCULAR MANIFESTATIONS

1. Lids
   - Trichiasis
   - Progressive keratinization of the tarsal conjunctiva
   - Entropion
   - Lagophthalmos
   - Abnormal blink
   - Ankyloblepharon
     - Due to conjunctival scarring and contraction, which pulls on the "insertion" of the conjunctiva at the eyelid margin, displacing the gray line inward, rotating the eyelashes and tarsus in
2. Lacrimal system
   - Severe aqueous-deficient dry eye results when the lacrimal gland orifices are obliterated by scarring.
3. Conjunctiva
   - Lacy subconjunctival scarring
   - Blunting of the forniceal angle
   - Symblepharon
   - Obliteration of the fornices
   - Ankyloblepharon
     - Due to progressive subepithelial fibrosis and contracture
   - Chronic conjunctivitis
   - Conjunctival epithelial defects from direct damage by autoimmune inflammatory process
   - Progressive, localized keratinization of the tarsal and eventually bulbar conjunctiva by migration of cutaneous epithelium from the eyelid margin
   - Dry, totally keratinized conjunctival surface
4. Cornea
   - Superficial punctate keratitis due to
     - Aqueous deficient keratitis sicca
     - Exposure
     - Lagophthalmos
     - Abnormal blink
     - Trichiasis

- Entropion
  - Direct central corneal epithelial cell damage by autoimmune inflammatory process
- Swirling corneal epitheliopathy of ocular surface failure due to failure of corneal limbal stem cells to adequately repopulate the central corneal epithelium
- Persistent corneal epithelial defects due to
  - Aqueous-deficient keratitis sicca
  - Exposure
  - Lagophthalmos
  - Abnormal blink
  - Trichiasis
  - Entropion
  - Failure of corneal limbal stem cells to adequately repopulate the central corneal epithelium
  - Direct central corneal epithelial cell damage by autoimmune inflammatory process
- Bacterial keratitis (actual infection or secondary colonization of a persistent corneal epithelial defect) may be due to the following predisposing conditions
  - Aqueous deficient keratitis sicca
  - Superficial punctate keratitis
  - Persistent corneal epithelial defects
- Corneal scarring and neovascularization (often focal or segmental) results from
  - Persistent corneal epithelial defects
  - Bacterial keratitis
- Total corneal opacification from multiple areas and episodes of corneal scarring and neovascularization
- Dry keratinized corneal surface from migration of cutaneous epithelium from the eyelid margin over the conjunctiva and then over the cornea

5. Intraocular pressure
- Open-angle glaucoma due to impaired facility of outflow by the inflamed, scarred, and contracted conjunctiva

6. Ocular motility
- Ocular motility restricted by ankyloblepharon

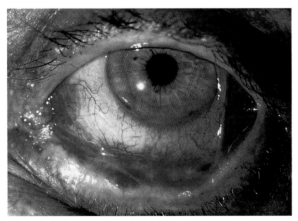

FIGURE 149.1. A patient with cicatricial pemphigoid; note subepithelial fibrosis, blunting of the angle, and symblepharon.

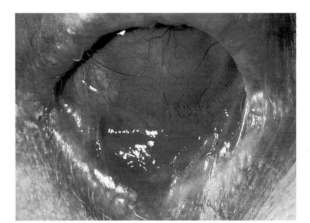

FIGURE 149.2. Scarred vascularized cornea with trichiasis and conjunctival keratinization in a patient with long-standing uncontrolled cicatricial pemphigoid.

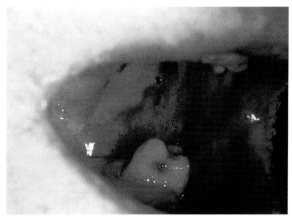

FIGURE 149.3. Oral ulcer in a patient with cicatricial pemphigoid.

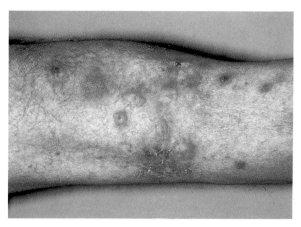

FIGURE 149.4. Tense bullous eruption and localized erythematous plaque in a patient with cicatricial pemphigoid.

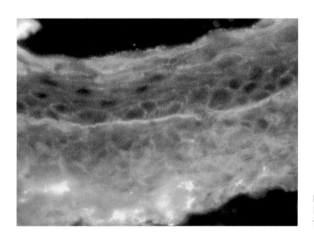

FIGURE 149.5. Immunofluorescence photomicrograph of conjunctival biopsy from patient in Fig. 149.1 demonstrating linear deposits of IgG at the conjunctival basement membrane.

SUGGESTED READINGS

Foster CS. Cicatricial pemphigoid. *Trans Am Ophthalmol Soc* 1986;84:527–663.

Mondino BJ. Cicatricial pemphigoid and erythema multiforme. *Ophthalmology* 1990;97:939–952.

Mondino BJ. Clinical immunologic diseases: Dermatologic diseases. In: Smolin G, Thoft RA, eds. *The Cornea: Scientific Foundations and Clinical Practice,* 3rd ed. Boston: Little, Brown; 1994:414–438.

Neumann R, Tauber J, Foster CS. Remission and recurrence after withdrawal of therapy for ocular cicatricial pemphigoid. *Ophthalmology* 1991;98:858–862.

Roat MI. Cicatricial pemphigoid: A scientific and practical approach to diagnosis and treatment. *Semin Ophthalmol* 1991;6:142–155.

Chapter 150

EPIDERMOLYSIS BULLOSA

Wing-Kwong Chan
Bartly J. Mondino

I. GENERAL

1. Epidermolysis bullosa (EB) is a heterogeneous group of rare heritable disorders characterized by mark fragility of the skin and mucosa and blister formation in response to insignificant trauma.
2. Onset of blisters is usually at birth or during early childhood.
3. Incidence ranges from 1/50,000 to 1/500,000 births.
4. Severity varies considerably depending on the specific type of EB, ranging from the occasional presence of blisters with little morbidity to widespread blistering that can be fatal.
5. Classification of the major subtypes is based on the anatomic location of blister formation. Multiple variants within the subtypes are based on clinical, genetic, histologic, and biochemical factors.
6. The blisters of EB simplex or nondystrophic type occur intraepidermally, superficial to the basement membrane complex, and rarely cause scarring. The blisters of the junctional or atrophic type occur within the lamina lucida of the basement membrane complex; scarring is uncommon but skin atrophy often occurs. Blisters of the dystrophic type occur in the superficial dermis below the lamina densa of the basement membrane complex and result in scarring.
7. The transmission of the nondystrophic types is autosomal dominant, the junctional or atrophic types is autosomal recessive, and the dystrophic types can be autosomal dominant or autosomal recessive. The recessive dystrophic variants of EB are more disfiguring than the others.
8. Ocular lesions occur in about 25% of all patients with EB, most commonly in recessive dystrophic EB and least commonly in EB simplex.
9. Mutation of keratin molecules or an increase in proteases is thought to be responsible for the pathogenesis of EB simplex; defective hemidesmosomes and abnormal anchoring fibrils result in the junctional or atrophic forms of EB; and increased collagenase activity and absent anchoring fibrils cause the dystrophic forms of EB.

II. SYSTEMIC MANIFESTATIONS

1. Mucocutaneous
   - Skin and mucosal surface blisters
   - Scarring of skin and mucosal surfaces
   - Paronychia and dystrophy of nails
   - Pattern baldness and scalp atrophy
   - Increased incidence of squamous cell carcinoma (in dystrophic EB)
2. Gastrointestinal
   - Esophageal strictures
   - Anal strictures
3. Genitourinary
   - Phimosis
4. Hematologic
   - Iron deficiency anemia
   - Anemia of chronic illness
   - Reduced clotting time
5. Musculoskeletal
   - Limb contractures
   - Resorption of distal terminal phalanges (mitten deformity)
6. Dental/oral
   - Microstomia
   - Ankyloglossia
   - Dysplastic teeth
   - Enamel defects
7. Otorhinolaryngologic
   - Stenosis of the larynx and trachea
   - Stenosis of the nares
8. Nonspecific
   - Malnutrition
   - Growth retardation
   - Reduced immunocompetence

III. OCULAR MANIFESTATIONS

1. Lids
   - Eyelid blisters and scars
   - Cicatricial ectropion and entropion
   - Trichiasis
   - Lagophthalmos
2. Cornea
   - Recurrent corneal erosions
   - Pannus formation
   - Corneal scar
   - Exposure keratopathy
3. Conjunctiva
   - Conjunctival blisters
   - Pseudomembrane formation
   - Symblepharon
4. Lacrimal system
   - Lacrimal duct obstruction
5. Lens
   - Cataract
6. Nonspecific
   - Refractive errors
   - Amblyopia

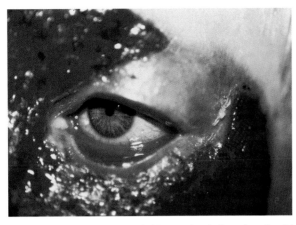

FIGURE 150.1. Ectropion and skin erosion in junctional epidermolysis bullosa. Courtesy of Andrew N. Lin, MD.

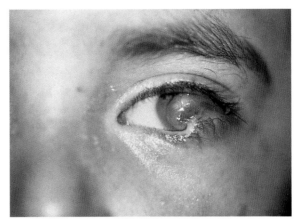

FIGURE 150.2. Corneal pannus and symblepharon in recessive dystrophic epidermolysis bullosa. Courtesy of Andrew N. Lin, MD.

SUGGESTED READINGS

Boothe WA, Mondino BJ, Donzis PB. Epidermolysis bullosa. In: Gold DH, Weingeist TA, eds. *The Eye in Systemic Disease.* Philadelphia: JB Lippincott; 1990:634–635. *A general review of the ocular and systemic manifestations of epidermolysis bullosa.*

Lin AN, Carter DM, eds.: *Epidermolysis Bullosa. Basic and Clinical Aspects.* New York: Springer-Verlag; 1992. *A comprehensive review of the basic science, clinical manifestations, and management of epidermolysis bullosa.*

Lin AN, Murphy F, Brodie SE, Carter DM. Review of ophthalmic findings in 204 patients with epidermolysis bullosa. *Am J Ophthalmol* 1994;118:384–390. *A good review of the ocular manifestations of epidermolysis bullosa.*

Chapter 151

ERYTHEMA MULTIFORME

Fiaz Zaman
Stefan D. Trocme

I. GENERAL

1. Acute inflammatory vesiculobullous reaction of the skin and mucous membranes
2. Associated with inciting drug or infectious agent
3. Occurs more commonly in children and young adults
4. Manfests a spectrum from mild to severe disease
5. Episodic, self-limited, mucocutaneous inflammatory disease

II. SYSTEMIC MANIFESTATIONS

1. Pulmonary
   - Upper respiratory tract symptoms
2. Mucocutaneous
   - Mucosal lesions are bullous and result in membrane or pseudomembrane cicatrization of mucosal lesions.
   - Mouth and conjunctiva are most commonly affected mucosal sites
3. Nonspecific
   - Prodrome of fever, malaise, sore throat, and arthralgias
   - Erythematous macular/papular skin lesions with vesicles

III. OCULAR MANIFESTATIONS

1. Lids
   - Entropion
   - Trichiasis
2. Conjunctiva
   - Diffuse conjunctivitis characterized as catarrhal, purulent, mucopurulent, hemmorrhagic, or cicatrizing membranes
   - Symblepharon
3. Cornea
   - Corneal vascularization
   - Corneal pannus
   - Corneal opacification
4. Nonspecific
   - Ocular involvement in 43% to 84% of patients with 36% experiencing permanent visual sequelae

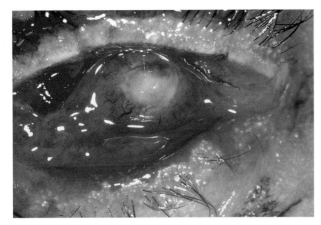

FIGURE 151.1. Erythema multiforme with symblepharon and chemosis.

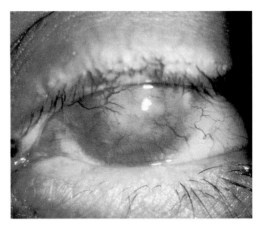

FIGURE 151.2. Erythema multiforme with corneal vascularization, thinning, and opacification.

SUGGESTED READINGS

Arffa R. *Grayson's Disease of the Cornea.* St. Louis: CV Mosby; 1997:603–607.

Hochman MA, Mayers M. Steven-Johnson syndrome, epidermolysis bullosa, staphylococcal scalded skin syndrome, and dermatitis herpetiformis *Int Ophthalmol Clin* 1997;37:77–92.

Smolin G. *The Cornea.* Boston: Little, Brown; 1994:421–425.

Chapter 152

PEMPHIGUS

Melvin I. Roat

I. GENERAL

1. Affecting men and women equally
2. Onset, usually in the fifth and sixth decade
3. In the past, pemphigus vulgaris was reported almost exclusively in Jews; now, however, pemphigus vulgaris has been documented in all ethnic groups.
4. The presence of the DR4 phenotype increases the risk for pemphigus vulgaris.
5. The lesions of pemphigus vulgaris are believed to result from an antibody-mediated cytotoxic response (type II hypersensitivity response) with abnormal production of a circulating autoantibody, the pemphigus vulgaris antibody, which binds to desmoglein 3, a protein of the desmosomes which produce the intercellular attachments of stratified squamous epithelial cells.
6. The autoantibody binding induces the upregulation of serine protease production leading to activation of plasinogen to plasmin, causing dissolution of intercellular attachments, loss of adherence of desmosomes, acantholysis, and subsequent blister formation.
7. In contrast to most autoimmune diseases, studies indicate that antibody binding alone, without complement or inflammatory cells, is sufficient for tissue injury in pemphigus vulgaris.
8. The intraepithelial nature of the disease does not lead to activation of subepithelial fibroblasts with subsequent scarring.
9. Most studies have found a positive correlation between circulating pemphigus vulgaris antibody titer and clinical disease activity.
10. Circulating pemphigus vulgaris antibody titer has been observed to fall or become undetectable with successful therapy.

II. SYSTEMIC MANIFESTATIONS

1. Pulmonary
   - Laryngeal erosions
2. Gastrointestinal
   - Anal erosions
   - Anal bleeding
   - Esophageal erosions
   - Esophageal deformity leading to dysphagia
3. Genitourinary
   - Vulval erosions
   - Cervix erosions
4. Cutaneous
   - Thin-walled, flaccid blisters on normal-appearing skin
   - The fluid in the blister is clear at first but may become hemorrhagic or seropurulent later.
   - Bullae may rupture spontaneously or with slight pressure.
   - Ruptured bullae leave painful, denuded areas that may ooze, bleed easily, crust, and enlarge peripherally.
   - Erosions and bullous lesions heal slowly and without scarring.
   - Postinflammatory hyperpigmentation is usually present at sites of healed lesions for some time.
   - Bullae and erosions typically involving the scalp, face, neck, axilla, and trunk.
   - In severe cases a substantial portion of the body surface may be denuded.
   - Rubbing normal-appearing skin will cause ready separation of the skin (Nikolsky's sign).
5. Ear/nose/throat
   - Short-lived oral bullae quickly rupture to form painful, raw erosions.
   - Intact oral bullae are rarely seen.
   - Oral erosions heal without scarring.
   - Pharyngeal involvement may result in hoarseness and difficulty with swallowing.
   - Oral mucosal involvement usually precedes cutaneous manifestation by many months.
   - Nasal erosions

III. OCULAR MANIFESTATIONS

1. Lids
   - Exposure or trichiasis due to distortion of the normal eyelid architecture by the crusting lesions
2. Conjunctiva
   - Bullae are transient leading to erosions.
   - Purulent or pseudomembranous conjunctivitis
   - Conjunctival scarring is very rare and does not progress or lead to decreased vision.

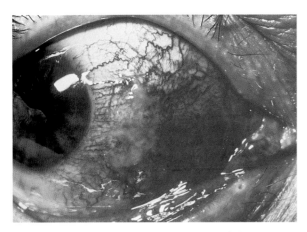

FIGURE 152.1. Conjunctival involvement with hyperemia and edema.

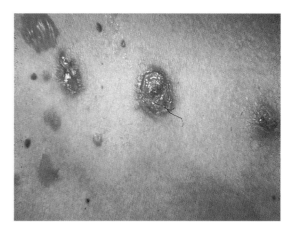

FIGURE 152.2. Erosions of flaccid bullae on normal-appearing skin. Courtesy of T. Abell, MD.

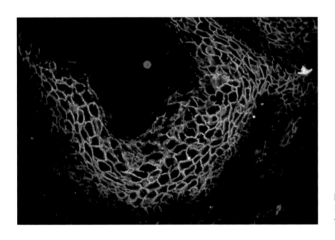

FIGURE 152.3. Binding of IgG to the epithelial intercellular substance in a skin biopsy, as demonstrated by direct immunofluorescence. Courtesy of T. Abell, MD.

SUGGESTED READINGS

Anhalt GJ, Labib RS, Voorhees JJ, et al. Induction of pemphigus in neonatal mice by passive transfer of IgG from patients with the disease. *N Engl J Med* 1982;306:1189–1196.

Bean SF, Holubar K, Gillet RB. Pemphigus involving the eyes. *Arch Dermatol* 1975;111:1484–1486.

Korman NJ, Eyre RW, Klaus-Kovtun V, Stanley JR. Demonstration of an adhering-junction molecule (plakoglobin) in the autoantigens of pemphigus foliaceus and pemphigus vulgaris. *N Engl J Med* 1989;321:631–635.

Michel B, Thomas CI, Levine M, et al. Cicatricial pemphigoid and its relationship to ocular pemphigus and essential shrinkage of the conjunctiva. *Ann Ophthamol* 1975;7:11–20.

Rees TD, Binnie WH, Wright JM, et al. Oral presentation of pemphigus vulgaris and its response to systemic steroid therapy. *Oral Surg Oral Med Oral Pathol* 1992;74:54–57.

PART 20.   VASCULAR DISORDERS

Chapter 153

ARTERIOSCLEROSIS

Ali M. Khorrami
Helen K. Li

I. GENERAL

1. Arteriosclerosis is a general term describing the thickening and hardening of arterial walls and includes three different processes, each affecting different sized blood vessels: atherosclerosis, focal calcific arteriosclerosis (Mönckeberg's sclerosis), and arteriolosclerosis.
2. Atherosclerosis affects large arteries and involves primarily the intimal layer with nodular lesions composed of variable combinations of lipid, fibrous tissue, and calcium. Mönckeberg's sclerosis is associated with degeneration of smooth muscle cells followed by calcium deposition in medium-sized arteries. Arteriolosclerosis affects smaller arteries and arterioles involving both intimal and medial layers, with endothelial hyperplasia, intimal and subintimal hyalization, medial hypertrophy, and fibrosis.
3. Atherosclerosis is a leading cause of morbidity and mortality of both sexes above age 65 in the United States.
4. Risk factors for atherosclerosis include cigarette smoking, aging, genetic predisposition, hypertension, hyperlipidemia, low levels of high-density lipoprotein, obesity, diabetes mellitus, physical inactivity, stress, and personality. Men are at a higher risk than women.
5. There are several theories of atherogenesis including endothelial injury, uncontrolled proliferation of smooth muscle cells, focal clonal senescence, and altered cellular enzyme functions.
6. Prevention of atherosclerosis is based on reducing risk factors.

II. SYSTEMIC MANIFESTATIONS

1. Cardiac
   - Coronary artery disease
   - Myocardial infarction
   - Arrhythmias
   - Angina
   - Syncopal episodes
   - Palpitation
   - Heart failure
2. Vascular
   - Decreased perfusion
   - Nonhealing ulcers
   - Gangrene
   - Refractory hypertension
3. Central nervous system
   - Strokes
   - Transient ischemic attacks
   - Dysarthria
   - Diplopia
   - Hemiparesis
   - Hemiplegia
   - Severe cognitive dysfunction
4. Renal
   - Hypertension
   - Decreased functional reserve
5. Genitourinary
   - Impotence

III. OCULAR MANIFESTATIONS

1. Anterior segment
   - Ocular ischemic syndrome (secondary to ipsilateral atherosclerotic carotid occlusive disease)
     - Iris neovascularization
     - Aqueous flare
     - Posterior synechiae
     - Anterior synechiae
     - Corneal edema
     - Cataract
2. Retina
   - Retinal emboli
     - Cholesterol (Hollenhorst plaque)
     - Fibrin platelet (Fisher plug)
     - Calcified
   - Retinal vascular occlusion
     - Branch or central retinal artery occlusion
       - Embolic—carotid atherosclerosis
       - Nonembolic—arteriosclerosis
     - Branch or central retinal vein occlusion
       - Associated with retinal arteriolosclerosis
   - Ocular ischemic syndrome (secondary to ipsilateral atherosclerotic carotid occlusive disease)
     - Midperipheral retinal hemorrhages
     - Microaneurysms
     - Neovascularization of retina and optic disc
     - Darkening of the retinal veins and narrowed arterioles
   - Age-related macular degeneration
3. Neuroophthalmologic
   - Ischemic optic neuropathy
   - Amaurosis fugax
   - Visual field defects
   - Cranial nerve palsies
   - Gaze disturbances
   - Diplopia
   - Nystagmus
   - Neuroparalytic keratopathy

SUGGESTED READINGS

Bierman EL. Atherosclerosis and other forms of arteriosclerosis. In: Isselbacher KJ, Braunwald E, Wilson D, eds. *Harrison's Principles of Internal Medicine,* 13th ed. New York: McGraw-Hill; 1994:1106–1116.

Breen LA. Atherosclerotic carotid disease and the eye. *Neurol Clin* 1991;9:131–145.

Chawluk JB, Kushner MJ, Bank WJ, et al. Atherosclerotic carotid artery disease in patients with retinal ischemic syndromes. *Neurology* 1988;38:858–863.

Kubota T, Von Below H, Holback LM, Naumann GOH. Bilateral cavernous degeneration of the optic nerve associated with multiple arteriosclerotic ischemic infarctions. *Graefe's Arch Clin Exp Ophthalmol* 1993;231:52–55.

Maves-Perlman JA, Brady WE, Klein R, et al. Dietary fat and age-related maculopathy. *Arch Ophthalmol* 1995;113:743–748.

Soukiasian S, Lahav M. Arteriosclerosis. In: Gold DH, Weingeist TA, eds. *The Eye in Systemic Disease.* Philadelphia: JB Lippincott; 1990:649–652.

Vingerling JR, Dielemans I, Bots ML, et al. Age-related macular degeneration is associated with atherosclerosis. *Am J Epidemiol* 1995;142(4):404–409.

Chapter 154

CARCINOID SYNDROME

Jacob Pe'er

I. GENERAL

1. Various age groups. Mean age of onset is fifth to sixth decade.
2. The name is "carcinoid" because of slow growth and homogenous and nonmalignant appearance of the carcinoid tumor cells, which leads to underestimation of their malignant potential.
3. Carcinoid tumors arise from neuroendocrine cells along the primitive endoderm, mainly (about 90%) along the entire gastrointestinal tract (where they are the most common endocrine tumors), about half of them in the appendix. Other sites are pancreas, pulmonary bronchi, thymus, biliary duct, Meckel's diverticulum, breast, and ovary.
4. The interval between onset of symptoms and diagnosis is long, averaging 4.5 years.
5. Appendiceal and colorectal tumors are usually benign and asymptomatic. Small bowel and bronchial carcinoid have a more malignant course, spreading by metastasis, and secreting hormones.
6. Carcinoid syndrome develops in about 5% of patients with carcinoid tumors, caused by a variety of hormones secreted by enterochromaffin cells.
7. Secretory products of carcinoid tumors are serotonine (the most important one), histamine, catecholamines, bradykinins, tachykinins, enkephalins, endorphins, vasopressin, gastrin, adrenocorticotrophin, prostaglandins, somatostatin, neurotensin, substance P, neurokinin A, and motilin.
8. The prognosis is highly dependent on the site and stage of the disease at diagnosis. Appendiceal and rectal carcinoids rarely affect survival.

II. SYSTEMIC MANIFESTATIONS

1. Gastrointestinal
   - Diarrhea
   - Abdominal pain or tenderness
   - Gastrointestinal bleeding
   - Intestinal obstruction (intussusception, mesenteric fibrosis)
   - Nausea
   - Malaise
   - Weight loss
   - Salivation
   - Mesenteric vascular insufficiency—infarction
   - Biliary obstruction
   - Protein malnutrition
2. Cardiac
   - Endocardial fibrosis
     - Right-sided valvular disease (tricuspid, pulmonary)
       - Secondary right-sided heart failure
     - Left-sided valvular disease
3. Mucocutaneous
   - Cutaneous flushing
   - Telangiectasias
   - Pruritis
   - Facial edema
   - Mild pellagra—in widely metastatic disease
4. Vascular
   - Paroxysmal hypotension
5. Pulmonary
   - Bronchoconstriction—wheezing
   - Dyspnea
   - Chronic coughing
   - Hemoptysis
   - Pneumonia

III. OCULAR MANIFESTATIONS

1. Intraocular manifestations
   - Yellow-orange mass in the choroid (most common)
   - Decreased visual acuity
   - Exudative retinal detachment
   - Visual field defect
   - Iris or ciliary body mass
2. Orbital metastasis
   - Pain
   - Diplopia
   - Proptosis
   - Ptosis
   - Impaired motility
   - Palpable mass
3. Manifestations due to carcinoid syndrome
   - Conjunctival hyperemia
   - Periorbital edema
   - Lacrimation
   - Changes in ocular fundus
     - Cyanotic reflex
     - Arteriolar narrowing
     - Venous dilatation
     - Intravascular sludging

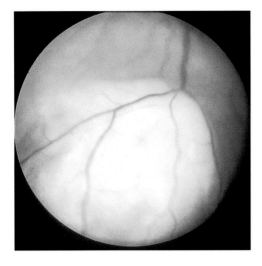

FIGURE 154.1. Elevated yellow-orange choroidal metastatic of carcinoid tumor. Courtesy of M. Seelenfreund, MD.

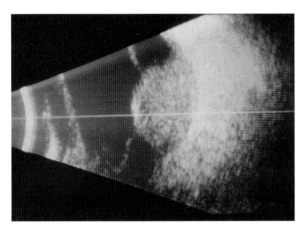

FIGURE 154.2. B-scan ultrasonography of choroidal metastasis of carcinoid tumor shows dome-shaped solid mass with exudative retinal detachment.

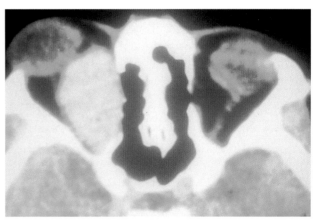

FIGURE 154.3. Orbital computed tomography scan shows a large metastasis of carcinoid tumor in the right orbit.

SUGGESTED READINGS

Fan JT, Buettner H, Bartley GB, Bolling JP. Clinical features and treatment of seven patients with carcinoid tumor metastatic to the eye and orbit. *Am J Ophthalmol* 1995;119:211–218.

Hajdu SI, Winawer SJ, Myers WP. Carcinoid tumors: A study of 204 cases. *Am J Clin Pathol* 1974;61:521–528.

Harbour JW, De Potter P, Shields CL, Shields JA. Uveal metastasis from carcinoid tumor. Clinical observations in nine cases. *Ophthalmology* 1994;101:1084–1090.

Riddle PJ, Font RL, Zimmerman LE. Carcinoid tumors of the eye and orbit: A clinicopathologic study of 15 cases, with histochemical and electron microscopic observations. *Hum Pathol* 1982;13:459–469.

Wong VG, Melman KL. Ophthalmic manifestations of the carcinoid flush. *N Engl J Med* 1967;277:406–409.

Chapter 155

CAROTID ARTERY INSUFFICIENCY

Sohan Singh Hayreh

I. GENERAL

1. Usually produced by atherosclerotic lesions of the internal/common carotid artery
2. Nonatherosclerotic lesions of the internal carotid artery producing insufficiency include fibromuscular dysplasia, spontaneous cervicocephalic dissection, aneurysm or radiation arteritis.
3. Manifestations of carotid artery insufficiency are cerebral or ocular or both.
4. Cerebral and ocular manifestations are produced by two mechanisms
   - Embolization
     - Emboli are produced by material from atheromatous or thrombotic lesions in the carotid arteries
     - Emboli are usually of three types: cholesterol, thrombotic (platelet-fibrin), and calcific.
     - In the eye the embolus may lodge temporarily or permanently in central/branch retinal artery or main/short posterior ciliary artery.
     - Retinal embolus produces ischemia of a segment or entire retina and that may be transient or permanent.
     - Embolus in the posterior ciliary circulation causes optic nerve head ischemia.
     - Transient ischemia of retina or optic nerve head produces amaurosis fugax.
     - Prolonged or permanent ischemia of the retina causes retinal infarction involving the corresponding retina.
     - Prolonged or permanent ischemia of the optic nerve head causes anterior ischemic optic neuropathy.
     - Transient embolization to cerebral cortex causes transient cerebral ischemic attacks.
     - Prolonged or permanent ischemia of the cerebral cortex causes ischemic stroke.
     - When a stenotic internal carotid artery becomes occluded, embolization may abate.
   - Reduction of blood flow
     - This is much less commonly seen than embolization.
     - Produced usually by occlusion or hemodynamically significant stenosis of the internal carotid artery
     - Also produced by stenosis or occlusion of ophthalmic artery or its ocular branches, and that may be seen in addition to or independent of the carotid artery disease
     - The blood flow in the eye is directly proportional to the perfusion pressure (mean blood pressure minus the intraocular pressure) and inversely proportional to the peripheral vascular resistance.
     - Thus, blood flow in the eye may be reduced by fall of mean blood pressure in the ocular arteries, rise of intraocular pressure, or increased vascular resistance, or by a combination of these factors.
     - Reduced blood flow in the eye produces chronic ocular ischemic syndrome.
     - Reduction of cerebral blood flow causes chronic cerebral ischemic changes.

II. SYSTEMIC MANIFESTATIONS

1. Cardiac
   - Majority of patients with carotid artery disease suffer from myocardial ischemia (angina, myocardial infarction).
   - Usually these patients eventually die from myocardial infarction and less often from cerebrovascular accident.
2. Vascular
   - Associated peripheral vascular disease common
   - Intermittent claudication common
3. Neurologic
   - Transient cerebral ischemic attacks
   - Ischemic strokes
   - "Silent" cerebral infarction
   - Cerebral atrophy
   - Dementia

III. OCULAR MANIFESTATIONS

1. Secondary to embolization
   - Amaurosis fugax
   - Asymptomatic retinal emboli
   - Central retinal artery occlusion
   - Branch retinal artery occlusion (Figure 155.1)
   - Cilioretinal artery occlusion
   - Anterior ischemic optic neuropathy
   - Choroidal infarction
2. Chronic ocular ischemic syndrome
   - Manifestations of anterior segment ischemia (Figures 155.2 and 155.3)
     - These are most important and seen commonly.
       - Iris neovascularization
       - Angle neovascularization
       - Neovascular glaucoma
       - Cataract

- Corneal/scleral necrosis
- Corneal neovascularization
- Manifestations of posterior segment ischemia (Figure 155.4)
  - Amaurosis fugax
  - Optic disc neovascularization
  - Retinal neovascularization

- Central retinal artery occlusion
- Anterior ischemic optic neuropathy
- Choroidal infarcts
- Central retinal vein occlusion—usually non-ischemic type
- Orbital pain

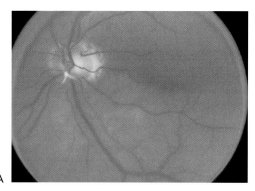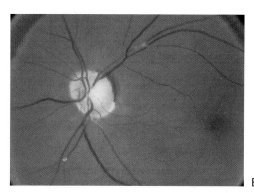

FIGURE 155.1. Fundus photographs showing retinal emboli. **(A)** Left eye shows an impacted thrombotic (platelet-fibrin) embolus in the inferior division of central retinal artery on the optic disc, resulting in infarction of lower part of the retina. **(B)** Left eye shows an impacted cholesterol plaque at bifurcation (typical site) of inferior retinal arteriole, with a sheathed segment of the superior temporal arteriole near the bifurcation (secondary to a temporarily impacted embolus in the past).

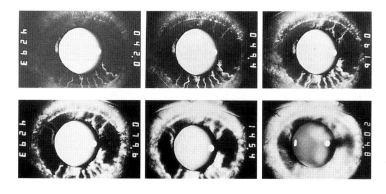

FIGURE 155.2. Fluorescein iris angiograms of an eye with chronic ocular ischemic syndrome showing markedly delayed, incomplete and patchy filling of the iris (see three top and two lower left angiograms from 42.0 to 145.4 seconds after injection of fluorescein), as well as iris neovascularization (shown by areas of fluorescein leakage, most marked in lower right late angiogram).

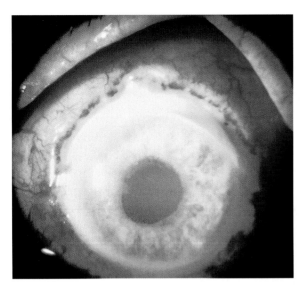

FIGURE 155.3. Peripheral corneal and limbal melting superiorly, with iris neovascularization at the pupil margin, in an eye with chronic ocular ischemic syndrome.

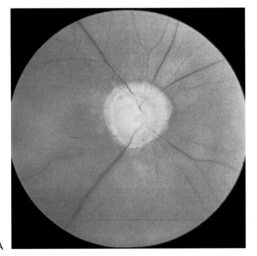

A

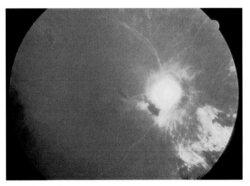

B

FIGURE 155.4. Fundus photographs show various manifestations of posterior segment ischemia in two eyes with chronic ocular ischemic syndrome. **(A)** Right eye shows signs of fresh central retinal artery occlusion (from very low perfusion pressure in it), optic atrophy (from previous anterior ischemic optic neuropathy), and optic disc neovascularization. **(B)** Right eye shows evidence of marked retinal and posterior ciliary artery circulatory collapse (from very low perfusion pressure), resulting in complete absence of filling of retinal vascular bed, optic atrophy (from anterior ischemic optic neuropathy in the past), and areas of chorioretinal degeneration (from choroidal infarcts). The chorioretinal degenerative lesion seen in inferior nasal sector in this eye is the tip of a large triangular lesion with its base at the equator. (This eye also had a number of other similar lesions in the periphery.)

SUGGESTED READINGS

Amaurosis Fugax Study Group. Amaurosis fugax (transient monocular blindness): A consensus statement. In: Bernstein EF, ed. *Amaurosis Fugax.* Heidelberg: Springer-Verlag; 1988:286–301.

Arruga J, Sanders MD. Ophthalmologic findings in 70 patients with evidence of retinal embolism. *Ophthalmology* 1982;89:1336–1347.

Hayreh SS. Chronic ocular ischemic syndrome in internal carotid artery occlusive disease: Controversy on "venous stasis retinopathy." In: Bernstein EF, ed. *Amaurosis Fugax.* Heidelberg: Springer-Verlag; 1988:135–158.

Hayreh SS, Podhajsky P. Ocular neovascularization with retinal vascular occlusion. II. Occurrence in central and branch retinal artery occlusion. *Arch Ophthalmol* 1982;100:1585–1596.

Mizener JB, Podhajsky P, Hayreh SS. Ocular ischemic syndrome. *Ophthalmology* 1997;104:859–64.

Chapter 156

CAROTID CAVERNOUS FISTULA

F. Jane Durcan

I. GENERAL

1. Occurs when there is communication between the internal carotid artery (ICA) and the cavernous sinus (CS)
2. There is shunting of arterialized blood into the venous system.
3. Symptoms are related to venous congestion and ischemia in the orbit, brain, and central nervous system.
4. Classification
   - Pathogenesis—traumatic versus spontaneous
   - Hemodynamics—high flow versus low flow
   - Anatomy—direct (ICA into CS) versus dural (dural branches of ICA into CS)

5. 75% of carotid cavernous fistulas (CCF) are traumatic and tend to occur most commonly in young men with basal skull fractures or deep penetrating orbital trauma.
6. 25% of CCFs are spontaneous and tend to occur in middle-aged and older women.
7. Risk factors for spontaneous CCF
   - Congenital vascular malformation
   - Atherosclerosis
   - Infectious agents (syphilis)
   - Connective tissue diseases
   - Pregnancy

II. SYSTEMIC MANIFESTATIONS

1. Headache
2. Orbital and periorbital pain
3. Subjective or objective bruit that stops on carotid compression
4. Facial pain or numbness
5. Transient seventh nerve palsy
6. Epistaxis
7. Enlarged venous loops may present as nasopharyngeal mass
8. Intracerebral hemorrhage
   - Seizures
   - Hemispheric dysfunctions
   - Death
9. Subarachnoid hemorrhage
10. High output cardiac failure—rare

III. OCULAR MANIFESTATIONS

1. Ipsilateral or contralateral to involved cavernous sinus or bilateral
2. External
   - Proptosis
   - Pulsation of globe
   - Orbital bruit
   - Episcleral or conjunctival vascular engorgement
   - Chemosis
   - Ptosis
3. Motility abnormalities
   - Sixth nerve palsy most common
   - Third nerve palsy
   - Fourth nerve palsy
   - Horner's syndrome
4. Glaucoma
   - Increased episcleral venous pressure
   - Neovascular glaucoma
   - Angle closure secondary to pupillary block
5. Anterior segment engorgement
   - Iris vessel engorgement
   - Conjunctival and episcleral vessel engorgement
6. Anterior segment ischemia
   - Corneal edema
   - Hypotony
   - Cell and flare
   - Cataract
   - Rubeosis iridis
7. Posterior segment
   - Disc edema
   - Congested tortuous retinal vessels
   - Retinal and vitreous hemorrhages
   - Slow flow retinopathy
   - Choroidal detachment
   - Serous and exudative retinal detachments
   - Central retinal artery occlusion
   - Central retinal vein occlusion
8. Optic neuropathy
   - Direct trauma
   - Ischemia
   - Glaucoma
   - Chronic hypoxia
   - Compression

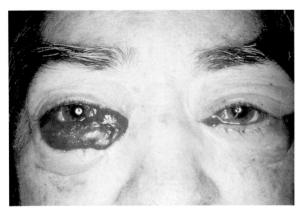

FIGURE 156.1. Proptosis and chemosis in a direct, high-flow, right carotid cavernous fistula following trauma. Courtesy of N. Schatz, MD.

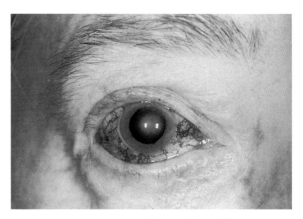

FIGURE 156.2. Woman, aged 82, with mild proptosis and epibulbar congestion from a spontaneous low-flow dural cavernous fistula. Courtesy of the Department of Ophthalmology, University of Iowa, Iowa.

SUGGESTED READINGS

Hamby WB. *Carotid-Cavernous Fistula.* Springfield, IL: Charles C. Thomas; 1966.

Phelps CD, Thompson HS, Ossoinig KC. The diagnosis and prognosis of atypical carotid-cavernous fistula (red-eyed shunt syndrome). *Am J Ophthal* 1982;93:423–436.

Slusher MM, Lennington BR, Weaver RG, Davis CH Jr. Ophthalmic findings in dural arteriovenous shunts. *Ophthalmology* 1979;86:720–731.

Sommer C, Mullges W, Ringelstein EB. Noninvasive assessment of intracranial fistulas and other small arteriovenous malformations. *Neurosurgery* 1992;30:522–528.

Zimmerman RD, Russell EJ. Angiography and the evaluation of visual disturbances. *Int Ophthalmol Clin* 1986;26:187–213.

Chapter 157

HEREDITARY HEMORRHAGIC TELANGIECTASIA

Elise Torczynski

I. GENERAL

1. This rare defect is inherited as an autosomal dominant trait with complete penetrance.
2. Males and females are equally affected; African-Americans uncommonly.
3. 30% of the vascular lesions arise in the first decade; 5% of new lesions appear every decade through the age of 70.
4. Three types of vascular malformations occur, sometimes congenitally
   - Flat spindle nevi with radiating vessels
   - Discrete, flat to slightly raised blue purple macules, up to 3 mm in diameter, beneath the epidermis and mucous membranes
   - Elevated, domed nodules filled with blood on the skin and mucous membranes
5. Mild trauma to vascular lesions initiates bleeding; epistaxis being the most common.
6. Pulmonary arteriovenous fistulas predispose to secondary polycythemia, clubbing of the fingers, cyanosis, and septic emboli (cerebral).
7. Severe bleeding may be lethal.

II. SYSTEMIC MANIFESTATIONS

1. Ear/nose/throat
   - Epistaxis (most common, onset often at puberty)
   - Repeated cautery may perforate nasal septum.
2. Gastrointestinal
   - Melena
   - Hemoptysis
3. Pulmonary
   - Hemoptysis
   - Polycythemia
   - Clubbing of fingers
   - Cyanosis
4. Genitourinary
   - Hematuria
   - Menometrorrhagia
5. Mucocutaneous
   - Surface bleeding
   - Vascular lesions of face, neck, fingers, chest, trunk, lips, tongue, nasal septum, gums, etc.
6. Hematologic
   - Secondary anemia
   - Normal bleeding and coagulation tests
7. Neurologic
   - Brain abscess
8. Vascular
   - Varicose veins
   - Hemorrhoids
9. Nonspecific
   - Any unexplained bleeding

III. OCULAR MANIFESTATIONS

1. Skin of lids
   - Telangiectasias
2. Conjunctiva
   - Telangiectasias, tarsal and bulbar
   - Tortuosities of blood vessels
   - Bloody tears
3. Retina (rare)
   - Telangiectatic tufts
   - Varices, tortuosities
   - Neovascularization
   - Hemorrhages, perivenous
   - Dilatations of distal veins
4. Vitreous hemorrhage
5. Neurologic (rare)
   - Visual field defects
   - Pupillary abnormalities
   - Ophthalmoplegia
   - Papilledema
   - Ptosis

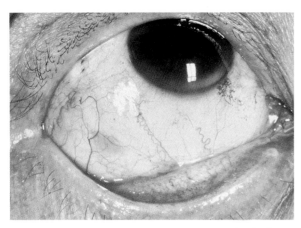

FIGURE 157.1. Conjunctival telangiectasia at the limbus. Angiomas inferotemporally and inferiorly. Courtesy of Robert A. Hardy, MD.

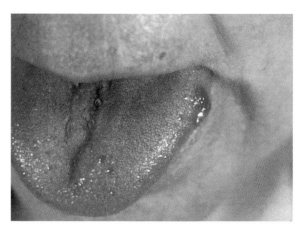

FIGURE 157.2. Domed, blood-filled vascular nodules on surface and lateral border of the tongue. Courtesy of Allan L. Lorincz, MD, University of Chicago, Chicago.

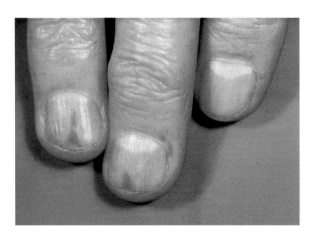

FIGURE 157.3. Subungal splinter hemorrhages. Courtesy of Allan L. Lorincz, MD, University of Chicago, Chicago.

SUGGESTED READINGS

Davis DG, Smith JL. Retinal involvement in hereditary hemorrhagic telangiectasia. *Arch Ophthalmol* 1971;85:618–623.

Reilly PJ, Nostrant TT. Clinical manifestations of hereditary hemorrhagic telangiectasia. *Am J Gastroenterol* 1984;79:363–367.

Chapter 158

HYPERTENSION

Sohan Singh Hayreh

1. Pathophysiologic mechanisms
   - Essential arterial hypertension is considered a multifactorial disease secondary to the interaction of many abnormalities, including the following
     - Abnormalities in cell membrane resulting in defective membrane control over intracellular calcium concentration
     - Abnormalities of calcium metabolism causing rise in cytoplasmic calcium, which in turn causes increased tone of the arteriolar smooth muscle
     - Abnormalities of sodium metabolism from inherited difficulty in the kidney's ability to eliminate sodium
     - Abnormalities of potassium metabolism affect biosynthesis of aldosterone and renin release
     - Abnormalities of renin-angiotensin-aldosterone system
     - Abnormalities of central nervous system including abnormal release of humoral factors (*eg*, natriuretic factor, vasopressin), increased sympathetic discharge, and increased neurogenic vasomotor tone
     - Abnormalities of prostaglandins
     - Abnormalities of vascular endothelial-derived vasoactive agents, such as endothelin-1 (a powerful vasoconstrictor) and nitric oxide (a vasodilator)
     - Genetic effects on blood pressure are polygenic in nature and play an important role in development of arterial hypertension.

2. The following factors produce specific types of hypertension
   - Renin-angiotensin system produces primary reninism, renovascular hypertension, and malignant hypertension.
   - Adrenal cortex through aldosterone produces primary aldosteronism and Cushing's syndrome.
   - Adrenal medulla and catecholamines produce pheochromocytoma.
   - Thyroid hormone produces thyrotoxicosis.
   - Increased plasma volume, as in terminal renal failure and possibly in acute glomerulonephritis, can produce hypertension.
   - Increased cardiac output in hyperkinetic persons with labile blood pressure may result in hypertension.
   - Loss of elasticity of the large vessels can result in atherosclerotic type of hypertension.
   - Proximal resistance to cardiac output may produce coarctation of the aorta and hypertension.
   - Atrophic pyelonephritic kidney and polycystic kidney disease can result from loss of renal tissue and of the antihypertensive function of the kidney.
   - Increase in red cell mass and blood viscosity results in polycythemia vera.
   - Excessive sodium intake in genetically predisposed individuals produces hypertension.

II. SYSTEMIC MANIFESTATIONS

1. Usually asymptomatic
2. Cardiac
   - Myocardial hypertrophy
   - Coronary artery disease
   - Myocardial ischemia and infarction
   - Congestive heart failure
3. Vascular
   - Arteriosclerosis
   - Aggravates atherosclerosis
   - Dissecting or saccular aneurysm of the aorta
   - Peripheral vascular disease
4. Neurologic
   - Headache—usually in severe arterial hypertension, coming on mostly in the morning and involving occipital region
   - Migraine—more prevalent in hypertensives
   - Aneurysms—berry aneurysms, Charcot-Bouchart aneurysms
   - Subarachnoid hemorrhages
   - Cerebrovascular accidents
   - Senile dementia
   - Hypertensive encephalopathy
   - Seizures
   - Coma
   - Cranial nerve paresis/palsy
5. Renal
   - Proteinuria
   - Oliguria
   - Microscopic hematuria
   - Renal failure
6. Ear/nose/throat
   - Epistaxis
   - Tinnitus
7. Hematologic
   - Microangiopathic hemolytic anemia
8. Pulmonary
   - Breathlessness

Fundus changes are the most common abnormalities seen and these fall into the following three distinct categories

1. Retinal lesions (hypertensive retinopathy)
   - Retinal vascular lesions
     - Focal intraretinal periarteriolar transudates (FIPTs) (Figure 158.1)
     - Inner retinal ischemic spots (cotton-wool spots) (Figure 158.2)
     - Retinal arteriolar changes
       - Arteriolar pseudo-narrowing (Figure 158.3)
       - Arteriolosclerosis
       - Arteriolar sheathing
       - Macroaneurysms
       - Central/branch retinal artery occlusion
     - Retinal capillary changes
       - Focal capillary obliteration
       - Microaneurysms
       - Inner retinal microvascular abnormalities
     - Retinal venous changes
       - Venous nipping at arteriovenous crossings
       - Central/branch retinal vein occlusion
       - Increased permeability of the retinal vascular bed
   - Extravascular retinal lesions
     - Retinal hemorrhages
     - Retinal and macular edema
     - Retinal lipid deposits ("hard exudates")
     - Retinal nerve fiber loss
2. Choroidal lesions (hypertensive choroidopathy)
   - Choroidal vascular bed abnormalities
     - Impaired choroidal arterial circulation
     - Choroidal vascular sclerosis
     - Occlusion of choroidal arteries, arterioles, and/or choriocapillaris
   - Retinal pigment epithelial (RPE) lesions
     - Acute focal RPE lesions (Figure 158.4)
     - RPE degenerative lesions (focal or diffuse)
   - Serous retinal detachment
3. Optic disc lesions (hypertensive optic neuropathy)
   - Optic disc edema (Figures 158.2 and 158.3)
   - Optic disc pallor
4. Miscellaneous
   - Cranial nerve palsies
   - Subconjunctival hemorrhages

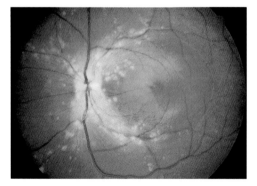

FIGURE 158.1. Fundus photograph of left eye of a rhesus monkey with malignant arterial hypertension showing multiple FIPTs (dull white punctate retinal opacities) situated along the major retinal arterioles and their main branches. It also shows mild optic disc edema and circular serous retinal detachment in the macular region with edema of the overlying macular retina. Published courtesy of *Ophthalmology* 1986;93:60–73.

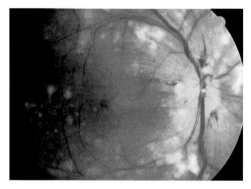

FIGURE 158.2. Fundus photograph of right eye of a rhesus monkey with malignant arterial hypertension showing optic disc edema, hemorrhages, multiple inner retinal ischemic spots (large bright retinal opacities), FIPTs (tiny dull white opacities along retinal arterioles), focal RPE lesions (depigmented, punctate RPE lesions temporal to fovea), macular retinal edema, and foveolar microcyst. Published courtesy of *Ophthalmology* 1986;93:74–87.

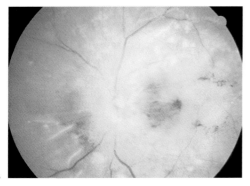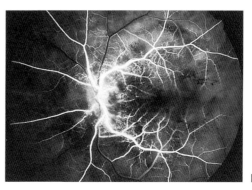

A   B

FIGURE 158.3. Fundus photograph (**A**) of left eye of a rhesus monkey with malignant arterial hypertension showing optic disc edema, retinal hemorrhages, many FIPTs, retinal and macular retinal edema, serous macular retinal detachment, and markedly attenuated retinal arterioles. However, fluorescein angiogram during the retinal arterial phase (**B**) shows normal caliber of the retinal arterioles (similar to that seen in prehypertensive normal angiogram). This shows that the arteriolar narrowing on ophthalmoscopy (universally considered a classical sign of hypertension) is simply a pseudo-narrowing and an ophthalmoscopic artifact. **A** published courtesy of *Ophthalmology* 1986;93:60–73; and **B** published courtesy of *Ophthalmologica* 1989;198:178–196.

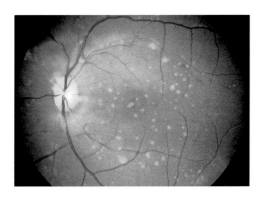

FIGURE 158.4. Fundus photograph of left eye of a rhesus monkey with malignant arterial hypertension showing multiple white acute RPE lesions, a few FIPTs (along the retinal arterioles), and foveal retinal edema. Published courtesy of *Ophthalmology* 1986;93:1383–1400.

SUGGESTED READINGS

Genest J, Kuchel O, Hamet P, Cantin M. Physiopathology of experimental and human hypertension. In: *Hypertension: Physiopathology and Treatment,* 2nd ed. New York: McGraw-Hill; 1983:3–675.

Hayreh SS. Hypertensive retinopathy. *Ophthalmologica* 1989;198:169–260.

Hayreh SS. Malignant arterial hypertension and the eye. *Ophthalmol Clin North Am* 1992;5:445–473.

Page IH. The mosaic theory of arterial hypertension—Its interpretation. *Perspect Biol Med* 1967;10:325–333.

Chapter 159

LYMPHEDEMA

Henry D. Perry
Anastasios J. Kanellopoulos
Alfred J. Cossari
Eric D. Donnenfeld

I. GENERAL

1. Lymphedema
- Milroy's disease (if onset at or near birth)
- Meige's disease (later onset)
- Can be associated with Turner's syndrome, but in this case usually disappears by the first year of life

II. SYSTEMIC MANIFESTATIONS

1. Lymphedema
- Lower extremity edema (marked)
- Upper extremity edema (may be unilateral or bilateral)
- Painless chronic edema
- Pleural effusions
- Obstructive jaundice
- Intestinal lymphagiectasia
- Primary pulmonary tension
- Cerebrovascular malformation

III. OCULAR MANIFESTATIONS

1. Lymphedema
- Conjuctiva—lymphedema
- Ocular motility—strabismus
- Amblyopia
- Eyelids—ectropion

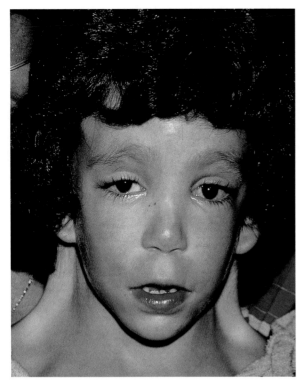

FIGURE 159.1. Clinical picture showing nasal conjuctival cysts and prominent webbed neck.

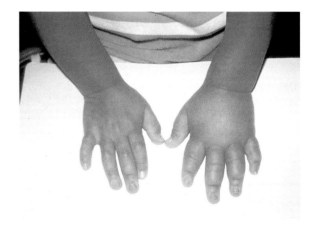

FIGURE 159.2. Clinical picture of upper extremities showing marked edema.

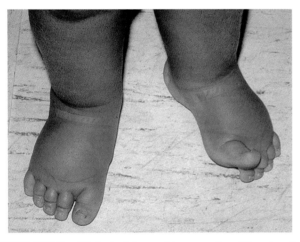

FIGURE 159.3. Clinical picture of lower extremities showing marked edema.

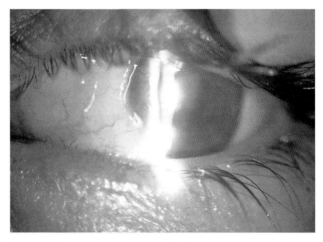

FIGURE 159.4. Clinical picture of left eye demonstrating significant conjuctival chemosis.

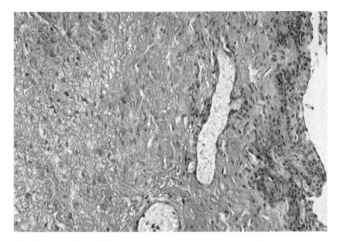

FIGURE 159.5. Histologic section of conjuctiva, demonstrating multifocal areas of dilated vascular channels in the substantia propria, with delicate septa lined on both sides with noncontiguous, flattened endothelial cells.

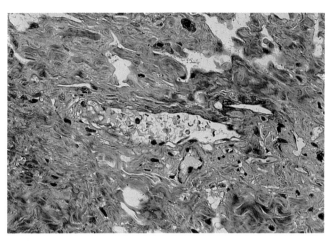

FIGURE 159.6. Histologic section of higher power demonstrating the same findings, also the surrounding collagen fibers are thickened and are strikingly different from normal conjuctiva.

SUGGESTED READINGS

Klein D, Doret M. Chronic hereditary lymphedema. *Modern Problems in Ophthalmology* 1957;1:576.

Kolin T, Johns KJ, Wadlington WB, et al. Hereditary lymphedema and distichiasis. *Arch Ophthalmol* 1991;109:980–981.

Perry HD, Cossari AJ. Chronic lymphangiectasis in Turner's syndrome. *Br J Ophthalmol* 1986;70:396–399.

Tabbara KF, Baghdassarian SA. Chronic hereditary lymphedema of the legs with congenital conjuctival lymphedema. *Am J Ophthalmol* 1972;73:531–532.

Turner HH. A syndrome of infantilism, congenital webbed neck and cubitus valgus. *Endocrinology* 1938;23:566–574.

Wheeler ES, Chan V, Wassman R, et al. A familial lymphedema praecox: Meige disease. *Plast Reconstr Surg* 1981;67:362–364.

Subject Index

Page numbers followed by f refer to figures. Page numbers followed by t refer to tables.